The Slow Death of the AIDS/Cancer Paradigm
and the Apocrypha of the Eukaryotic Cell

The Slow Death of the AIDS/Cancer Paradigm and the Apocrypha of the Eukaryotic Cell

Nancy Turner Banks MD

Copyright © 2016 by Nancy Turner Banks MD.

Library of Congress Control Number:		2016915607
ISBN:	Hardcover	978-1-5245-4423-2
	Softcover	978-1-5245-4422-5
	eBook	978-1-5245-4421-8

All rights reserved. No part of this book may be reproduced or transmitted in any form or by any means, electronic or mechanical, including photocopying, recording, or by any information storage and retrieval system, without permission in writing from the copyright owner.

Any people depicted in stock imagery provided by Thinkstock are models, and such images are being used for illustrative purposes only.
Certain stock imagery © Thinkstock.

Print information available on the last page.

Rev. date: 10/14/2016

To order additional copies of this book, contact:
Xlibris
1-888-795-4274
www.Xlibris.com
Orders@Xlibris.com
741665

This book is dedicated to Dr. Heinrich Kremer, The Perth Group and all of the courageous men and women who had the courage and integrity to speak truth to power.

Contents

Preface ix
Introduction xv

Part 1

1. Understanding "AIDSPEAK"—When a Virus Is Not a Virus......................1
2. When Isolation Is Not Isolation—Why p24, without Reverse
   Transcriptase, Is Not Evidence of HIV 16
3. When an HIV Antibody Test Is Not an HIV Antibody Test 36
4. When Viral Load Is Not Viral Load..58

Part 2

5. Volatile Nitrites, Folic Acid Inhibitors, and AZT—
   a Lethal Combination...84
6. Nitric Oxide: The Multifaceted Mighty Mouse of Molecules 110
7. Biological Evolution of the Endosymbiotic Event..................................134
8. The Versatility of the Mitochondrial Endosymbiont Is Consistent
   with Its Evolutionary Heritage 164
9. The Binary Strategy of Human Immune Defense—The Essential
   Absurdity of Counting Total CD4+T cells 186

Part 3

10. Cell Dis-Symbiosis: Reversal of the Trend of the Chimeric
    Genome, Reassessment of the Appropriate Clinical Marker for
    an Acquired Energy Deficiency Syndrome 213
11. Therapeutic Considerations..244

Preface

And the light shineth in darkness; and the darkness comprehended it not.

—Jn. 1:5

Medical interns and residents develop a language all their own. It is not meant for public consumption. It speaks to the train of horrors that they see while learning to seem professionally aloof—in a state of constant awareness, rising instantly to the next disaster. The language is not always pretty or sophisticated, but it is evocative. It makes sense in the context of the senselessness of the emergency room or the quiet of the morgue at midnight. It is the shorthand language that battles the fatigue of long hours and little sleep, of finding humor in the macabre. This current work uses some of that shorthand language that attempts to convey the meaning of complex concepts without raising them to the threshold of the divinely inspired. AIDS has been turned into a religion.

The AIDS tragedy did not have to happen, but it did. It was made to happen. The people who underwrote this tragedy do not deserve respect, honor, rewards, or even the banter of polite scientific conversation. This includes scientists, physicians, pharmaceutical company executives, journalists, and paid activists who knowingly blocked the science and scientists who could have saved millions from the scourge of the desired "human experimentation" of toxic chemotherapy and the obscene death profits engendered from the ninth level. Added to that list are members of the Epidemic Intelligence Service and the gutless wonders in the various governmental and educational bureaucratic hierarchies who knew and remained silent, who knew and took the death dollars as a reward for their silence. They deserve nothing less than a new round of Nuremberg-type trials. The so-called AIDS dissident movement has been addressing this issue with solemnity and respect for thirty years. The HIV/AIDS paradigm deserves neither solemnity nor respect. It deserves nothing less than outrage and ridicule as the awareness increases that it is based purely on myth and the magic of technological razzmatazz and has nothing to do with the logic of scientific truth.

Hannah Arendt was sent by the *New Yorker* to observe the Adolf Eichmann trial, out of which came the phrase "the banality evil" because Eichmann was an ordinary man. In fact, he was an "everyman." His life was boringly ordinary, but he was caught up in an international script of the political state that he had neither the inclination nor the mental resources to comprehend. His response was that of a trained animal, just following, following—never thinking an original thought or doing an original deed. He learned how to get along. So it has been in the hallowed halls of the National Cancer Institute (NCI), National Institute of Allergy and Infectious Diseases (NIAIDS), the Centers for Disease Control (CDC), the World Health Organization (WHO), and the Food and Drug Administration (FDA) all the way down to the private doctor's office. Thousands of people are making their living by not exactly lying but not exactly telling the truth—just following, following. The groupthink mentality has had deadly consequences. It defies honor. And because it is a delusional and deadly fantasyland, I call it AIDSworld. AIDSworld is a mythical land where diminutive minds and shrunken souls have been given billions in blood money sucked from the corpses of the AIDS dead to create an illusion of a virus that has never been found. However, it is the opening round in the death-knell scenario for the obsolete and disproven theory of genetic determinism.

Western culture is bereft of any conscious theory of balance and harmony. Whether in words or action, the manner in which Western culture is structured and how it has construed a world view is vis–à–vis the pyramidal conceptualization—a few at the top essentially parasitizing the great herd at the bottom. Thus, every structure created from this paradigm becomes hierarchical, including the hypothesis of how the eukaryotic cell is structured, in which the theory of genetic determinism has claimed that the central nucleus is the top controlling element essentially transferring information unidirectionally and linearly in the creation of the micro-gaian life dance of the cell. This theory has proved wrong on so many levels, but it has not deterred its adherents from pressing forward with outrageously dangerous genetic manipulations of both plants and animals. In fulfilling the Western cultural logos of domination and destruction of harmonious elements in the pursuit of the will to dominate, it has also inhibited the development of a life science that works with nature rather than against it.

Other cultures have developed different world views based not on the principle of hierarchy but balance and harmony. In Taoism, it is known as the principle of yin and yang. The ancient Africans lived by the principles of ma'at—the concept of balance by harmonizing the male and female principle manifest in all living things. In Confucianism, there is the "doctrine of the mean"; and in Buddhism, there is the principle of the "middle way." From Hinduism comes the concept of balancing the chakras. Thus, the willingness and ability to develop scientific theories congruent with the laws of nature is a human potential.

In cell physiology, the concept of balance has become known as homeostasis. Homeostasis of the eukaryotic cell has an evolutionary foundation. It is estimated that primitive life first occurred on planet Earth four billion years ago. During the first two billion years, the basic cellular anatomy and metabolic functions of microorganisms began to evolve. DNA and the glycolytic energy pathways developed in an almost oxygen-free atmosphere but an oxygen-positive ocean. Some of these early organisms learned how to use the free energy of the oxygen atom in a limited way. Two billion years ago in an Earth that had begun to increase the oxygen content of the atmosphere, two different bacteria, the Archaea and the proteobacteria, united to eventually become the eukaryotic cell. The theory of the process of that ancient syntrophic marriage is now known as endosymbiosis. As a result of this association, the central genome of eukaryotes is now a chimera. It contains genes from both the archaea and the proteobacteria, which have transitioned into a mitochondria. Almost all the mitochondrial genes have been transferred to the central nucleus with the exception of some of those that code for proteins in the electron transport chain.

After two billion years, the genes in the chimeric nucleus and their respective proteins continue to have segregated but *cooperative* functions. Although fewer in number, the human genes of archaebacterial origin tend to encode for shorter and more central proteins in the protein-protein interaction network, are less likely to be involved in heritable human disease, and tend to be involved in informational processes: translation, transcription, and replication—the life process that evolved during the first two billion years. On the other hand, the operational genes have principally come from the proteobacteria and are involved in amino acid synthesis, biosynthesis of cofactors, cell envelope, energy metabolism, intermediary metabolism, fatty acid and phospholipid biosynthesis, nucleotide biosynthesis, and regulatory functions—the life process that developed and/or matured after the fusion event.

The theory of endosymbiosis postulates that the combining and cooperating of two different ancient organisms for survival to eventually become eukaryotic cells was a unique evolutionary biological event. Heinrich Kremer's theory of cellular dis-symbiosis postulates that the endosymbiotic trend of eukaryotic cells can unravel in an evolutionary biologically predictable manner under stressful conditions. Living cells may react to external stimuli in only a few specific ways: they may be induced to perform their specialized function, they may change their specialized functions by differentiation or dedifferentiation, they may enter into the mitotic cycle and proliferate, or they may proceed to apoptosis or necrosis. The manner in which the information to proceed with particular functions is transmitted is by the process of redox signaling—the energetics of living systems based on excitation-de-excitation dynamics, which is also the basis of chemical bonding.

> *The day science begins to study non-physical phenomena, it will make more progress in one decade than in all the previous centuries of its existence*
>
> —Nikola Tesla

Cellular dis-symbiosis predicts that under an avalanche of acute reactive oxygen and nitrogen species (RONS) leading to a deficit of the reducing agent glutathione and the thiol pool, there will be a breakdown in the counterregulatory homeostatic capability, which leads to a chain of predictable events including a decrease in the mitochondrial membrane potential, increased mitochondrial calcium cycling, and concomitant release of mitochondrial proteins, a degradation of nuclear DNA and structural proteins and depending on the rapidity of the insult—apoptosis or necrosis. This is known as type I overregulation and clinically presents as acute infections, inflammatory processes, and autoimmune reactions and illnesses.

With long-term chronic RONS stressors, the system has developed evolutionarily conserved mechanisms for survival in a reduced energy environment. Nitrosylation of thiol proteins occurs with a feedback reduction in the production of these stressors—which are not only "stressors" but also play a fundamental role in the energy kinetics of the entire cell. As a result, the energy that is stored in the space-time structure of the cell itself begins to thermalize, the mitochondrial membrane becomes hyperpolarized, and there is a decrease in the mitochondria permeability transition channel, a decrease in mtCalcium cycling, and a decrease in the number and activities of the mitochondria. The evolutionary "hybrid impulse" of the eukaryotic cell reverses, and the cycling of hydrogen ions from the cytoplasm to the mitochondria via the malate aspartate and the glycerol phosphate shuttles decreases. This leads to a decrease in a supply of hydrogen ions needed for electron transport chain for the production of mitochondrial ATP but simultaneously an increase of the reductive signals that are necessary to upregulate the enzymes for glycolysis. If there is an adequate supply of reducing agents, the cell is able to exit the late

S phase of the cell division cycle, divide, and enter the G1 phase. Under stress conditions, the signals change. This process has become known as the Warburg effect. The aberrant redox signals produced by these changes allow the cell to become trapped in a mitotic repetitive cycle under the control of the archaeal part of the genome.

AIDS is not magic or mystery. It was the predictable evolutionary biological response to a historical onslaught of identifiable environmental stressors and lifestyle choices. The AIDS dissident movement has spent thirty years telling the world what HIV/AIDS is not which has certainly been helpful but not generally clinically applicable. The theory of cell dis-symbiosis presents clinically actionable and practical information on reversing the proton and other underlying metabolic deficits that characterize the syndrome.

Do many people die from AIDS? No. In the United States, it is not even listed in the top twenty mortality category, but there are more than twenty-five diseases that define the syndrome, several of which are cancers. This, of course, makes the study of the biology of AIDS relevant to a significant part of the population as according to the U.S. Centers for Disease Control, cancer is the second leading cause of mortality in this country. Thus, while AIDS might be a yawn for many people, understanding the electrochemical reordering of cellular processes of what is being called AIDS is also a way of understanding the electrochemical reordering in cancer. Thus, this is a topic of relevance to a wide international audience. Further, an understanding of the corruption in the "science" around the topic of AIDS is a gateway to a better understanding, in spite of the horrendous cancer statistics, why proven cancer cures (of which there have been many) are not now and will not in the near future be coming to a mass market.

The Richard Nixon War on Cancer project essentially suppressed the early work of Nobel laureate Otto Warburg who established that cancer cells undergo a metabolic transformation in energy production from using mostly the oxidative phosphorylation system of the mitochondrial symbiont to the less-efficient enzymatic production of ATP by glycolytic enzymes in the cytoplasm. Since the obvious failures of the Nixon War on Cancer and the effort to prove that cancer is an infectious disease, the resources of the country have been directed to those researchers who have claimed that cancer is primarily a genetic disease. This has likewise proven another dead end as it has not led to any therapeutic interventions that have been able to reduce the cancer death rates. The primary cause of cancer is neither infectious nor genetic. Infections and genetic abnormalities that are often associated with various cancers are the effects of evolutionarily conserved electrochemical changes in the retrograde and antigrade communication networks between the mitochondrial symbiont and the chimeric nucleus. Cancer, as Warburg was attempting to establish, is fundamentally a metabolic process. What Warburg did not understand, as the research had not yet been done, is that the development of cancer follows an ancient evolutionarily conserved electrochemical pattern of behavior of the eukaryotic cell.

I have kept much of Dr. Kremer's theory of cell dis-symbiosis intact. Where he discusses the quantum depths of the micro-gaian milieu, I directly address this concept by delving into recent research into how structured water, one-electron oxygen reduction, the role of reactive oxygen species in the production of biophotons, and the electronegative potential of ATP all contribute to the cells-stored energy in the space/time continuum. Unfortunately, most biologists are steeped in nineteenth-century dogmas evoked in the theory of genetic determinism while physicists have roundly entered this new era of twenty-first century science. Hopefully, this work will start a much-needed dialogue and will be seen not as an end but as a beginning. If we, as a species, don't change and soon, not only will our planet continue to suffer, but we may reach a point of no return. We thought ourselves into this predicament. We must have the spiritual and intellectual integrity to think ourselves out of it.

The book is divided into three parts. Part I translates into English what I have termed *AIDSpeak*. I analyze the meaning of HIV, of virus, of HIV antibody test, and of viral load. Once there is a common language established, part 2 delves into the metabolic response patterns that resulted at a particular time from a particular set of oxidative stressors and establishes the foundational principles of cell dis-symbiosis. Finally, part 3 outlines in detail the metabolic response patterns of cell dis-symbiosis and, using the concepts of cell dis-symbiosis, addresses the appropriate markers for evaluating and predicting the potential worsening of the thiol deficiency syndrome that clinically presents as an imbalance in the immune system characterized by a diminished capacity of the cell-mediated response to upregulate sufficient nitric oxide to kill intracellular parasites as well as a concomitant compensation of humoral immunity demonstrated by an elevated output of various antibodies. Finally, healing therapeutic interventions are suggested based on measurable deficits.

INTRODUCTION

AIDS has been defined as an acquired immune deficiency syndrome. This has some limited validity, but it is at best the superficial exploration of a bigger story. It is an unfortunate truth that the context that gives rise to the HIV/AIDS theory and many other extant medical theories of disease causation has been too little explored. The foundational principles of modern molecular biology have become moribund, and while there are alternative solutions to the current crisis in biology and medicine, change is slow in coming. The principles and practices of modern medicine derive from the theory of genetic determinism. The theory of genetic determinism—which claims that the code of life is exclusively written in DNA sequences, selected by chance in the course of the evolutionary struggle for existence—has proven that it lacks the essential feature of a genuine scientific theory: predictive power.

The root cause of what has come to be known as AIDS is not buried in the numerical oscillations of cells of the immune system or in disparate pieces of unidentifiable floating RNA or "proviral DNA" fragments quantified by the polymerase chain reaction. It is, however, evidenced in the fluctuations of the quanta and electrodynamics of the self-organized living state. Cells are large complex dynamically structured ensembles of thousands of different molecules in which a cascade of increasingly macroscopic changes occur by the mobilization of stored energy in the space-time structure. The various ways in which the eukaryotic cell maintains its homeostatic balance and responds to external cues in an effort to maintain that balance have been accumulated over time in the evolutionary biological memory of the chimeric genetics of the central genome and its interaction with the energy modulation functions of the mitochondria. This energetic and molecular cooperation is the result of the great fusion event and the massive prokaryotic gene transfer(s) that followed the formation of the eukaryotic cell.[1] This fusion event occurred

---

[1] Rivera, MC., et al, (1998), "Genomic evidence for two functionally distinct gene classes," *Proc Natl Acad Sci, USA;* 95: 6239-6244

more than two billion years ago when two separate bacteria, the archaea and the proteobacteria, combined to eventually become the eukaryote.[2] It is the energetic conversation between the chimeric genome, which includes genes from both of these ancient organisms, and the descendant of the proteobacteria, the mitochondria, that has transferred almost all but the genes that support the electron transport chain to the central genome that determines the complex stress response patterns. That ancient fusion event has come to be called endosymbiosis.

Before the evolution of free O_2, there was an excess of reducing equivalents on Earth's surface. The first traders in the planetary electron market were reductants and oxidants that were globally traded—consumed electrons from the growing population of potential donors, including H_2, H_2S, and CH_4.[3] Because all redox reactions are paired, the resulting protein networks became an integrated system of elemental cycles in which a forward reaction in one area is complemented by a reverse reaction in another. The nonrandom nature of the charge distribution in proteins[4] indicates that proteins evolved not only to serve various functions in cells but also to meet the principle of lowest energy.

Over the first two billion years of Earth's history, the major life metabolic pathways that became biochemical cycles that facilitate all electron transfers evolved in this reducing atmosphere.[5] It is likely that nitric oxide (NO), which accumulated in Earth's atmosphere before oxygen, contributed to the development of redox control of protein functioning as evidence points to a system that is preserved throughout phylogeny. Further, as will be stressed in the core of this work, cysteine has evolved specifically as an NO sensor: it is conserved in all mammals but absent from microorganisms that do not possess a recognizable nitric oxide synthase.[6]

Although these primitive organisms developed oxidases belonging to oxygen, nitrate, sulfate, and sulfur respiratory pathways, which were all characterized by their iron-sulfur (Fe-S)[7] centers, it was not until the rising

---

[2] Lane, N., Martin W., (2010), "The energetics of genome complexity," *Research Hypothesis;* 467: 929–934

[3] Falkowski, PG., (2006), "Tracing oxygen's imprint on earth's metabolic evolution," *Science;* 311: 1724–1725

[4] Soda, K, Kakuyama, K, Miki, Y., (1997), "Non-random ionic-charge distribution responsible for the structural stability and molecular recognition of proteins," *Biosystems;* 43(3): 199–204

[5] Falkowski, Ibid.

[6] Stamler, JS., et al., (2001), "Nitrosylation: the protypic redox-based signaling mechanism," *Cell;* 106: 675–683

[7] Castresana, J, Moreira, D., (1999), "Respiratory chains in the lat common ancestor of living organisms," *J Mol Evol;* 49:453–460

levels of oxygen in the atmosphere began to radically change the exchange marketplace and put a survival pressure on these organisms that the driving of the evolution of the endosymbiotic event became a possibility. Organisms that were strictly anaerobic and organisms that were facultative anaerobes eventually combined and developed a chimeric central nucleus. In this manner, they were able to adapt and integrate the old pathways that evolved in a reducing environment and continue the development of the new pathways that evolved in a more oxidative atmosphere.[8] It was a functional energetic adaptation. The old pathways that formed in a more reducing atmosphere continued to use the ancient signaling modalities and to control informational processes involved in translation, transcription, and replication. The newer pathways, which evolved in a more oxidative atmosphere and developed a different signaling system, were involved in higher order operational processes and were largely responsible for the development of complex organisms, including humans.[9] This fusion event continues to operate at the edge of energetic chaos. Under biologically stressful conditions, the cooperative trend has the potential to unravel. The dissolution of the cooperative trend is not random. It is orchestrated using a series of stochastically predictable metabolic patterns that have been evolutionarily preserved and is known as dis-symbiosis.

When the organism is confronted with either a massively acute or a prolonged oxidative/nitrosative stress load that results in a deficit of available reducing equivalents, there arises a cellular crisis. This energetic crisis leads to a dissolution of the symbiotic trend—a dis-symbiosis, which is an energetic unwinding and disassociation of the endosymbiotic cooperative trend of the chimeric genome and its energetic relationship with the mitochondria.[10] The cell, having lost a portion of its stored structural energy, either dies or reorganizes its metabolic functions into a survival mode. With the conserved genetic memory from the initial reducing atmosphere of the early earth, the operational functions that primarily use the oxidative phosphorylation energy system decrease while the informational functions (transcription, translation,

---

[8] Falkowski, PG., Godfrey, LV., (2008), "Electrons, life and the evolution of Earth's oxygen cycle," *Phil Trans R. Soc.;* 363: 2705–2716

[9] Alvarez-Ponce, D, McInerney, JO, (2011), "The human genome retains relics of its prokaryotic ancestry: human genes of archaebacterial and eubacterial origin exhibit remarkable differences," *Genome Bio & Evolution;* dol:10.1093/gbe/evr073

[10] Alvarez-Ponce, D, McInerney, JO, Ibid

and replication) that are still largely under the control of the cytosolic glycolytic energy system increase.[11,12,13]

The condition being called AIDS occurred as a result of a massive electron deficit expressed clinically as a significant reduction in the important antioxidant tripeptide molecule, glutathione, which contains a cysteine molecule, and a generalized exhaustion of other antioxidant systems.[14,15] When it is recognized in the context of the evolutionary biology of the eukaryotic cell, it can be understood that AIDS is not primarily a complication of the immune system but a fundamental systemic problem of energy deficiency. This energy-deficiency state manifested not only as a predictable evolutionarily programmed imbalance in cellular immune defense but also in an alteration in systemic homeostatic mechanisms. Therefore, it requires a more appropriate redefinition: AEDS, an acquired energy deficiency syndrome. The implications of this altered view profoundly reorient the way this dilemma has been positioned in the marketplace of ideas. If, in fact, the key factor in cellular homeostasis is energy deficiency—a decrease in energy storage under energy flow as early on in the AIDS crisis was indicated by the consistent finding of reduced glutathione and its precursor, cysteine, in the lung mucosa, plasma and T helper immune cells of HIV positive patients[16,17]—then by this change of focus from the immune system to the cells energy metabolism, AEDS becomes a problem that is noninfectious, will never lead to the predicted pandemics, will never have a vaccine, and is reversible.

How modern medical science used an acute environmental episode to define a situational crisis of immune cell and vascular endothelial cell homeostasis to create both an international panic and a profit center was described in *AIDS, Opium, Diamonds, and Empire: The Deadly Virus of International*

---

[11] Alverez-Ponce Op Cit.

[12] Brand, Karl, (1997), "Aerobic glycolysis by proliferating cells: protection against oxidative stress at the expense of energy yield," *J Bioenergetics & Biomembranes;* 29(4): 355–364

[13] Rivera, M.C., et al., (1998), "Genomic evidence for two functionally distinct gene classes," *PNAS, USA.,* 95: 6239–6244

[14] Eck, HP, et al.,(1989) "Low concentrations of acid-soluble thiol (cysteine) in the blood plasma of HIV-1-infected patients," *Biol Chem Hoppe Seyler;* 370(2): 101–108

[15] Buhl, R, et al., (1989), "Systemic glutathione deficiency in symptom free HIV seropositive individuals," *Lancet;* 334(8675): 1294–1298

[16] Buhl, R., Holroyd, K. J., Mastrangell, A. et al. (1989), Systemic glutathione deficiency in symptom-free-HIV seropositive individuals. Lancet, 11, 1294-1297.

[17] Eck, HP, et al., (1989), "Low concentrations of acid globule thiol (cysteine) in the blood plasma of HIV-1 infected patients," *Biol Chem Hippe-Seyler;* 370: 101–108

Greed.[18] How this problem can be repositioned, understood, and resolved in the context of knowable cellular biology is the focus of this treatise. How were we so led astray?

For most of the past century, biological advancement has been constrained by the narrow dictates of the masters of an economic system who were not so much interested in compelling ideas as they were in the advancement of a particular shared vision of developing various ways in which they could use science to control society. By a coordinated arrangement of patronage, the focus of biology, the study of life, was constricted to the study of macromolecules—molecular biology, which is a term coined in 1938 by Warren Weaver. Weaver was the director of the Rockefeller Foundation's natural science division[19] and was charged with the power to direct funding to those people and institutions that voluntarily conformed to the eugenics principles. As stated in the division's 1934 progress report, "the challenge . . . is obvious. . . Can we develop so sound and extensive a genetics that we can hope to breed, in the future, superior men?"[20]

Water, which gives life both its context and matrix and by far is the most important and abundant constituent of all living organisms, has been completely ignored by the molecular biologists except to assume that it acts solely as a solvent. Nothing could be further from consistent observations.[21,22] Ninety-nine percent of the cell's molecules are water,[23] and most of it is structured in such a way that it is an active participant in all redox reactions.[24,25] Yet scientists trained with an orientation to molecular biology have spent almost a century ignoring this fact and trying to construct a paradigm of life based on the examination of less than 1 percent of the cell's molecules removed from their

---

[18] Banks, NT., (2010) "AIDS, Opium, Diamonds and Empire. The Deadly Virus of International Greed," iUniverse

[19] Kay, LE, 1993, The Molecular vision of life, Caltech, the Rockefeller Foundation and the rise of the new biology, Oxford University Press, N.Y. pp.4–5

[20] Franks, M, (2005), "Margaret Sanger's Eugenic Legacy: The Control of Female Fertility," p. 156 McFarland Co., North Carolina

[21] Pollack, G., (2001), "Cells, Gels and the Engines of Life," Ebner & Sons,

[22] Voeikov, VL, (2009), "Water Respiration—the basis of the living state," *Water;* 1: 52-75

[23] http://www.tetonnm.com/pics/IndependentSamplePages/1-893441-42-3.pdf Chemical composition of living cells, downloaded 12 June 2014

[24] Del Giudice, E., et al., (2010), "Water dynamics at the root of metamorphosis in living organisms," *Water;* 2: 566-586

[25] Voeikov, V., (2001), "Reactive oxygen species, water, photons and life," *Riv Biol;* 94(2): 237-258

milieu—polarized water and polarized water, protein and ATP interactions, and the resultant arising electromagnetic fields.[26,27]

Lily Kay received her doctorate in the history of science from Johns Hopkins. In 1993, she published an exposé of the history of modern molecular biology, *The Molecular Vision of Life*. The basic premise of her thesis was that this biology project funded by several financial titans in the early part of the twentieth century was not fundamentally a scientific idea but issued from the social orientation of the Rockefeller Foundation's Science of Man project. The stated purpose of this project was an effort to socially engineer humanity to weed out those targeted as "undesirable." Eugenic objectives played a significant role in the conception and design of the molecular biology program at a time when the violence of the old eugenics had to become more subtle and surreptitious to give the illusion of scientific validity to new methods of mass control. The focus of this control was via the dissemination, as fundamental truths, of ideas that held a prescribed world view. This new program created a space that claimed to place the study of human heredity and behavior on rigorous grounds. This new biology became mesmerized with genetics while simultaneously ignoring the fundamentals of cell physiology. It was an effort at cementing a different type of social control at the moment in history when it became publicly unacceptable to advocate social control based on crude racist eugenic principles and hostile racial theories.[28]

Molecular biology has gained enormous technological and social power, even with the increasing realization of the bad science on which it is based, including a multitude of weak points in genetic and evolutionary theory.[29] Yet this has not prevented its advocates from attempting to direct the world into such sophomoric, unpredictable, and life-threatening ventures as genetic engineering, biotechnology in agriculture and medicine and the Human Genome Project. The deeper nature of this project is exposed by its association with the scientific descendants of the Department of Energy's Atomic bomb endeavor[30] and the use of the military reference of the "Manhattan Project of life sciences."

---

[26] Cifra, M, (2009), "Study of electromagnetic oscillations of yeast cells in kHz and GHz region," Doctoral Thesis, Czech Tech. Univ. in Prague, Faculty of Electrical Engineering

[27] Ling, GN., (2001), Life at the cell and below-cell level, Pacific Press, New York, NY

[28] Kay, Op cit p 9

[29] Ho, MW, (1999) Genetic Engineering—Dream or Nightmare? 2nd rev ed. Dublin Gateway

[30] Trewhella, J., (2013), "The human genome project: an adventure in research that has delivered great benefit," http://sydney.edu.au/news/research_support/2C379.html?newsstoryid=11666 12 June 2014

The Slow Death of the AIDS/Cancer Paradigm
and the Apocrypha of the Eukaryotic Cell

The so-called war on cancer initiated during the Nixon administration was an outgrowth of the molecular biology project. When that effort was on the verge of total collapse, the AIDS crisis arose and repositioned the barren landscape called virology in such a way that it had the effect of resurrecting the careers of the cancer researchers from the ashes of another failed "war" initiative that had wasted billions of dollars and thousands of man-hours on the fruitless search for an infectious cause of the genetic defects often found in cancer cells.

Molecular biology, as it exists today, and because of its foundational reductionism, should be regarded more as an engineering discipline rather than science. It is pragmatic instrumental knowledge that relies heavily on technological wizardry and that arrogantly and irrationally seeks to overwhelm nature rather than attempting to understand nature by understanding the language that nature has provided.[31] As this technology takes into account neither the evolutionary biology nor the energetic and quantum underpinnings of the self-organizing processes that characterize life, it does not constitute a scientific theory of life able to give us orientation to live rationally with nature. At best, it can only provide specious and ultimately destructively futile attempts at technological control over life.[32] Thus, contemporary molecular biology has become a scientific technology that has lost contact with the epistemological sciences. It has avoided addressing the fundamental issues of living matter—the problems that are at the very core of biological organization and development: homeostasis, ontogenesis, and phylogenesis.[33]

To unravel the AIDS mystery, one has to begin a journey that has been sidestepped by the dogma of molecular biology and examine questions of a more profound quality, namely, not just how living matter came into existence but exactly what the nature of living matter is.

The effort to understand the processes of life without undertaking an investigation of the processes that animate life has been both a great folly and beset with human tragedy. The fruits of following the tenets of molecular biology became abundantly clear by the year 2000 when an article in *JAMA*[34] asked, "Is US Health Really the Best in the World?" It made the startling claim that the health care system itself is the third leading cause of death totaling 225,000 deaths annually of which 106,000 deaths per year are from

---

[31] Primas, H., (1982), Chemistry and Complementarity, *Chimia*; 36: 293–300
[32] Primas, H. et al., (eds) (1999), "On quanta, mind and matter, Hans Primas in Context" Lecture notes in Chemistry, 24, Dordrecht, Kluwer
[33] Rosen, R., (1967) "Optimality Principles in Biology" Plenum Press, NY
[34] Starfield, B., (July 26, 2000), "Is US health really the best in the world," *JAMA*; 284(4):483–485

nonerror, adverse effects of medications. A more recent study has revised this number upward to 400,000.[35] This is the direct cost of trying to quantify the unquantifiable by measuring life by abstracting and counting its fundamental parts and measuring lives by an economic measure of a "cost/benefit" ratio[36] all the while ignoring the basic question of the nature of living matter.

Living beings are not machines as some are still claiming.[37,38,39] They have key fundamental and profound differences. Work performed by a machine is not aimed at preserving its structure or its ability to function. The machine structure acts only as the transformer into work of free energy that it receives from the external sources. It is true that the possibility of dismantling a machine to understand how it functions is a process that has been repeatedly successful. Although the dismantling of a cell to study its parts has given us much useful information, this laboratory activity undertaken without a fundamental concept of the nature of the living state cannot and never will lead to a successful understanding of the complex nonlinear self-organizing processes in a living cell in its dynamic state. The instant a molecule is separated from its context, both the molecule and the network are irretrievably altered.

The Nature of the Living State According Albert Szent-Györgyi

A major characteristic of living systems is that the work they perform is done at the expense of their own structural energy. The Nobel laureate and discoverer of vitamin C, Albert Szent-Györgyi, observed that [molecular] biologists might not be able to formally distinguish between "animate" and "inanimate" things because they concentrate on studying the substances (macromolecules) to the neglect of two matrices without which these substances cannot perform any functions: water and electromagnetic fields.[40] "Biology has forgotten water

---

[35] James, JT., (2013) "A new, evidence-based estimate of patient harms associated with hospital care," *J Patient Saf;* 9(3): 122–128

[36] Gruber, J., et al., (1997), NBER working paper 6034, "Abortion legalization and child living circumstances: who is the marginal child?" Nat. Bureau of Economic Research: http://www.nber.org/papers/w6034.pdf

[37] Michael Polanyi, "Life transcending physics and chemistry," *Chemical and Engineering News,* 45(35): 54-66 (August 21, 1967).

[38] Bruce Alberts, "The Cell as a Collection of Protein Machines: Preparing the Next Generation of Molecular Biologists," *Cell,* Vol. 92: 291 (February 6, 1998).

[39] Piccolino M., "Biological machines: from mills to molecules" *Nat Rev Mol Cell Biol.* 2000 Nov;1(2):149-53.

[40] Voeikov, VL, DelGiudice, E.,(2009) "Water Respiration—the basis of the living state," *Water;* 1:52–74

or never even thought of it."[41] In point of fact, it has been demonstrated that water is the actual basis of biological organization.[42,43] Recent studies have demonstrated oscillatory modes of photon emissions that spontaneously arise in water solutions of simple sugars or other carbonyl compounds and amino acids.[44] Processes, with the participation of reactive oxygen species (when radicals recombine, a quanta of energy is released equivalent to the energy of photons of visible or even UV light), demonstrate a propensity to self-organize.[45] Szent-Györgyi then postulated that life could be considered as the interposition between two energy levels of an electron: the excited state and the ground state.[46] It is organized water existing close to biomolecular surfaces that is able to induce long-lasting electronic excitation of the different molecular species present, making their activation possible.[47,48] The fundamental issue is to establish a suitable explanation and an overarching framework for understanding the energetic nature of the living state.

While molecular biology has spent decades studying gene mutations, it has been observed by wiser players that it is not gene mutations—which are, in essence, the material traits of energy fluctuations—but the thermodynamic fluctuations of energy themselves that alter both the informational and operational molecular structures of the network. Thus, to begin to fashion any understanding of the network, one must begin at the beginning, and the beginning is to establish the basic conditions of the framework that nature has established to carry out these functions.

---

[41] Szent-Gyorgy, A. (1956), Bioenergeitcs. *Science,* 124:873-875

[42] Del Giudice, E., (2007), "The organization of water as the basis of the biological organization: the special role of the ELF magnetic fields," Presentation given 17 Dec. 2007 Conference, Venice, Italy, *Foundations of bioelectromagnetics: towards a new rationale for risk assessment and management*

[43] Winfree, AT., (1984), "The prehistory of the Belousov-Zhabotinsky oscillator," *J Chem Educ;* 61(8): 661-663

[44] Kondrashova, et al., (2000), "The primary physico-chemical mechanism for the beneficial biological/medical effects of negative air ions," *IEEE Transactions on Plasma Sci;* 28(1): 230-237

[45] Kummer, U, et al., (1996), "Oscillations in the peroxidase oxidase reaction: a comparison of different peroxidases," *Biochim Biophys Acta;* 1289: 39-403

[46] Voeikov, DelGiudice (2009) op cit.

[47] Szent-Gyorgi, A., *Introduction to a supramolecular biology;* Academic Press: New York, NY, USA, 1960

[48] Mallamace, F, et al., (2014), "The role of water in protein's behavior: the two dynamical crossovers studied by NMR and FTIR techniques," *Computational Structural Biochtech J;* 13: 33–37

The Nature of the Living State According to Ervin Bauer

While the molecular biologists favored by the Rockefeller Science of Man project were being well funded to advance a particular point of view, antithetical to the true form of observational science from which derived their hypotheses and theories, on the other side of the world, a Russian biologist of Hungarian origin, Ervin Simonovich Bauer, was constructing an altogether different perspective. Bauer—rather than attempting, for reasons of political or social control, to impose his will upon nature—was observing the natural world and formulating a set of fundamental principles by which to distinguish animate from inanimate systems. Living systems, according to Bauer, have unique properties: metabolism, growth and development, multiplication, adaptability, excitability and reactivity, senescence, and evolution. All these, Bauer described as innate laws of the development of living matter on Earth. Bauer expounded on three fundamental postulates:

1. All living systems are always in stable-nonequilibrium condition and therefore have *energy* to perform work. This energy is used to sustain the nonequilibrium state; therefore, they are purposeful (stable nonequilibrium).
2. Living systems are preforming internal work and external work (interaction with the environment, obtaining of food, etc.). This postulate states that the proportion of the energy used in external work to that used in internal work increases in development (augmentation and homeostasis).
3. Nonequilibrium in living systems consists of molecular compounds in whose conformation the metabolic energy is used to form them is stored[49] (energy storage under energy flow).

The Principle of Stable Nonequilibrium

According to Bauer, "All and only living systems are never in equilibrium. At the expense of their free energy, they ceaselessly perform work against sliding toward equilibrium [entropy] demanded by the physical and chemical laws appropriate to the actual external conditions."[50] The nonequilibrium

---

[49] Integrative Biophysics Biophotonics, edited by Fritz-Albert Popp and Lev Beloussov 2003, Kluwer Academic Publishers, Boston; p 49
[50] Bauer, ES., *Theoretical Biology;* Reprint of the 1935 edition with a preface, a biographical and critical essay, Akadémiai Kiadó, Budapest 1982

state is thus an inherent quality at all levels of a living system's organization including (1) the sustaining of chemical gradients and (2) electrical gradients across membranes, (3) as well as other phase boundaries.[51] Because matter's nonequilibrium state is equivalent to its excited state, as opposed to its ground state, Bauer defined the energy of an excited (nonequilibrium) state of matter as "structural energy."[52] This has been confirmed by observations on the properties of the cytoskeleton, especially microtubules, which fulfill the prerequisites for the generation of quasi-coherent electromagnetic fields as they are highly electrically polar, have an energy supply, and possess nonlinear properties that may convert random thermal energy to quasi-coherent.[53] Bauer further observed that all work performed by living systems is executed by its excited structures, which transit from the excited state to the ground state (see above Szent-Györgyi). This also implies that living systems have the need for an excess of available electrons or reducing equivalents for redox reactions.[54]

In relation to AIDS, given that the energy fluctuations in these patients transition from the predominate use of the more efficient oxidative phosphorylation system to in end stages, the less efficient aerobic glycolysis, the opportunistic infections, degenerative patterns, and wasting syndrome will be shown to be understandable evolutionarily conserved consequences of this energetic transformation as the result of a deficit of reducing equivalents. The trap from which the AIDS paradigm has not been able to extricate itself is that no matter how many studies indicate that there is a significant reduction of glutathione in the microcellular compartments, or how it has been shown that a deficiency of this molecule in the blood, plasma, immune cells, and mucosal surfaces is associated with impaired survival in HIV positive patients,[55] and how much is known and knowable about this electron deficit and its role in creating

---

[51] Voeikov, VL., Del Giudice E., Op Cit. 2009

[52] Ibid

[53] Cifra, Michal, (2009), "Study of electromagneitc oscillations of yeast cells in kHz and GHz region" Doctoral Thesis, p. 3, Czech Technical Univ., Prague, Faculty of Electrical Engineering

[54] oxidation may be defined as the addition of oxygen, the loss of electrons, or the loss of hydrogen atoms (but not hydrogen ions, H$^+$); conversely, reduction can be defined as the removal of oxygen, the addition of electrons, or the addition of hydrogen atoms.

Oxidation–reduction reactions only occur when there are pairs of substrates, forming pairs of products:

Aox + Bred ⇔ Ared + Box mnemonic: LEO says GER= meaning "loss of e- = oxidation and gain of e- = reduced

[55] Herzenberg, L.A., (1997), "Glutathione deficiency is associated with impaired survival in HIV disease," *Proc Natl Acad Sci USA;* 94: 1967–1972

the biological responses leading to cellular imbalances, which will be called dis-symbiosis,[56] the obvious energetic imbalances and the resultant metabolic after effects are willfully ignored.

A conditional principle of the nonequilibrium state is that "all the work that may be performed by living systems is done only at the expense of structural energy [of its excited elements that transit from the excited to the ground state]—that is, by forces generated by a living system itself."[57] This implies that the living system is intrinsically active and that this assembly cannot emerge by the passive elements as acclaimed by conventional molecular biology. The living state emerges from the transition of these components into a new state. The new state has properties different from those elements in isolation.[58,59] Claude Bernard,[60] Walter Cannon,[61] and Hans Selye[62] all later incorporated this idea into their various hypothesis of the coordinated physiological processes that maintain a steady state (nonequilibrium) in the organism—observations that, until recently, had insufficient biophysical correlates to institute rational clinical therapies.

Living systems use their own structural energy to extract chemical energy from food or light energy in the case of photosynthesis. This energy is converted to structural energy of the molecular components of living matter. This structural energy is then able to be converted into work. To avoid energy loss through heat, the energy is stored within extended regions (e.g., cytoskeleton and other molecules in the excited state) able to keep it as the continuous agent of long-lived excited states of the extended region.[63] The work of theoretical physicist Herbert Fröhlich was crucial in elucidating this feature of the living state by consideration of how longitudinal vibrations in the microwave frequency range (10^{11} and 10^{12} Hz) arise from the dipole properties of cell membranes, macromolecular bonds such as hydrogen bonds, and delocalized electrons. In a 1968 paper, he observed that "the non-equilibrium state created by the

---

[56] Kremer, H., (2008), "The Silent Revolution in Cancer and AIDS Medicine," XLibris
[57] Bauer, Op Cit
[58] Ling, GN., *Life at the cell and below cell level, the hidden history of a fundamental revolution in biology*, 2001 Pacific Press, NY
[59] Pollock, GH., *Cells, gels and the engines of life, a new, unifying approach to cell function*, 2001, Ebner & Sons, Seattle, Washington
[60] Bernard, C. (1974) Lectures on the phenomena common to animals and plants. Trans Hoff HE, Guillemin R, Guillemin L, Springfield (IL): Charles C Thomas
[61] W. B. Cannon; Physiological Regulation of Normal States: Some Tentative Postulates Concerning Biological Homeostatics; IN: A. Pettit (ed.); A Charles Richet: ses amis, ses collègues, ses élèves; p. 91; Paris; Éditions Médicales; 1926.
[62] Selye, H. (Oct 7, 1955). "Stress and disease." Science 122: 625–631.
[63] Voeikov, VL, DelGuidice, E., Op cit.

continuous supply of a certain minimum of energy should . . . bring about a stationary state in which energy is not completely thermalized, but stored in a highly ordered fashion."[64] This order then gives rise to long-range phase correlations—coupling forces that bind particles together in pairs separated by hundreds of atomic diameters.[65] These are the energetic patterns of the living state at the quantum level of cellular organization that have been assiduously ignored by molecular biology.

This stored energy, being capable of doing work, is also mobilizable energy or coherent energy. Coherent energy comes and goes together so it can do work as opposed to incoherent energy that goes in all directions and cancels itself out.[66] Since work is performed against an equilibrium, free energy is consumed. Thus, each excited element of a living system performing its job inevitably slides toward equilibrium and if unabated will ultimately manifest as altered homeostatic levels. This decrease in the supply of electrons can lead to the dis-symbiosis of the trend of the chimeric genome, a decreasing ability to supply protons to the electron transport chain of the mitochondria, a general switch in the high-efficiency energy production in the mitochondria away from oxidative phosphorylation to the relatively low-efficiency energy production by the cytosolic aerobic glycolytic process. Clinically, these cellular processes are what manifest as either "acute" or "chronic" and/or "incurable" diseases. If left unbalanced, as is currently the practice in all allopathic medical disciplines (with the exception of some gross vitamin deficiencies), it eventually leads to death.

To preserve the nonequilibrium state, a living system continuously repairs or substitutes its exhausted structural elements. Energy is needed for this work, and this energy comes from the inherent nonequilibrium structures in the living system. Of course, this implies that if the energy is not available, both the structural integrity and the functional capacity of the cell become less than optimal. In principle, Bauer was already intuitively understanding that the structural energy of the living state was more than that which could be supplied by the hydrolysis of ATP.

---

[64] Frolich, H., (1968), "Long range coherence and energy storage in biological systems," *Int J Quantum Chemistry;* 2: 641-649
[65] Popp, FA., Beloussov, L., (2003), "Integrative biophysics, biophotonics," Kluwer Academic Publishers, Boston, Mass p 52
[66] Ho, MW., *The Rainbow and the Worm* 2008 World Scientific Publishing, Hackensack, NJ

The Principle of Augmentation of External Work Performance and Homeostasis

A living system gradually loses its free energy and the matter "charged" with it and needs to replace them with new matter and energy (chemical energy of food, energy of light, etc.) consumed from the environment.[67] This energy is then used for reexcitation or substitution of exhausted structural elements. These structural elements function as disposable instruments for the performance of active life. Understanding this process becomes vitally important in the context of AIDS research. It will be demonstrated that the disposal of these oxidized expendable structural elements have unfortunately often been misconstrued by electron microscopy as "virus" or "virus-like particles." They have also been misconstrued as the cause of cellular changes when, in fact, they will be demonstrated to be the consequence of the cell's disposal of oxidatively damaged molecules.

However, the transformation of this external energy cannot happen without external work being performed. The dominant mode of energy *extraction* from organic compounds by living systems is respiration, which, in eukaryotic cells, takes place mostly in the mitochondria. It is more efficient than glycolysis because it requires less substrate to produce more ATP.[68] During the performance of this external work, a living system loses its structural energy and tends toward equilibrium.[69] Before equilibrium (death) is reached, depending on the rapidity of changes, there can be a transition from oxidative phosphorylation to glycolysis. It will be noted here that, currently, biology teaches that the process of mitochondrial respiration is an energy-supplying process and downplays the energy-using extractive processes necessary to turn the energy from sun/food into utilizable structural energy. Bauer's theory underscores that it must first work to extract this energy from organic compounds before the energy can then be supplied back to the system. This understanding becomes crucial in the clinical setting.

The clinician then must consider the multiple ways in patients with AIDS that the energy extraction process may be subverted. AIDS patients may have bowel inflammation from trauma, infectious processes, or use of antibiotics, which alter the microflora/and or the cellular absorptive surfaces in such a way to interfere with normal absorption patterns as well as immunological

---

[67] Voeikov, VL, Del Guidice, E., Op. cit.
[68] Brand, K, (1997), "Aerobic glycolysis by proliferating cells: protection against oxidative stress at the expense of energy yield," *J Bioenergetics Biomembranes;* 29(4): 355–364
[69] Voeikov, VL, Del Guidice, E., Op cit.

responses; the lung tissue may be deficient in glutathione, which will be shown to alter the level of oxidative phosphorylation. If there is a history of inhaled nitrate use, methemoglobinemia may be a problem for the exchange of oxygen; if there is an increase in aerobic glycolysis as a result of either chronic oxidative stressors or iatrogenic use of antiretroviral drugs, this will bring about a change in the mitochondrial membrane potential, and a decrease in the efficiency of the electron transport chain will ensue. Long term, as the result of increased substrate requirement because of the upregulation of glycolytic enzymes, there will be a breakdown in the peripheral muscle tissue sufficient to supply the cytosolic enzyme system with substrate for the aerobic glycolysis process—resulting in classic muscle wasting and a severe nitrogen imbalance. If there is an electron deficit in the T helper and other immune cells, they will be propelled toward a type 2 cytokine dominance pattern and away from a type 1 pattern in which the immune and other cells can no longer upregulate inducible nitric oxide synthase to mount a nitric oxide intracellular gas attack against invading organisms. As the AIDS proponents seldom address these global metabolically critical issues, rather than understand that the organism cannot provide internal work for its own maintenance if the extraction processes (external work) are blocked, they continue to give drugs that actually block the extraction processes while at the same time fail to replenish the cysteine/glutathione and other nutrient deficiencies, thereby creating a downward spiral of the patient that they continue to defend and define as the natural consequence of the HIV virus infection. None of the so-called antiretroviral drugs sufficiently answer the fundamental issue of glutathione deficiency.

Living organisms are thermodynamically open systems that are operating far from thermodynamic equilibrium in an environment in which they exchange energy and matter and are able to decrease their own entropy as a consequence of their dynamics. This is what has been termed as a *dissipative structure*.[70] Since reduction of the nonequilibrium state of a living system, resulting from its own efforts, contradicts the principle of stable nonequilibrium, and since a living system cannot violate the principle of its existence, it may perform external work only by infringing on the nonequilibrium of its structures under the influence of external impulses.[71] Therefore, external influences, irritations that infringe on the nonequilibrium of a living system, have the effect that the energy freed is spent to perform external work rather than internal work—which, is in fact, in the context of AIDS; and the recognized electron deficits

---

[70] Prigogine, I., *Introduction to Thermodynamics of Irreversible Processes*, John Wiley & Sons, NY 1962

[71] Op cit, Voeikov

can then be understood to be not an acquired immune deficiency syndrome but an acquired energy deficiency syndrome by virtue of the these deficits.

This is one of the fundamental differences between the living state and inanimate objects. Machines are passive acceptors of energy that flows through them and is converted to work. Outside sources charge the inanimate system with energy, which can then be changed into work. However, in the living system, neither chemical nor solar energy can be gained from the environment and transformed into structural energy without external work being performed. Other sources of structural energy of the living cell come from one-electron oxygen reduction in what has been termed the *fourth phase of water*,[72] the reactive oxygen species produced at a steady state in the mitochondrial network, and not as currently considered, by the hydrolysis of ATP, but by the electronegative energy transduction of ATP as a force multiplier transmitted through the water/protein/ion matrix,[73] including the cytoskeleton, especially microtubules that are highly electrically polar and possess nonlinear properties that have the ability to convert random thermal energy to a quasi-coherent electromagnetic field.[74]

Water in Living Systems as the Primary Source of Structural Energy

When biomolecules are separated from living matter or from catalysts, they are able to interact with many other molecules thereby producing a great number of reactions. But in the context of living matter, the biomolecule behaves very differently. Each biomolecule lives inside of each particular biochemical cycle in an almost-monogamous condition (at least within definite time intervals)—that is, a biomolecule (in the confined space of subcellular compartments) interacts with only well-defined partners and ignores the other biomolecules, with which interaction would have been possible in empty space. Living matter therefore produces a "context" that is capable of preventing a great number of chemical interactions that would theoretically be possible.[75] It is this "context" that will be directly addressed in part 2 of this book.

---

[72] Pollack, GH., The Fourth Phase of Water, beyond solid liquid vapor, 2013 Ebner & Sons, Seattle, WA

[73] Ling, G, (2001), Life at the cell and below level, the hidden history of a fundamental revolution in biology; Pacific Investment Research, Inc.,

[74] Cifra, Op Cit.

[75] Del Giudice, E., "The Role of water in living organisms" http://www.heavylight.de/publish_en/hl_article_delgiudice_tedeschi_1_09.php

One of the most significant discoveries over the past three decades has been that water has quantum properties under ambient conditions and forms what have been termed *exclusion zones* or *coherent domains* next to protein surfaces.[76] This revolutionary observation has greatly altered our understanding of redox chemistry, especially since all living systems gain energy from oxidation-reduction reactions—electron transfers from substances that can hold them more weakly to ones that can hold them more strongly. Ordinarily, water is considered a very poor electron donor. However, in a series of recent papers, Gerald Pollack[77] has pointed out that water-hydrating hydrophilic surfaces is very different from bulk water in viscosity, density, freezing temperature, relative permittivity—so different that it has been termed the fourth phase of water.[78] It appears that the thickness of this layer may reach hundreds of microns and that these water molecules may then oscillate in unison within extended coherent domains (CD) between two configurations: the first is where all electrons are tightly bound to their molecule; in the second configuration, one electron per molecule is almost free. In this way, a CD includes a reservoir of vortices of the plasma of quasi-free electrons. Since the vortex motion is coherent and frictionless (cannot decay thermally), its potential lifetime could be extremely long (weeks, months).[79] Consequently, CDs become systems able to store large amounts of energy, transforming it from high-entropy to low-entropy energy. This stored energy can be released to nonaqueous molecules when the frequency of oscillation of these molecules matches the frequency of oscillation of the CD. Thus, these water networks are able to transmit information around the proteins and act as a control mechanism for protein dynamics. In this way, selected molecules get activated, facilitating the self-organizing biochemical processes that are the hallmark of living organisms.[80]

This coherent domain/exclusion zone of water, or EZ water, has some unexpected properties: EZ water has negative electrical potential with respect to the bulk water adjacent to it (down to -150 mv), protons concentrate at the boundary between EZ water and bulk water, and EZ-water has a prominent peak of light adsorption at 270 nm, and it emits fluorescence when excited with

---

[76] Del Giudice, Ibid

[77] Pollack, GH., *Cells, gels and the engines of life, a new unifying approach to cell function,* 2001 Ebner and Sons, Seattle, Washington

[78] Pollock, GH., *The fourth phase of water, beyond solid liquid vapor,* 2013 Ebner & Sons, Seattle, Washington

[79] Del Giudice, E., "Formation of dissipative structures in liquid water," lecture 4th annual conference on the physics, chemistry and biology of water Oct 22-25, 2009 http://www.waterjournal.org/uploads/vol2/supplement/WATER-vol2-Suppl.pdf

[80] Del Giudice, E., Ibid

this wavelength. The thickness of the EZ-water layer increases when illuminated with visible and especially IR radiation.[81] Generally, a water molecule is considered a poor electron donor; however, all these listed features strongly suggest that electrons in EZ water are much less bound—they reside at a much higher state of excitation—than electrons in bulk water. Therefore, a much lower energy of excitation is needed to free them. As radiation, especially light in the IR part of the spectrum, increases the thickness of the layer of EZ water. It increases its electron-donating capacity. The H bonds in these structures last only a few picoseconds. The rapid fluctuations of this electrically charged structure are actually making it an antenna having an oscillation frequency in the infrared region.[82] The wavelength of this oscillation is large enough to cover a huge number (in the millions) of molecules, producing a collective motion that cannot be reduced to the sum of two body scatterings.[83]

EZ water then becomes an almost-inexhaustible source of electrons and may therefore be considered as residing in a stable nonequilibrium state with respect to bulk water. To convert the potential energy of quasi-free electrons in EZ water into free energy capable of performing work, an acceptor of these electrons is needed. Oxygen is always available, and water is the ultimate source of oxygen on Earth. If EZ water is in contact with bulk water in which oxygen is dissolved, EZ water will donate electrons to oxygen.[84] When EZ water (the excited state) reverts to bulk water (the ground state), high-grade, high-potential energy may be donated by this reaction for every fully reduced O_2 molecule. This release of energy from excited to bulk phase is the "structural energy" (Bauer's analogy) of EZ water that is released when two water molecules belonging to this stable nonequilibrium structure revert to ground state water molecules.[85]

EZ water or coherent domains are thus able to give rise to significant electron transfer, which is very useful in biological systems where it supplies redox reactions. The probability of electron transfer is higher when the CDs are completely surrounded by the noncoherent state.[86]

The importance of this is that water in the coherent domain is a process able to collect low-grade energy in the environment having high entropy and

---

[81] Voeikov, Del Guidice, op cit
[82] Ibid
[83] Ibid
[84] Ibid
[85] Ibid
[86] Del Giudice, et al., Op Cit role water in living organisms

convert it, by exciting coherent vortices of almost-free electrons, into high-grade energy with low entropy.[87]

What happens to an organism over time when, because of chronic oxidative/nitrosative stressors leading to a significant electron deficit, the structural energy of electronic excitation combined with the decreased production of ATP is no longer sufficient to maintain the integrity and biorhythms of the dynamic cellular networks? What happens when the external cues are aberrant or absent? Is there a predictable way in which cells react under optimal and suboptimal conditions? Living cells may react to external stimuli in only a few evolutionary biological programmed specific ways:

1. They may be induced to perform their specialized function.
2. They may change/alter their specialized function by differentiation, dedifferentiation, or degeneration (see # 5 below for dedifferentiation and degeneration).
3. They may enter into the mitotic cycle and proliferate.
4. They may proceed to necrosis or to apoptosis (programmed cell death). This will be further defined under the theory of cellular dis-symbiosis as type 1 overregulation.
5. They may counterregulate to establish a new lower energy homeostatic level. This will be further defined under the theory of cellular dis-symbiosis as type 2 counterregulation, which leads to degeneration or dedifferentiation, depending on the cell type.

Both type 1 overregulation (leading to apoptosis/necrosis) and type 2 counterregulation (leading to dedifferentiation and degeneration) have recurring predictable metabolic patterns based on principles of nonlinear quantum dynamics, redox chemistry, and evolutionary biology that answer many of the conundrums the AIDS theory has failed to address and to unify into a coherent theoretical model. Cellular dis-symbiosis[88] has the aspect of a theory lacking in the theory of HIV/AIDS--predictive power. The essence of the HIV/AIDS theory is not that HIV causes AIDS, but that HIV causes AID, an acquired immune deficiency that has been defined as a decrease in CD4+T cells. It is the decrease in these immune cells that is said to be the cause the syndrome, "S". This will be shown to be both a tenuous and unfounded

---

[87] Ibid
[88] Kremer, H., The Silent Revolution in Cancer and AIDS Medicine, 2008, Xlibris Corp.

proposition as a decrease in CD4+T cells is a common finding in many disease states or no disease state whatsoever.

Under the theory of cellular dis-symbiosis, AEDS is redefined as thiol deficiency and has three identifiable stages:[89]

1. *The clinically mute phase: reserve capacity of cell respiration at a critical threshold*
2. *The clinically compensated phase: type 1 and type 2 cytokine dysregulation, type 1 to type 2 switch, type 1 overregulation of cell dis-symbiosis, and/or type 2 counterregulation of cell dis-symbiosis, the point in time of a possible "HIV" test reaction.*
3. *The clinically manifest phase: Opportunistic diseases, Kaposi's sarcoma, lymphomas, myopathies, encephalopathies, wasting syndrome, etc.*

In the case of AIDS, the initial phase 3 patients presented with two identifiable diseases that only developed after long-term exposure to well-known oxidative stressors that led to the electron deficit manifested by the consistent finding of glutathione deficiency:

1. Prolonged nitrate inhalation
2. Uncontrolled antibiotic consumption
3. Analgesics
4. Recreational drugs
5. Chronic antigen stress as a result of multiple and or recurrent infections
6. Alloantigenic stress via resorption of foreign proteins[90,91]
7. Psychological stress induced by lifestyle choices

The hallmark diseases were: pneumocystis (PCP) and Kaposi's sarcoma. Kaposi's sarcoma is a pattern in which vascular endothelial cells are, after sustained electron deficits, beginning a "dis-symbiosis" of the cooperative trend of the chimeric genome and the mitochondria expressed as a dedifferentiation and a repetitive proliferative mitotic cycle—it is called cancer. PCP, a fungus, arose because of the glutathione deficit that led to the development of a counterregulation in immune cells to a type 2 cytokine predominance with an increased production of antibodies and away from the specialized function of

---

[89] Ibid, p 320
[90] Pifer, LL, Wang, YF., et al, (1987), "Borderline immunodeficiency in male homosexuals: Is lifestyle contributory?, *South Med J.*, 80: 687-697
[91] Root-Bernstein, RS., (1991), Rethinking AIDS, The tragic cost of premature consensus, The Free Press, New York

the type 1 subset of the CD4+T immune cells and other immune cells that were no longer able to produce enough nitric oxide gas to kill attacking intracellular pathogens. That both the endothelial cells and the CD4+T immune cells acted in an evolutionary biological predictable manner to long-term harmful external stimuli that created persistent electron/proton deficits was not thirty years ago and is not now well understood by either researchers or clinicians and those who are still looking for viruses.

CHAPTER 1

Understanding "AIDSPEAK"— When a Virus Is Not a Virus

When George Orwell wrote his visionary dystopian novel 1984, he introduced a new form of imagined language created by the totalitarian state of Oceania. This language was devised to meet the state's ideological needs. The language was called Newspeak. It superseded standard English, which was called Oldspeak. It was a linguistic tool that was designed with intention to promote a particular world view and at the same time to remove the possibility of creative or inventive thought—thought considered to be heretical by state authority. It accomplished this goal by eliminating certain words from the language and by giving other words new meaning. The vocabulary was divided into sections. The A vocabulary was for business, the B vocabulary was to be used for politics and finally, the C section vocabulary included words that related specifically to science and the technical fields. It was a language created in such a way that the individual cipher lost the facility to contemplate the connections among the various disciplines and draw any meaningful conclusions. It was the language of manipulation and deception.

Today it might fall under the rubric of "political correctness" as it defines the sanctioned boundaries within which it is permissible to have any discourse, political or scientific or the scientific that has become politicized. For example, much of science that reaches the general public is no longer the science done by individuals raising questions and seeking answers. Much of what passes for current science addresses itself to solving preformed notions of desired outcomes. It works backward to find a solution rather than forward to an honest outcome that might contradict the desired solution. The public (including physicians) is then given the dumbed-down version of a duplicitous process[92,93] that has been filtered through self-appointed committees who decide by consensus what they want and do not want the public to know. Almost thirty years ago, there was a committee convened[94] that constructed what I shall call the AIDSworld view. AIDSworld has been, with malicious intent, linguistically structured in such a way that it has generated years of fear and confusion in the public mind. The strategy has been successfully accomplished by the clever manipulation of scientific language to construct a new genre of obfuscation that I shall call AIDSPEAK. AIDSpeak lacks the essential fundamental characteristic of scientific language: precision.

I begin this treatise on the HIV/AIDS paradigm with a reference to Orwell because the language of HIV/AIDS has become so dense that the need for a way to elucidate rather than obscure and to begin to have a commonly understood vocabulary is one of the most paramount issues in this matter. The predominate question to be initially addressed is the following: what is really meant in the AIDS literature with the use of words such as virus or isolation or viral load? In AIDSpeak, a virus is not a virus, isolation is not isolation, an HIV antibody test is not an HIV antibody test, viral load is not viral load, and immune deficiency turns out to have its origin in the objectively decreasing amounts of available energy. More importantly, the term AIDS has been used as if it were a singular disease. In fact, not only is there not a singular-disease AIDS, the theory is not even that HIV causes AIDS but that HIV causes AID, which causes S. Thus, the first order of business is to deconstruct the language by reference to and analysis of the research in this area and to clarify the intentional vagueness by translating AIDSpeak into English.

To simplify the complexity of AIDSpeak, I will review a brief history of word corruption that has been used to convince the world that a new unique virus was discovered and classified and called by the flagrant misnomer: the human immunodeficiency virus (HIV). As asserted by Robert Gallo[95] and Luc Montagnier,[96] the two researchers most associated with the HIV/AIDS paradigm, although not demonstrated by their published work, HIV (HTLV-III

---

[92] Jain, A., et al., (2014) "Corruption: medicine's dirty open secret," *BMJ;* 348 editorial; http://www.bmj.com/content/348/bmj.g4184

[93] Ioannidis, JPA., (2005), "Why most published research findings are false," *PLoS Med;* 2(8): 0690-0701

[94] Duesberg, P, (1994), "Infectious AIDS—Stretching the germ theory beyond its limits," *Int Arch Allergy Immunol;* 103: 118–126

[95] Gallo, R., et al, (1984), "Frequent Detection and isolation of cytopathic retroviruses (HTLV-III) from patients with AIDS and at Risk for AIDS," *Science;* 224: 500–502

[96] Barre-Sinoussi, F., (1983), "Isolation of a T-lymphotropic retrovirus from a patient at risk for acquired immune deficiency syndrome (AIDS)," *Science;* 220: 868–871

and LAV) is the cause of AID, not AIDS. The distinction is crucial. AID is defined as a decrease in the number of CD4+T cells circulating in the periphery. It was alleged that the demise of circulating CD4+T cell lymphocytes by this virus is the "acquired deficiency" by sex and/or blood that dooms an individual to a future of disease mayhem and the development of one or more of the twenty-nine listed conditions as defined by the Centers for Disease Control: the S or syndrome.[97] This assumption of a killer virus as the sole cause of AID (decrease in circulating lymphocytes) was made even though it was already known by work completed in the 1970s by one of the major AIDS cheerleaders and leading bureaucrats, Little Anthony Fauci, long-time NIAID director, who seems to have conveniently forgotten his own early work that demonstrated that these immune cells leave the periphery under various stressful conditions.[98,99] By the early 1980s, it was already common knowledge among immunologists that the vagaries of lymphocyte levels in disparate diseases made their enumeration a "waste of time"[100] and counting their numbers in the bloodstream had little if any clinical significance. There was even a commentary in August 28, 1981, edition of JAMA that stated: "The T and B cell measures, having run through the sick, the elderly, the young, the pregnant, the bereaved, had finally run out of diseases. Each condition was the subject of many reports; so that now, to give but one example, we can conclude with some assurance that T cell numbers are up, down, or unchanged in old folks . . . and now it's starting all over again, this time with T cell subsets. . . . My strongest argument is this: Measurement of T and B cells and their subsets in diseases has no clinical meaning. . . . Nonimmunologists have naturally assumed that any subject occupying so much space must be relevant in some way—a logical but incorrect assumption.[101] This was an early warnings against using these unreliable cell counts as a measure of morbidity. No matter. It was AIDSworld that took flow cytometry, an unreliable cell-counting technique, from the obscurity of the research laboratory[102] and introduced it to the mass market to support the notion of a cytocidal virus, all the while ignoring the known and predictable behavior of lymphocyte movements to multiple and varied external biological stressors. Ignoring the

---

[97] http://www.cdc.gov/MMWR/PREVIEW/MMWRHTML/rr5710a2.htm

[98] Fauci AS, Dale DC. The effect of in vivo hydrocortisone on subpopulations of human lymphocytes. J Clin Invest 1 974;53:240-246

[99] Fauci AS, Dale DC. The effect of hydrocortisone on the kinetics of normal human lymphocytes. Blood 1 975;46:235-243.

[100] Goodwin, JS., (1981), "OKT3, OKT4, and all that," *JAMA;* 246(9): 947–948

[101] Goodwin, Ibid

[102] Banks, N., Baker, C.,(2011) "The Alchemy of Flow Cytometry," http://www.omsj.org/corruption/the-alchemy-of-flow-cytometry

obvious, this non-specific finding of a decrease in CD4+T cells conveniently became HIV disease.

AIDSworld has steadfastly ignored the fact that only 2 percent of the lymphocyte pool is at any one time in the peripheral blood[103] and that low CD4+ T cell counts are not uncommon and can be found in patients in a variety of clinical settings: the intensive care unit, various human infections (AIDS patients were found to often be positive for CMV, hepatitis, and other viral pathogens), pneumonia, pyelonephritis, infected wounds, cellulitis, sepsis, malaria, mononucleosis, pulmonary tuberculosis, injection of foreign proteins, exposure to opiates and cocaine, injuries and burns, normal human pregnancy, overexercising, malnutrition, diurnal variation, psychological stress and social isolation, antiretroviral drugs, and unexplained low counts defined as Idiopathic CD4 T lymphopenia.[104] In essence, what the AIDS proponents have known since the beginning of this crisis is that AID as defined by a decrease in the number of circulating T helper cells is not an uncommon finding in many diseases (or no disease at all) and thus, as was warned, is an essentially useless test for making important therapeutic clinical decisions. This is a glaring clue to the intentional fraud of the entire HIV/AIDS debacle as well as the power of mass media programming. This is why the more honest actors were warning clinicians against relying on this variable and therefore unreliable parameter as a measure of the patient's clinical status.

Virus is a word that derives from the Latin virus, meaning poison, sap of plants, or slimy liquid. By the fourteenth century, the meaning was somewhat transformed to venomous substance or poisonous fluid. By the late nineteenth century, the dogma of bacterial disease causation was well established. However, certain disease entities eluded the microscope; and so not having an understanding of how the cell functions under normal conditions let alone under duress or a cogent theory of cell metabolism, the Western mind, locked into the "life as war" (Darwinian "survival of the fittest") conceptual framework, transformed the notion of poisonous fluid into the dogma of infectious virus—an infectious agent that was too small to be seen with the light microscope. The notion that these little elements were the cause of disease was an idea that originated well before there were electron microscopes or isolation techniques (ultra-high-speed centrifugation) and biochemical methods for the characterization of the structural elements to describe fully such entities. It was

---

[103] Westerman, J., Pabst R., (1990), "Lymphocyte subsets in the blood: a diagnostic window on the lymphoid system?" *Immunol Today;* 11:406-410

[104] Irwin, M., (2001), "Low CD4+T lymphocyte counts, a variety of causes and their implications to a multifactorial model of AIDS" http://www.virusmyth.com/aids/hiv/milowcd4.htm 12 June 2014

also well before it was clear how the cell actually functions at the microscopic or the electron microscopic level.

Oncoviruses, which became retroviruses after the discovery of the enzyme reverse transcriptase, were simply a way for virologists to explain cell phenomenon they did not fully comprehend. It filled a void but at an immense cost. It has recently been demonstrated that noncoding RNAs and the reverse transcriptase enzyme that moves them, rather than being infectious agents as claimed by virology, are actually a fundamental mechanism by which complex life on planet Earth evolved.[105] The early interpretation of cellular metabolic processes (moveable RNA) as viruses, of course, left the description and assumed function of these laboratory preparations to the imaginations of the observer. Nevertheless, viruses as causative agents of disease became the dogma that allowed for the development of the vaccine industry; and for a brief period of time during the Nixon War on Cancer, there was an attempt to define oncoviruses as infectious agents that caused cancer.

A virus has been defined by both its structure and metabolic functions. It is said to be a tiny packet of genetic information (either DNA or RNA, single or double stranded) surrounded by a covering that consists of repeats of the same protein that is called the capsid. They lack interstitial water or an energy source. Depending on the species, the genetic material should all be the same length. The HIV genome has variously been described as being 9.1 to 9.2 kb (9193)[106,107] to as long as 9749 kb.[108] However, since, as will be shown in the coming chapters, no distinct particle has ever been isolated and characterized separate from cellular debris, it is unclear from where these fragments of genetic material originate.[109,110]

It is postulated that the only way that viruses can reproduce themselves is by infecting a suitable host and somehow taking over its operating system. Each virus is said to have a unique gene and protein structure characteristic to that species.

---

[105] Mattick, JS., Makunin, IV., (2006), "Non-coding RNA," *Hum Mol Genet*, 15 Spec No1:R17-29

[106] Wain-Hobson, et al., (1985), "Nucleotide sequence of AIDS virus, LAV," *Cell;* 40:9–17

[107] Alizon, M, et al., (1984), "Molecular cloning of lymphadenopathy associated virus," *Nature;* 312: 757–760

[108] Ratner L, eta la. "Complete nucleotide sequence of the AIDS virus HTLV-III" *Nature* 1985;313:277–284

[109] Bess, J.W., et al., (1997), "Microvesicles are a source of contaminating cellular proteins found in purified HIV-1 preparations," *Virology;* 230: 134–144

[110] Gluschankof, P, et al., (1997), "Cell membrane vesicles are a major contaminant of gradient enriched human immunodeficiency virus type-1 preparations," *Virology;* 230: 125–133

The protein composition gives rise to the specific size and shape of a given virus particle. Retroviruses are said to be about 100–120 nm in diameter and contain two identical strands of RNA. This size requirement will be important to remember as will be demonstrated (in chapter 3) from AIDS research. The only pictures of "HIV isolates" to claim a demonstration of "HIV particles" show particles more than twice this size! The surfaces are "studded with projections [spikes, knobs]."[111] Although the "HIV experts" concur that these knobs are an essential part of the mechanics of HIV infection,[112] it has been attested to by other researchers that cell-free supernatants with viral particles (which are used to "infect" other cultures) contain no knobs or spikes,[113,114] making their ability to infect new cultures, by their own definition, structurally impossible. No matter.

Retroviruses have been further categorized into families. HIV has been variously called a C particle (with a cylindrical core),[115] then a C particle (with a conical core),[116] then a D particle,[117] and finally, as the time definition of AIDS changed and people were actually living long term, it became a lentivirus.[118] The major genetic material consists of env gene, which codes for the envelope; the gag (group-specific antigen) region that codes for major components of the capsid; and pol, which codes for enzymes.

To complicate the situation further, in these laboratory culture mixes, there are also other particles that look like viruses but are not viruses and are referred to as virus-like particles. These particles are not rare and are commonly found in human placentas[119] and in the artificial environment of laboratory cell cultures,[120] especially after activation with mitogens and cytokines. Gallo

---

[111] Gelderblom HR, ᵀᴹzel M, Hausmann EHS, et al. Fine Structure of Human Immunodeficiency Virus (HIV), Immunolocalization of Structural Proteins and Virus-Cell Relation. Micron Microscopica 1988;19:41–60.
[112] Wain-Hobson S., "One on one meets two"; *Nature* 1996:384:117–118
[113] Hausmann EHS, et al, "Detection of HIV envelope specific antibodies by immunoelectron microscopy and correlation with antibody titre and virus neutralizing activity" *J Virol Meth* 1987;16:125-137
[114] Gelderblom H, et al, "MHC antigens: constituents of the envelopes of human and simian immunodeficiency viruses," *Zeitschrif fr Naturforchung* 1987;42C:1328–1334
[115] Gallo, RC., et al, (1986), "First isolation of HTLV-III," *Nature;* 321:119
[116] Brown, P., (1991), "The strains of the HIV war," *New Scientist:* (25 May): 14–15
[117] Bohannon, RC., (1991), "Isolation of a type D retrovirus from B-cell line of a patient with AIDS," *J Virology;* 5663-5672
[118] Coffin, JM., (1995)"HIV population dynamics in vivo: implications for genetic variation, pathogenesis and therapy; *Science;* 267: 483-489
[119] Nelson, J, et al, "Normal human placentas contain RNA-directed DNA polymerase activity like that in viruses"' *Proc Natl Acad Sci* Dec. 1978;72:12 pp. 6263-6267
[120] Lua, LHL, et al, "Bioengineering virus like particles as vaccines," *Biotech & Bioeng* 2013, peer reviewed and accepted for publication

The Slow Death of the AIDS/Cancer Paradigm
and the Apocrypha of the Eukaryotic Cell

used an immortal H9 (HUT78) cell line in his culture mix, which is known to release virus-like particles when not infected with HIV.[121] Further, under normal metabolic conditions, the cell has a large-scale endocytic-exocytic cycle in which membrane-bound particles are moved through the various organelles and some are extruded from the cell by exocytosis.[122] Unfortunately, these virus-like particles, which can be frequently seen by electron microscopy escaping from the cell membrane, have commonly been defined as HIV and have been part of the confusion of the definition.

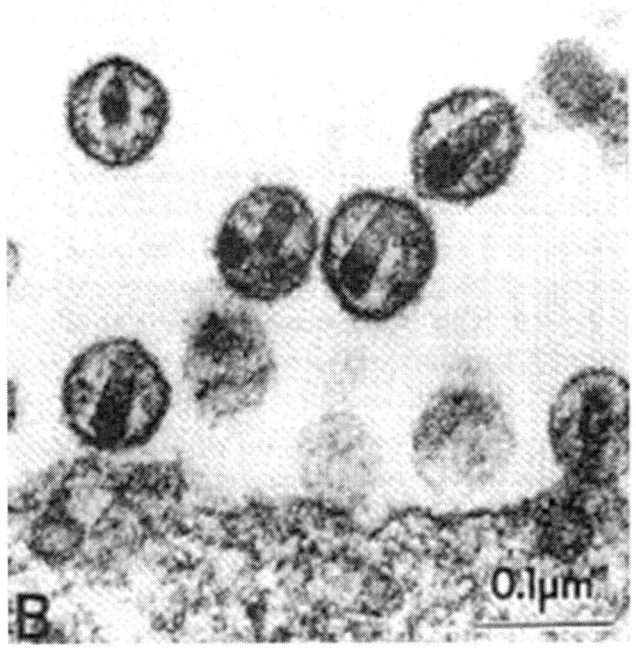

EM photo of small particles in ultrathin cell-line section. The particles are claimed to be HIV but are cellular and not viral particles (they are normally referred to as virus-like particles, microvesicles, and microsomes). The debris on the lower part of the photo indicates that the particles are not purified or isolated. These photos are always published without any evidence that the particles are of viral origin.[123]

---

[121] Dourmashkin, RR., et al, (1991), "The presence of budding virus like particles in human lymphoid cells used for HIV cultivation" VIIth International Conference on AIDS, Florence:122

[122] von Grafenstein, H, et al., (1986), "Kinetic analysis of the triggered exocytosis/endocytosis secretory cycle in cultured bovine adrenal medullary cells," *J Cell Biol*; 103: 2344–2352

[123] Lanka, Stefan, (1995), "HIV pictures, what they really show," http://www.virusmyth.com/aids/data2/slvirusphotos.htm 12 June 2014

How it is possible that these tiny packets of genetic material that are not quite living can overwhelm structures that are three orders of magnitude larger, are genetically and energetically superior, and have evolved sophisticated multifaceted systems of defense is still not well defined by the viral research establishment.

DNA viruses are thought to be cytocidal. RNA viruses are not.[124] HIV is said to be an RNA virus. Thus, by the logic of virology, if employed, would negate the possibility of HIV as the cause of AID. Because AIDSworld has adopted an Alice in Wonderland logic, a virus that is not cytocidal is after thirty years still claimed to be the culprit in the mystery of the disappearing lymphocytes. A paper coauthored by Fauci[125] (who has been at the helm of the National Institute of Allergies and Infectious Diseases since 1984) stated that "the primary mechanisms of CD4+T cell depletion in vivo remain unclear; there is no direct evidence that HIV is cytopathic in vivo, despite the fact that cytopathicity can be readily demonstrated in the artificial milieu of culture."

While the dogma of viral disease causation has been widely accepted, it is unclear, if one reads the early literature, if what is being described as "viruses" are indeed a prophenomenon or an epiphenomenon of stressed cell metabolism and laboratory isolation methodology or simply the agreed consensus that arose from the frustrations of the failure to isolate as defined by the scientific literature.[126]

Because HIV is said to be a retrovirus, which has as its genetic material RNA, I will focus on this issue.

In classical genetic theory, DNA is the center of the cellular universe and controls all heritable expressions of phenotypic change. It was posited under this theory that information transfer at the cellular level was unidirectional. That is that DNA transcribed into messenger RNA, which then follows with what is defined as translation, the ribosomal assembly of amino acids into proteins.[127] In 1970, an enzyme was discovered that contradicted the basic tenets of the unidirectional principle of the theory of information flow from DNA to

---

[124] Duesberg, PH, "Inventing the AIDS Virus," 1996 Regency Publishing, Inc., Washington, D.C. pg 117

[125] Pantaleo, G., Fauci, AS, (1996), "Immunopathogenesis of HIV infection," *Annu Rev Microbiol;* 50: 825–854

[126] Ostrom, N, (2001), "Will the poliovirus eradication program rid the world of childhood paralysis? with so little poliovirus detected around the world, with is causing today's outbreaks of acute flaccid paralysis," http://homeoint.ru/pdfs/polioeradication.pdf

[127] Lehninger, AL, The molecular logic of living organisms, Part I and Part 4, In Lehninger AL (ed): "Biochemistry. The molecular basis of cell structure and function" New York: Worth, 1981: 3-14, 17-360, 854-1056

RNA to protein.[128] The enzyme was reverse transcriptase. It was ascertained that this enzyme was able to transfer information in the other direction by catalyzing RNA into DNA. Given that in molecular biology circles, DNA was seen as the immutable driver of cell function, this was a startling and surprising discovery because it challenged the prevailing idea of the cellular hierarchical relationships. However, rather than reconfigure the theory, it was erroneously posited by some researchers that this enzyme could be used as an indirect marker for an oncovirus because the cells in which it was found were being used to study cancer.[129] Therefore, the conjecture was made that cells became cancerous by being infected by a virus. So instead of revisiting a dogma about the stability and central role of DNA in the cell and the unidirectional flow of information, the ad hoc idea of a cancer-causing virus was used to explain this new discovery; and oncoviruses became retroviruses, thereby creating more confusion about the genomic response to stress. The explanation given was that the viral RNA would be converted into DNA by the RT enzyme and the proviral DNA could then be inserted into the genome, thus initiating cancerous transformation. After the discovery of reverse transcriptase, virologists again by consensus, mistakenly began to use and to convince themselves that finding reverse transcriptase in cell culture was the definitive indication of the presence of a retrovirus. However, this time, the same entity no longer caused cell immortality but caused cell death. This highly speculative assumption without scientific proof has become virology dogma.

The RNA tumor virus idea was short lived because cancer could not be shown to be transmissible. Neither could it suggest a remedy in the form of a vaccine.[130] At this time, which was just a little over a decade before the outbreak of disease clusters in subpopulations of urban homosexuals, the spread of cancer by viruses was being blamed on homosexuals, prostitutes, and black people, the same AIDS target groups thirteen years later.[131]

Reverse transcriptase was also known by its discoverers (David Baltimore and Howard Temin)[132] not to be unique to retroviruses. Reverse transcription

---

[128] Nobel Prize, Oct. 1975 http://www.nobelprize.org/nobel_prizes/medicine/laureates/1975/press.html
[129] Gerald B. Dermer. 1994. The Immortal Cell: Why Cancer Research Fails. Avery Publishing Group, Garden City Park, NY. Gerald B. Dermer. 1994. Another Anniversary for the war on Cancer. Bio/Technology 12: 320.
[130] Beardsley, T, "A war not won," Jan. 1994 *Scientific American;* Vol. 270, p. 130–138
[131] Ellison BJ & Duesberg, PH, 1994 "Why we will never win the war on AIDS"; Inside Story Communications, El Cerrito, CA.
[132] Temin HM, Baltimore D. RNA-Directed DNA Synthesis and RNA Tumor Viruses. Adv Vir Res 1972;17:129–186

can be found in leukemic T cells,[133] normal spermatozoa,[134] and—according to Harold Varmus, another Nobel laureate—in the uninfected cells of yeast, insects, and mammals.[135] As it stands, RT is not a unique feature of retroviruses but is a ubiquitous enzyme involved in the repair of not only the DNA but also the telomere, a region of repetitive nucleotide sequences found at the end of each chromatid, which protects the end of the chromosome from deterioration as well as from fusion with neighboring chromosomes. It can commonly be found in stressed cells under laboratory conditions after the addition of mitogens and cytokines to the cell mix.

To identify RT in culture media, a synthetic template primer $A(n).dT_{15}$ is used.[136] However, it is well understood that this template primer can be transcribed not only by RT but by all cellular DNA polymerases.[137] RT is an RNA-dependent DNA polymerase.[138] Instead of using the natural genetic messenger material, the RNA genome of the virus, which should be there if the virus existed and had been isolated, always, without explanation, this synthetic template is used.[139] Although it is understood that this template is not specific for the process of reverse transcription, in AIDSpeak, even reverse transcription may not be reverse transcription.

In 1973, a decade before the AIDS crisis erupted, it was Robert Gallo (one of the initial proponents along with Luc Montagnier and Jay Levy[140] of the HIV/AIDS theory) who was the first to show that RT can be found in mitogen-stimulated (but not unstimulated) normal human blood lymphocytes.[141] In 1975, at an international conference on eukaryotic DNA polymerases, which

---

[133] Gallo RC, Sarin PS, Wu AM. On the nature of the Nucleic Acids and RNA Dependent DNA Polymerase from RNA Tumor Viruses and Human Cells. In: Silvestri LG, ed. Possible Episomes in Eukaryotes. Amsterdam: North-Holland Publishing Company, 1973:13-34.

[134] Whitkin SS, Higgins PJ, Bendich A. Inhibition of reverse transcriptase and human sperm DNA polymerase by anti-sperm antibodies. Clin Exp Immunol 1978;33:244-251.

[135] Varmus H. Reverse Transcription Sci Am 1987;257:48-54.

[136] Mercer, JF, Naora, H., (1975), "A comparison of the chromatographic properties of various polyadenylate binding materials," *J Chromatogr;* 114(1): 115-128

[137] Sarngadharan MG, et al, 1978 "DNA polymerases of normal and neoplastic mammalian cells" *Biochim. Biophysica. Acta.;* 516, 419-487

[138] Tzertzinis, G., et al., (2008), "RNA dependent DNA polymerases," *Curr Protoc Mol Biol;* Chapter 3: Unit 3.7

[139] Brian WJ, et al. "Virology Methods Manual," Academis Press, 1996

[140] Levy, JA., (1993), "Pathogenesis of human immunodeficiency virus infection," *Microbiol Rev;* 57(1): 183-289

[141] Op Cit Gallo et al, 1973

both Baltimore and Gallo reportedly attended,[142] DNA polymerase γ was defined as "a component of normal cells"[143] and "found to be widespread in occurrence," "whose activity can be increased by many factors including PHA (phytohaemagglutinin) stimulation"[144] and as "the enzyme which copies A(n). dT$_{15}$ with high efficiency but does not copy DNA well."[145]

Because these researchers were aware of the information about reverse transcriptase not being specific to retroviruses and had knowledge about the nonspecificity of the template primer used to transcribe it, in that the primer could also identify other DNA polymerases that might be found in cell culture, Montagnier's group at the Pasteur Institute and Robert Gallo's laboratory at the National Cancer Institute by claiming that they discovered a new retrovirus because they were able to find reverse transcriptase using that very same synthetic template primer A(n).dT$_{15}$ in mitogen-stimulated mixed cultures was a scientific fraud. Montagnier's group cultured cells from a "high risk" patient who clinically did not have AIDS but did have cervical lymphadenopathy. His cells were mixed with fetal cord blood cells to which mitogens were added. Instead of cord blood cells, Gallo's group used the H9 leukemia cell line, also stimulated with mitogens and type 1 cytokines. Since Gallo had already published that RT can be found in mitogen-stimulated normal human blood lymphocytes, it is simply inconceivable that he could use the finding of this same enzyme to claim he had discovered a new virus. Thus, one of the code words for HI virus in AIDSpeak is finding (maybe) reverse transcriptase using a nonspecific template primer in mitogen-stimulated complex cell cultures. The 1983 Montagnier, Barré-Sinoussi paper in Science[146] for which these two were awarded the 2008 Nobel Prize in Physiology or Medicine unequivocally equates finding reverse transcriptase in cell culture as "virus production." Every clinician needs to be clear that, in AIDSpeak, finding RT in stimulated complex mixed cell cultures with a few other "indirect markers" has, by consensus, come to be called a virus.

---

[142] Weissbach, A., Baltimore D, Bollum F., (1975) "Nomenclature of eukaryotic DNA polymerases," *Science,* 190, 401--402

[143] Robert'Guroff, M et al, (1977) "DNA polymerase gamma of human lymphoblasts; *Biochem.;* 16, 2866-2873

[144] Lewis, BJ, et al, (1974) "Human DNA polymerase III (R-DNA): Distinction from DNA polymerase I and reverse transcriptase"; *Science,* 183, 867–869.

[145] Op Cit, Weissbach A.

[146] Barré-Sinoussi, F., et al., (1983), "Isolation of a T-lymphotropic retrovirus from a patient at risk for acquired immune deficiency syndrome (AIDS)," *Science;* 220(4599): 868–871

REPETITIVE ELEMENTS, RETROTRANSPOSONS, ENDOGENOUS "RETROVIRUSES" A.K.A. RETROID ELEMENTS

To confuse the issue of retroviruses further, new words have been added to the lexicon of DNA mysteries. Eukaryote DNA including that of humans contains large portions of noncoding sequences. If the copies of a sequence lie adjacent to one another in a block or an array, they are said to be tandem repeats. The repetitive sequences dispersed throughout the genome as single units flanked by unique sequences are interspersed repeats. Most of these repeats originate by a process of transposition, which is the "jumping" of a DNA segment to another place on the genome. This already was described by Barbara McClintock in the 1940s when she began to publish her work on maize where she demonstrated that when DNA was exposed to external stressors (she used X-rays), that was able to produce moving or transposable elements in response to that stress. These moving segments ultimately became known as jumping genes. In a Nobel lecture delivered in 1983, she stated that "We do not know when any particular element [of the genome] will be activated. Some responses to stress are especially significant for illustrating how a genome may modify itself when confronted with unfamiliar conditions. Changes induced in genomes when cells are removed from their normal locations and placed in tissue culture surroundings are outstanding examples of this."[147] Virology researchers, when reverse transcriptase was discovered as the mover of these elements, were either ignorant of her work or simply ignored its significance when they posited a new class of organism to explain the bidirectional flow of genetic information, which she had already described thirty years earlier.

Retrotransposons are the most important transposable elements in the human genome. First, they are abundant, directly forming at least 45 percent of the human genome[148,149] (the estimations vary, but most researchers believe that it must be even more since ancient retrotransposons that have been inactivated have diverged by mutation to the point where they are unidentifiable). Second, retrotransposons are still active in the human genome.[150] For jumping, they require an RNA polymerase. All retroviral reverse transcriptases have both

---

[147] McClintock, B., "The significance of responses of the genome to challenge" Nobel lecture 8 December, 1983

[148] Lander ES, et al, "Initial sequencing and analysis of the human genome" *Nature* 2001;409:860-921

[149] Venter JC, et al, "The sequence of the human genome" *Science* 2001, 291:1304-1351

[150] Wicker, T., (2007), "A unified classification system for eukaryotic transposable elements," *Nature Rev; 8:* 973–982

DNA polymerase and RNase H activities. The synthesis of retroviral DNA requires both activities. Genetic studies and homology alignments made between various polymerases and RNases H provided evidence that the DNA polymerase and RNase H activities of RT are separate domains of a single polypeptide.[151,152] Thus, RT can be considered first and foremost as a DNA polymerase, which in both structure and function is similar to cellular DNA polymerases.[153] The RNA copy is reverse transcribed into DNA, and this DNA segment is inserted into the genome at a new location. Retrotransposons can be further classified as autonomous and nonautonomous. Autonomous retrotransposons are coding for proteins necessary for their transposition, although they are also dependent on host RNA polymerases and DNA repair enzymes (RT) for successful jumping. Nonautonomous retrotransposons do not code for any protein and must hijack other transposons' enzymes to be able to transposition.

RNA is a central player in natural genetic modification at the core of living processes that alter genetic information of cells and organisms in response to their environments. These modifications assure survival, and some may be passed on to future generations.[154] It has been considered that noncoding RNA holds the key to the development and evolution of complexity. Recent evidence suggests that the majority of genomes of mammals and other complex organisms are, in fact, transcribed into noncoding RNAs (ncRNAs), many of which are alternatively spliced and/or processed into smaller products. These RNAs appear to comprise a hidden layer of internal signals that control various levels of gene expression in physiology and development, including chromatin architecture/epigenetic memory, transcription, RNA splicing, editing, translation, and turnover. It is currently thought that RNA regulatory networks may determine most of our complex characteristics.[155]

As an example, the human genome contains only about twenty thousand protein-coding genes, similar to nematodes that have only one thousand cells compared to humans' 10^{14} cells.[156] Nonprotein-coding DNA increases

---

[151] Johnson V.A., Byington R.E., Kaplan J.C. 1990. Reverse transcriptase (RT) activity assay In Techniques in HIV research (ed. A. Aldovini and B.D. Walker), pp. 97–102. Stockton Press, New York.

[152] Tanese N., Goff S.P. Domain structure of the Moloney MuLV reverse transcriptase: Mutational analysis and separate expression of the polymerase and RNAse H activities. Proc. Natl. Acad. Sci. 1988;85:1777–1781. [PMC free article] [PubMed]

[153] Coffin, JM, Hughes, SH, Varmus, HE., editors, (1997) "Retroviruses," Cold Spring Harbor Laboratory Press, Cold Spring Harbor, NY

[154] Ho, MW., (2014), "Non-Coding RNA and Evolution of Complexity," *ISIS*

[155] Mattick, Makunin, Op. Cit.

[156] Ho, op cit

in complexity, reaching 98.8 percent of the human genome, much of which has been referred to as junk DNA until geneticists discovered that most of these sequences (greater than 80 percent, according to latest estimates[157,158]) are dynamically transcribed, primarily into noncoding, ncRNAs, apart from ribosomal RNAs and transfer RNAs. What current research is demonstrating is that RNA is emerging as a major component of the regulatory circuitry that underpins the development and physiology of complex organisms. In fact, RNA may supplement endocrine and paracrine signaling by small molecules and proteins and act as an efficient and evolutionarily preserved flexible source of sequence-specific information transfer between cells, both locally and systemically. Therefore, RNA signaling may play a pivotal role in multicellular ontogeny, homeostasis, and transmitted epigenetic memory.[159] Thus, genetic modification is a natural response to external cues—but in AIDSworld, it became "rapidly mutating HIV."

To hold on to the idea that retro elements are infectious agents rather than an epiphenomenon of cell metabolism under various biological stress conditions and to add to the further distraction, virologists have posited the existence of another transposable entity known as human endogenous retroviruses, or HERVs. Around 8 percent of the genome is said to be derived from sequences with similarity to "infectious retroviruses" (HIV), which are also recognized by three genes—gag (encoding structural proteins), pol (viral enzymes), and env (surface envelope proteins)—as well as long terminal repeats (LTRs). The existence of HERVs has been known for many years.[160] It is claimed that HERVs represent the remnants of ancestral retroviral infections that became fixed in the germ-line DNA. They are found commonly in the human placenta.[161]

A more plausible postulate, however, is that RNA was the initial genetic material.[162] The unique potential of RNA molecules to act both as information carrier and as catalyst forms the basis of the RNA world hypothesis. Evidence that RNA arose before DNA in evolution can be found in the chemical differences between them. Ribose, like glucose and other simple carbohydrates,

---

[157] Palazzo, AF., Gregory, TR, (2014), "The case for junk DNA," *PLOS Genetics;* 10(5): e1004351. doi:10.1371/journal.pgen.1004351

[158] Bernstein, BE, et al., (2012), "An integrated encyclopedia of DNA elements in the human genome," *Nature* 489: 57–74 doi:10.1038/nature11247.

[159] Dinger, ME, et al., (2008), "RNAs as extracellular signaling molecules," *J Mol Endocrinol;* 40: 151-159

[160] Boeke, JD & Stoye JP, "Retrotransposons, endogenous retroviruses, and the evolution of retroelements" *Retroviruses* Edited by Coffin, Hughes, and Varmus, Cold Spring Harbor; Cold Spring Harbor Laboratory Press:1997:343–435

[161] http://www.ncbi.nlm.nih.gov/pubmed/15033302

[162] http://www.ncbi.nlm.nih.gov/books/NBK26876/

can be formed from formaldehyde (HCHO), a simple chemical that is readily produced in laboratory experiments that attempt to simulate conditions on the primitive Earth. The sugar deoxyribose is harder to make and in present-day cells is produced from ribose in a reaction catalyzed by a protein enzyme, suggesting that ribose predates deoxyribose in cells.[163]

If this hypothesis proves correct, then the idea of retroviruses as exogenous, infectious entities will prove moot and HERVs and retrotransposons will no longer be considered ancient parasites that were somehow added to the mammalian genome by an infectious process but will be viewed as the underlying mechanism of increasing eukaryotic evolution and complexity. What is important to the current discussion is that all these transposable elements make use of reverse transcriptase. Many of them translate elements that cross-react with what are called "HIV proteins"[164] and have the same or similar genetic sequences commonly identified as HIV.[165]

Although AIDSpeak continues to use reverse transcriptase as an identifying marker for the presence of HIV, it can be understood from the above examples that the enzyme RT is not unique to HIV and can be expressed by cells under a multiplicity of internal and external conditions. There is also evidence that during evolution, the symbiont mitochondrial genes were transferred to the nucleus through reverse transcription (i.e., as double-stranded reverse transcribed mitochondrial mRNA).[166] Therefore, finding RT in cell cultures cannot be used as a substitute marker for HIV or any other virus. If the RNA as the original genomic material proves to be correct, then the idea that complex life-forms developed vis-à-vis a series of viral infections will be lauded for the peculiarity of the assertion.

---

[163] Ibid
[164] Garrison, KE, et al, "T cell responses to human endogenous retroviruses in HIV-1 infection'" *PLoS Pathogens*; Nov. 2007, Vol3:11:1617-1627
[165] Nelson, PN., et al., (2003), "Demystified...human endogenous retroviruses," *Mol Pathol;* 56(1): 11–16
[166] Henze, K., Martin, W., (2001), "How do mitochondrial genes get into the nucleus?," *Trends Genetics;* 17(7): 383–387

CHAPTER 2

When Isolation Is Not Isolation—Why p24, without Reverse Transcriptase, Is Not Evidence of HIV

Well over a century ago, a great debate was being waged among European scientists as to whether microscopic organisms were monomorphic or pleomorphic—[167,168] whether these organisms were the cause of disease or the result of an altered biological terrain lacking proper oxygenation and/or nutrients, thereby creating the conditions for more rapid cell death and turnover. To those who saw organisms as pleomorphic, they were the harbinger of news of nutritional deficits or increased toxicity. The notion was advanced that these unwelcome parasites functioned to vacuum the resulting elevated levels of dead and dying nutrient-starved tissue. To those who promoted the monomorphic idea of microbial existence, there was the possibility of a vaccine or drug to attack the target, leaving the biological terrain to its own devices. It has been since the time of those important debates that allopathic medicine, while claiming to acknowledge deleterious lifestyle and environmental impacts on health, has done little to understand the underlying metabolic aberrations except in the context of either extreme nutritional deficiencies or offering a drug, a vaccine, surgery, or radiation therapy. Detoxification and replacement therapy is still considered the purview of nontraditional medicine, and the bioterrain is all but ignored by allopaths until crisis.

---

[167] Kritschewski, IL, Ponomarewa, IW., (1933), "On the pleomorphism of bacteria, I on the pleomorphism of B paratyphi B.," *Micbiol Inst. People's Comm Ed. Moscow;* pp111–126

[168] http://jcm.asm.org/content/40/12/4771.long "Are there naturally occurring pleomorphic bacteria in the blood of healthy humans?"

The Slow Death of the AIDS/Cancer Paradigm
and the Apocrypha of the Eukaryotic Cell

Needless to say, Louis Pasteur, who espoused the monomorphic idea of the germ theory of disease causation, has become renowned as one of the leaders of modern biology while Antoine Béchamp, the author of the pleomorphic idea and from whom Pasteur is charged *with* plagiarizing much of his work, has been lost to obscurity.[169,170] It has been documented that Pasteur may have pirated many of Béchamp's ideas about microbes but simultaneously failed to understand their complete significance. It seems that Pasteur, as are many of today's "top doctors and scientists," rather than being the best and brightest in his field, was politically well connected and was aided in his triumphal career of pronouncements upon disease-germs not only by his high-placed establishment connections but also by the conclusions of Heinrich Hermann Robert Koch, a German researcher who also espoused the monomorphic theory of disease causation. Koch developed a series of laboratory techniques for the isolation of microorganisms thought to be the causative disease agents. These techniques are known as Koch's postulates; and because they are still the rules subscribed to, to this day, by bacteriologists and, with special addenda, by virologists, I will revisit these rules so as to secure the concept of what biologists/virologists claim to mean when they say that a bacteria or virus has been isolated.

The Merriam-Webster Dictionary defines isolation as "the act of separating something from other things, the act of isolating something." The word originally arises from the Latin insula, meaning island; and an island, is of course, a piece of land surrounded by water, separate from other landmasses. There is no part of the English language in which one can ascertain that nonspecific markers that are not unique to the condition/entity under consideration can be substituted and/or interpreted as the isolation of the unknown entity. As an example, although palm trees are commonly found on many tropical islands, finding a palm tree and claiming that the presence of the palm tree is evidence of an island would be ludicrous, especially if standing, for example, in the middle of Cancun, Mexico. But not in AIDSworld, where finding indirect markers that are not unique to the entity under consideration allows one to claim the viral island for God and country. In AIDSworld, isolation takes on an entirely different meaning.

In biology, when the concept of isolation is alleged, it is understood that the scientist has committed his/her work to the application of Koch's postulates conceived and published in 1890 that consist of four criteria designed to

---

[169] Pearson, RB; "The Dream and Lie of Louis Pasteur" http://www.desireerover.nl/wp-content/uploads/2011/10/The-Dream-Lie-of-Louis-Pasteur.pdf

[170] Hume, ED, "Pasteur Exposed, germs, genes, vaccines, the false foundations of modern medicine" 1989 Bookreal, Australia

establish a causal relationship between a microbe and a particular disease entity:

1. The microorganism must be found in abundance in all organisms suffering from the disease.
2. But should not be found in healthy organisms.
3. The microorganism must be isolated from the diseased organism and grown in pure culture.
4. The microorganism must be reisolated from the inoculated diseased experimental host and identified as being identical to the original specific causative agent.

The astute reader will immediately discern that the first postulate (and therefore the third) cannot be universally proven. It is well established that microorganisms that are said to cause disease can be found in the tissues of perfectly healthy people (e.g., 5 to 10 percent of the U.S. population harbor mycobacterium tuberculosis;[171,172] Pneumocystis jirovecii [173,174] was found in 80 percent of Spanish children by the age of thirteen[175] or cytomegalovairus in 50 percent[176] of asymptomatic carriers and herpes in 25 to 50 percent[177]) who never express any symptoms of these "disease-causing agents." That modern medicine has overlooked the conditions (changes in homeostasis or the biological terrain as espoused by Béchamp) that allow *microorganisms to* take hold is an understatement.[178] However, I will use the internal logic of modern biology that still uses Koch's postulates as a baseline from which to evaluate whether or not Montagnier or Gallo ever "isolated" a unique virus HIV and what AIDSpeak really means when they say that they have "isolated."

---

[171] https://www.clinicalkey.com/topics/pulmonology/tuberculosis.html#111217

[172] Evans, A.S., & Feldman, H.A., eds. (1982) Bacterial Infections of Humans: Epidemiology and Control (Plenum, New York/London).

[173] Ponce, CA et al, "*Pneumocystis* colonization is highly prevalent in the autopsied lungs of the general population" *Clinical Inf Dis;* 4 Jan 2010:50 pp. 347-353

[174] Beard, CB, et al, "Genetic differencesin *Pneumocystis* isolates recovered from immunocompetent infants and from adults with AIDS: epidemiological implications:, *J Inf Dis* 13 Oct. 2005:192 pp. 1815-1818

[175] Respaldiza, N, et al.,(2004) "High seroprevalence of pneumocystis infection in Spanish children," *Clin Microbiol Infec;* 10:1029–31

[176] Evans, A.S., ed. (1982) Viral Infection of Humans: Epidemiology and Control (Plenum, New York/London).

[177] Ibid

[178] Hume, D., (1932), Bechamp or Pasteur: A lost chapter in the history of biology" Kessinger Publishing, LLC (Sept. 10, 2010)

The Slow Death of the AIDS/Cancer Paradigm
and the Apocrypha of the Eukaryotic Cell

Procedures for isolating and purifying retroviruses (RNA tumor viruses or oncoviruses) were developed as early as 1964.[179,180] Further, the rules for isolation of retroviruses were elaborated in greater detail at the Pasteur Institute, Paris, in 1973 and are considered to be the logically consistent minimal requirements for establishing the independent existence of an infectious retrovirus.[181,182]

1. Culture of the putatively infected tissue
2. Purification (isolation) of specimens by density gradient high speed ultracentrifugation
3. Electron micrographs of particles exhibiting morphological characteristics and dimensions (100-120 nm) of retroviral particles at the sucrose (or percoll) density of 1.16 gm/ml and **containing nothing else.**
4. Analysis and characterization of the particles for physical, chemical or biological properties desired[183]
5. Proof that the particles contain reverse transcriptase
6. Proof that 1-5 are a property only of putatively infected tissues and can not be induced in control cultures. These are identical cultures, that is, tissues obtained from matched, **unhealthy** subjects and cultured under identical conditions differing only in that they are not putatively infected with a retrovirus.
7. Proof that the particles are infectious, that is when **pure** particles are introduced into an uninfected culture or animal, the identical particle is obtained as shown by repeating steps 1-5.

Although these rules were designed to bring some order and precision to the discipline of virology, when, by following the protocols, it became increasing difficult to obtain the desired results, the protocols were then expediently ignored and or violated by orthodox cancer/AIDS researchers as they began to construct the parameters of AIDSworld. In their quest first to find the viral

---

[179] O'Connor TE, Rausher FJ, Ziegel RF. Density gradient centrifugation of a murine leukemia virus. Science 1964; 144: 1144-1147.

[180] de Harven E. Viremia in Friend murine leukemia: the electron microscope approach to the problem. Pathologie-Biologie 1965a; 13: 125-134.

[181] Toplin I. Tumor Virus Purification using Zonal Rotors. Spectra 1973; 4:225-235.

[182] Sinoussi F, Mendiola L, Chermann JC. Purification and partial differentiation of the particles of murine sarcoma virus (M.MSV) according to their sedimentation rates in sucrose density gradients. Spectra 1973;4:237-243.

[183] Beard JW. Physical methods for the analysis of cells. Annals of the New York Academy of Sciences 1957;69:530-544.

cause of cancer and then to assert that HIV was the cause of AID, they began to use a shorthand with which every clinician should become familiar.

In a 1997 interview with French journalist Djamel Tahi,[184] Luc Montagnier who has been credited as the one who "isolated" HIV, repudiated these procedures and claimed that an assemblage of nonspecific properties—reverse transcriptase, pictures of budding (of virus like particles from the cell membrane), and morphology—were enough to stake the claim of isolation. Although he stated emphatically in this interview, "You cannot purify it,"[185] he illogically added, "If you know somebody who has antibodies against the proteins of the virus, you can purify the antibody/antigen complex. That's what one did. And thus one had a visible band, radioactively labelled, which one called protein 25, p25. And Gallo saw others. There was the p25 which he called p24."[186] Of course, the issue here is from whence comes p24 if it is not from a purified culture?

It is important for the clinician to understand from the above discussion that, at some unspecified point in time, virologists collectively decided not to follow their own rules and began to assert that finding reverse transcriptase and a few other nonspecific indirect markers in mitogen- and cytokine-stimulated mixed cell cultures (mixed with cells that are known to produce reverse transcriptase and virus-like particles, e.g., cancer cells and human cord blood cells) was called isolation. This deception has such far-reaching consequences to the practice of medicine that by the confusion in terminology, there has been done incalculable harm to millions of patients. By choosing not to expose this disinformation, because clinicians rely on scientists to exhibit some level of integrity, the fundamental Hippocratic values of the discipline are completely subverted.

In 1983 Montagnier's group at the Pasteur Institute in Paris found a homosexual male who did not have AIDS and was clearly in phase 2 of thiol deficiency:[187] he had a recent history of multiple infections including CMV, Epstein-Barr and herpes simplex viral infections, gonorrhea, and syphilis. He reported over fifty sexual partners in the previous year and presented with "cervical lymphadenopathy and asthenia." T lymphocytes were taken from this patient to be stimulated and cocultured with human cord blood cells. This work became the basis for a paper "Isolation of a T-lymphotropic retrovirus

---

[184] Tahi, D., (1997), "Interview Luc Montagnier," *Continuum*, Winter
[185] Ibid.
[186] Tahi, Op cit.
[187] See introduction page 17

The Slow Death of the AIDS/Cancer Paradigm
and the Apocrypha of the Eukaryotic Cell

from a patient at risk for acquired immune deficiency syndrome (AIDS),"[188] which, along with four papers published one year later in the same journal from the laboratory headed by Robert Gallo at the U.S. National Cancer Institute, became the foundational papers for the HIV/AIDS theory. The Pasteur researchers stated that, "After 15 days of culture, a reverse transcriptase activity was detected in the culture. . . . Virus production continued for 15 days and decreased thereafter."[189] In essence, this AIDSworld paper claims that finding reverse transcriptase was the unconditional evidence for the presence of "virus production." This virus production, however, did not occur spontaneously; but only after laboratory manipulations could this "virus production" be transmitted, with the use of cord blood cells (Montagnier) or with the use of H9 cancer cells (Gallo), to uninfected cells. This was said to be proof of infection.[190] This, and this alone, is the primary evidence on which the entire HIV/AIDS paradigm has been structured. The other indirect markers are equally nonspecific. It should be noted, contrary to Koch's postulates and the Pasteur rules for isolation, no "infection" of uninfected cells occurred before the addition of rapidly dividing cells (H9 cancer cells or cord blood cells) and mitogenic stimulation.

This Pasteur Institute paper published images of the budding of virus-like particles from a cell membrane, which are claimed to be "characteristic of retroviruses." However, it was already well-known, as discussed in the previous chapter, that this is a nonspecific finding that in no way can be claimed as a marker for the discovery of a new retrovirus.[191,192] Evidence has emerged that many microvesicles contain RNA and are involved in cell-to-cell communication.[193,194] Generally, microvesicles are also enriched in various bioactive molecules and may directly stimulate cells as a kind of "signaling

---

[188] Barré-Sinoussi, F., (1983), "Isolation of a T-lymphotropic retrovirus from a patient at risk for acquired immune deficiency syndrome (AIDS)," *Science*; 220:(4599): 868–871

[189] Ibid.

[190] Barré-Sinoussi, Op cit.

[191] Nelson, J, et al, "Normal human placentas contain RNA-directed DNA polymerase activity like that in viruses'" *Proc Natl Acad Sci* Dec. 1978;72:12 pp. 6263-6267

[192] Lua, LHL, et al, "Bioengineering virus like particles as vaccines," *Biotech & Bioeng* 2013, peer reviewed and accepted for publication

[193] Baj-Krzyworzeka, M, et al., (2006), "Tumour derived microvesciles carry several surface determinants and mRNA of tumour cells and transfer some of these determinants to monocytes," *Cancer Immunol Immnuother;* 55:808–818

[194] Ratajczak, J, et al., (2006a) "Membrane derived microvesicles: important and underappreciated mediators of cell to cell communication," *Leukemia;* 20: 1487–1495

complex" or are able to transfer membrane receptors, proteins, mRNA and organelles (e.g., mitochondria) between cells.[195] Further, the only electron micrograph in the Montagnier study is of these virus-like particles budding from a cell membrane. There is no EM as required by the isolation protocols of the spun sediment at 1.16 gm/ml in sucrose (condition three under virus isolation protocol). When Tahi inquired of Montagnier in the 1997 interview why the EM photographs came from the culture and not from purification (the sediment at 1.16 gm/ml), Montagnier responded that (a) there was not enough virus and (b) the particles seen did not have the morphology typical of retroviruses. "We did not have, and I have always recognized it, was that it was truly the cause of AIDS."[196] No matter. In AIDSworld, this is what it takes to identify a new virus and win a Nobel Prize.

The first Gallo paper (**main author M. Popovic**) published in **Science** in May 1984[197] attempting to both isolate and establish the cytopathology of T cells from AIDS patients claiming that the virus can "selectively kill T cells" curiously observed that when the T cells from these patients were put in culture with normal T cells, the cells did not respond as anticipated, i.e., nothing happened to the uninfected cells. Neither were there any "AIDS-like diseases" that developed when HIV was inoculated into chimpanzees or healthy humans.[198,199,200]

Without the prompting from laboratory stimulation, the cells combined with the cells from AIDS patients did not express the indirect markers considered to be indicative of viral infection. They did not become cytopathic or immortal or cause symptoms of an infection when injected into another host. The Popovic paper claimed a "transient" expression (of what? RT) was their main obstacle to isolation. Essentially, there was no evidence that the cells from the AIDS patients were infectious. To remedy this "transient expression" problem and to express the indirect markers that they would claim as HTLV-III (HIV), they then began to use an immortal lymphoid leukemia cell line combined with the cells from AIDS and pre-AIDS patients to which were added the type 1 cytokine

---

[195] Ratajczak, Ibid
[196] Tahi, Op cit.
[197] Popovic, M., et al., (1984), "Detection, Isolation and continuous production of cytopathic retroviruses (HTLV-III) from patients with AIDS and pre-AIDS," *Science;* 224(4648): 497–500
[198] Duesberg, PH.,(1987) "Retroviruses as carcinogens and pathogens: expectation and reality," Can Research; 47, pp. 1199–1220
[199] Curran, JW., et al., (1988), "Epidemiology of HIV infection and AIDS in the United States," *Science;* 239(4840): 610-616
[200] Friedland, GH, Klein, RS., (1987), "Transmission of the human immunodeficiency virus" *NEJM;* 317: 1125-1135

The Slow Death of the AIDS/Cancer Paradigm and the Apocrypha of the Eukaryotic Cell

IL-2 and mitogens. They had used these same techniques and this same cell line previously to produce the earlier HTLV variants. Gallo claimed that his first two HTLVs, I and II, were cancer causing. HTLV-III, containing the same level of genetic information, would be positioned as cytocidal, although, to date, there is no concrete evidence of this in any published AIDS literature.[201,202,203]

It was an established fact from previous cancer cell research by Gallo[204] and others that virus-like particles and reverse transcriptase could often be found in their culture preparations and in no way indicated evidence for the "isolation" of a new virus. The particles were known not to be viruses because they lacked the ability to replicate. However, Gallo threw caution to wind, and even though there was no evidence of isolated particles in the debris field that banded in the sucrose gel at 1.16 gm/ml after ultracentrifugation, because there was evidence of reverse transcriptase in the supernatant and the banded material after laboratory manipulation with mitogens and cytokines and because it was claimed that there were reactions between the culture proteins and some non-specific antibodies in the AIDS patients' sera, but not from healthy controls, he proclaimed this evidence for the discovery of a new virus HTLV-III-HIV. This series of nonspecific findings was construed as having isolated a new retrovirus. In essence, like the Pasteur Institute a year before, the researchers at the National Cancer Institute likewise abandoned both Koch's postulates and the viral isolation protocols, and the era of antiscience became the accepted pattern of thinking and operation. It was the beginning of the tyranny of AIDSworld and a scientific black hole from which the world has not yet recovered.

In the second 1984 Science paper[205] in which Gallo is the lead author, these indirect markers were said to be found in eighteen of twenty-one pre-AIDS patients, but in only twenty-six of seventy-two patients claimed to have full-blown AIDS. This, of course, defies the first Koch postulate of finding the putative infectious agent in all those infected. The paper asserted without

---

[201] Duesberg, PH.,(1987) Op cit.
[202] Duesberg, PH.,(1988), "HIV is not the cause of AIDS," *Science;* 241: 514–517
[203] Zagury, D., Bernard, J., Leonard, R., Cheynier, R., Feldman, M., Sarin, P. S. & Gallo, R. C., (1986), "Long-Term Cultures of HTLV-III-Infected T Cells: A Model of Cytopathology of T-Cell Depletion in AIDS" *Science;* 231:850–853.
[204] Gallo, R. C., Wong-Staal, F., Reitz, M., Gallagher, R. E., Miller, N. & Gillepsie, D. H. 1976. Some evidence for infectious type-C virus in humans. pp. 385-405, in Animal Virology, edited by D. Balimore, A. S. Huang and C. F. Fox, Academic Press Inc., New York.
[205] Gallo, R., et al., (1984), "Frequent detection and isolation of cytopathic retroviruses (HTLV-III) from patients with AIDS and at risk for AIDS," *Science;* 224 (4648): 500-3

explanation as to the nature of this oddity that "these results and those reported elsewhere in this issue suggest that HTLV-III may be the primary cause of AIDS." In this, he echoed the conclusion of the 1983 Montagnier paper that observed, "The role of the virus in the etiology of AIDS **remains to be determined.**"[206] *(emphasis added)* However, the subjunctive mood became the declarative mood in the national press, and the HIV/AIDS paradigm was born an unnatural birth, repeated incessantly into a created reality.

In AIDSpeak, the rules have been shortened in such a way that when the literature claims to have "isolated HIV," what they are saying is that they have evidence in the culture mix of virus-like particles, reverse transcriptase (discussed in the previous chapter, determined by transcription of not an HIV pro-viral DNA template but the nonspecific template A(n).dT15) and have detected a protein, p24, which is claimed to be the HIV gag protein.[207]

The Montagnier paper claiming to distinguish his "isolate" from HTLV-1 used a "polyclonal goat antibody to p24."[208] What this implies is that the reader is assumed to be unfamiliar with an earlier 1981 paper to which Gallo's name is attached[209] that had already identified this same protein from the HTLV line associated with human T-cell lymphoma. "A protein of molecular weight 24,000, p24, was purified from this virus (HTLV). Several results indicate that this p24 is an internal core protein of HTLV."[210] However, p24 is really the approximately the weight of the two light chains of the ubiquitous myosin molecule. One can almost feel Gallo's desperation for glory as he was already trying to stake the claim of discovery in the moribund effort of finding cancer-causing viruses by using this p24 protein. When that didn't pan out, it didn't stop the virus hunters from using it again in an entirely different metabolic process. That AIDS patients had not a proliferative T cell response but an increase in apoptosis was irrelevant, and so was the fact that p24 clearly was not unique to HIV! No matter. The use of p24 as a marker for isolation of HIV has become part of

---

[206] Barré-Sinoussi, Op cit.

[207] Please be aware that the counter-argument to the template question has to do with identifying RT vs polymerases by using different pH buffers in the culture medium—however, there is still no evidence that finding RT in a culture mix of this nature is evidence for the discovery of a new retrovirus. On the contrary, it is evidence for creating cell stress and the need for the up-regulation of repair enzymes.

[208] Barré-Sinousssi, F., Op Cit.

[209] Kalyanaraman, VS., et al, (1981), "Immunological properties of a type c retrovirus from cultured human T lymphoma cells and comparison to other mammalian retroviruses," *J Virol;* 906–915

[210] Ibid

the dogma and has the same integrity as selling the identical piece of land to multiple buyers.

P24 has been used as an identifier of HIV because in AIDSworld, in spite of this old cancer research, it is now claimed to be unique to this entity. However, there are some serious problems with this particular assertion including dissension in the ranks of the HIV advocates. Other than a joint publication with Montagnier where they assert that the HIV p24 is unique, Gallo and his colleagues have repeatedly stated that the p24s of HTLV-I and HIV immunologically cross-react.[211] HTLV-I is the second "retrovirus" identified by Gallo, which he declared as the cause of adult T-cell leukemia. Why is this such a problem? Because Gallo used an immortal adult T-cell leukemia cancer cell line in his culture mix, H9 (HUT-78), which actually turned out to be H9, the cancer cell that he claimed contained the HTLV-1 proviral sequences.[212] In addition to this Gallo trick, Montagnier used umbilical cord lymphocytes in his culture mix. Cord blood lymphocytes had been previously studied because retroviruses were said to be transmitted vertically (in the germ cell line) and were thought to play a role in differentiation. Cells in which retroviruses were commonly claimed to be found included sperm, ova, placenta, and fetal and embryonic tissue as well as umbilical cord lymphocytes.[213,214,215]

If p24 is a unique HIV protein, then it must be present in all AIDS patients if not all seropositive patients and not in persons not at risk of developing AIDS. This however, is not the case. Antibodies to p24 have been detected in 1 out of 150 healthy individuals, 13 percent of randomly selected otherwise healthy patients with generalized warts, 24 percent of patients with cutaneous T-cell lymphoma and prodrome, and 41 percent of patients with multiple

---

[211] Wong-Staal, F. and Gallo, R.C. 1985. Human T-lymphotropic retroviruses. Nature 317:395-403.

[212] Wong-Staal F, Hahn B, Manzuri V, et al. A survey of human leukemias for sequences of a human retrovirus. *Nature* 1983;302:626-628.

[213] Johnson PM, Lyden TW, Mwenda JM. Endogenous retroviral expression in the human placenta. Am J *Reprod Immunol* 1990;23:115-120.

[214] Cohen M, Powers M, O'Connell C, et al. The nucleotide sequence of the env gene from the human provirus ERV3 and isolation and characterization of ERV3-specific cDNA. *Virol* 1985;147:449-458.

[215] Thiry L, Sprecher-Goldberger S, Hard RC, et al. Expression of retrovirus-related antigen in pregnancy. I. Antigens cross-reacting with simian retroviruses in human fetal tissues and cord blood lymphocytes. J *Reprod Immunol* 1981;2:309-322

sclerosis[216] and organ transplant patients,[217] up to 36 percent of patients with systemic lupus erythematosus,[218] and in patients who received HIV negative UV irradiated blood.[219]

Conversely, the p24 is not found in all HIV positive or even AIDS patients. In another study, "in half of the cases in which a subject had a positive p24 test, the subject later had a negative test without taking any medications that would be expected to affect p24 antigen levels. . . . The test is clinically erratic and should be interpreted very cautiously."[220] Another paper questioned the accuracy of p24 antigen testing when the study cohorts were found to be HIV antibody positive on initial screening and were described as having "chronic HIV infection," yet 82 percent were negative for p24 antigen![221] In one study that measured HIV-1 RNA against p24 in thirty patients, they found that sixteen of the sera did not have detectable p24 antigen.[222]

The HIV research group from Perth, Australia, have published two papers that are highly technical but are recommended as mandatory reading for every clinician who desires a deeper understanding of the minutiae of these controversies. The first paper, "The Isolation of HIV—Has it Really Been Achieved? The Case Against,"[223] outlines in detail the prescribed methodology of isolation and how and why it has been violated. They observed that, "It is important to note that although all groups, Montagnier's, Gallo's and Levy's, refer to the material from the culture supernatants which in sucrose density gradients bands at 1.16 gm/ml as viral particles, virions and to the RNA and proteins at that density as 'particle-associated' RNA or proteins, not one of the groups presented evidence for the existence at this density of any particles, retroviral-like or otherwise, pure [isolated] or otherwise. Instead

---

[216] Ranki, A., Johansson, E. and Krohn, K. 1988. Interpretation of Antibodies Reacting Solely with Human Retroviral Core Proteins. NEJM 318:448-449.

[217] Vincent, F., et al., (1993), "False positive neutralizable HIV antigens detected in organ transplant recipients, *AIDS,* 7:741-742

[218] Barthel, HR, Wallace, DJ., (1993), "False positive human immunodeficiency virus testing in patients with lupus erythematosus," *Semin Arthritis Rheum;* 23(1):1–7

[219] Kozhemiakin, LA., Bondarenko, IG, (1992), "Genomic instability and AIDS," *Biochimiia;* 57:1417–1426

[220] Todak, G., Klein, E., Lange, M. et al. 1991. A clinical appraisal of the p24 Antigen test, p326. In:Vol. I, Abstracts VII International Conference on AIDS, Florence.

[221] Darr, ES., Little, S., et al.,(1.2. 2001) "Diagnosis of primary HIV-1 infection," *Ann Intern Med;* 134(1);25-29

[222] Semple, M., et al., (1991), "Direct measurement of viremia in patients infected with HIV-1 and its relationship to disease progression and zidovudine therapy," *J Med Virol,* 35:38–45

[223] http://www.virusmyth.com/aids/hiv/epreplypd.htm

these researchers cultured lymphocytes from AIDS patients and stimulated [activated] them with a wide variety of agents. Reverse transcription of the A(n). dT15 template in the culture supernatant was considered proof for infection with a retrovirus or even proof of isolation."[224]

In another Perth paper, "Is a positive western blot proof of infection?"[225] a follow-up to "The Isolation of HIV," it makes the argument that if there is scant evidence of isolation as they defined in the first paper, free of contaminants, then any test designed to identify the putative HIV will be neither sensitive nor specific, which, in fact, has been the case. From the Gallo and Montagnier research papers came the impetus for the development of the "HIV antibody tests." These are the tests that clinicians are expected to use in practice to determine the fate of their patients. Since the source of these antigens has never been identified, physicians are using tests that the CDC claims have greater than 99 percent sensitivity and specificity, but, in fact, have zero sensitivity and zero specificity—to tell patients that they have a deadly disease (See chapter 3— "When an Antibody Test Is Not an Antibody Test").

Several years after those initial papers from the Pasteur Institute and the National Cancer Institute were published in Science, another paper written by researchers from Gallo's laboratory revealed the startling fact that hydrocortisone was added to the original culture medium. That paper stated, "Isolation of virus from cultured cells was also substantially facilitated by inclusion of hydrocortisone in the culture media."[226] This was an important and shocking revelation that had been left out of the original published papers. Cancer cell virus researchers had over the years come to the consensus that finding RT in the cell culture mix would be the de facto definition of viral isolation. Over time, these same researchers learned subtle esoteric laboratory manipulations that could increase the yield of RT produced by the culture medium. One of these tricks insightfully elucidated by Heinrich Kremer in his book The Silent Revolution in Cancer and AIDS Medicine[227] was the addition of hydrocortisone to the mitogen-stimulated culture mix. It had been discovered that the addition of hydrocortisone, a glucocorticoid, could have specific actions on human T helper cells, and that was to inhibit mitogen-induced proliferation while simultaneously increasing the production of reverse transcriptase, which

---

[224] Ibid
[225] http://www.virusmyth.com/aids/hiv/epwbtest.htm
[226] Ibid.
[227] Kremer, H, (2008), The Silent Revolution in Cancer and AIDS Medicine, XLibris pp. 211-212

was described in the Gallo papers as "the continuous and high level production of HTLV from patients with AIDS and pre-AIDS."[228]

In 1987, two members of the Gallo team reported on the manner in which they had treated the T helper cells of the AID and AIDS patients. They admitted, "Stimulation in vitro could be provided by mitogen or added cells [allogenic antigens]. . . . Certain manipulations of culture conditions were found to improve the outcome, e.g., cocultivation of patient cells with mitogen stimulated peripheral blood leukocytes from uninfected donors. Isolation of virus from cultured cells also was substantially facilitated by inclusion of hydrocortisone in the culture media."[229]

During recent decades, it became evident that the neurological, endocrine, and immune systems have significant interactions and feedback loops and that glucocorticoids are hormones possessing powerful and far-reaching neuroimmunoregulatory activity. Glucocorticoids inhibit the increase and proliferation of human T helper cells.[230] They suppress cell-mediated immunity while at the same time enhancing antibody production.[231] They transmit their effect via the interactions of the neuro-endocrine-immune systems acting as an effective immune suppressor.[232,233] If there are true retroviruses in human T helper cells then they can only proliferate when the enzymes (DNA polymerases) for the duplication and division of the DNA are present and active.[234] Since glucocorticoids inhibit the synthesis and activation of the DNA polymerases of

---

[228] Popovic, Op cit.

[229] Sarngadharan, MG, Markham PD, (1987), "The role of human T-lymphotropic retroviruses in leukemia and AIDS" in: Wormser, GP (ed.) *AIDS acquired immunodeficiency syndrome—and other manifestations of HIV infection;* Noyes, Park Ridge, NJ (pp. 197-198

[230] Gabrielsen, AE, Good, RA, (1967), "Chemical suppression of adaptive immunity," *Adv Immunol;* 6: 91-229

[231] Bucala, R., (1996) "MIF rediscovered: cytokine, pitutary hormone, and glucocorticoid-induced regulator of the immune response," *FASEB J;* 10: 1607-1613

[232] Gabrielsen AE., et al 1967, "Chemical suppression of adaptive immunity" *Adv Immunol* 6:91-2229

[233] http://www.ncbi.nlm.nih.gov/pubmed/15265777 Overview of the actions of glucocorticoids on the immune response: a good model to characterize new pathways of immunosuppression for new treatment strategies.Ann N Y Acad Sci. 2004 Jun;1024:124-37.

[234] Levin J.G., Hatfield D.L., Oroszlan S., Rein A. 1993. Mechanisms of translational suppression used in the biosynthesis of reverse transcriptase In Reverse transcriptase (ed. A.M. Skalka and S.P. Goff), pp. 5–31. Cold Spring Harbor Laboratory Press, Cold Spring Harbor, New York. (double check this ref.)

the T helper cells, this makes the replication of any virus highly unlikely.[235,236] Glucocorticoids also inhibit the expression of inducible NO synthase for the production of cytotoxic NO at the genetic transcription level and at the translation stage of RNA transcripts in the biosynthesis of proteins.[237] However, glucocorticoids can promote the synthesis of repair enzymes (including reverse transcriptase) and the repair process in T helper cells.[238,239] The essential prerequisite for the production of "HIV" in T helper cells is the stimulation by the type 1 cytokine IL-2[240] and mitogens. However, glucocorticoids block the effects of IL-2 and mitogens.[241] Therefore, the cultivation of retroviruses from human T helper cells is blocked by the glucocorticoid hydrocortisone. Furthermore, glucocorticoids are used clinically to treat type 1 cytokine overreactions exhibited by many inflammatory and autoimmune diseases and some cancers and to prevent organ transplant rejection.[242]

It is evident that what Gallo and his researchers found was not a virus but the coercion of an increase in the repair enzyme reverse transcriptase and then overcoming the hydrocortisone blockage of cytokine synthesis with the addition of cytokines, interleukin 2, which activates interferon-γ,[243] which in turn stimulates cytotoxic nitric oxide (NO). The culture medium included the H9 cancer cells, which are highly counterregulated and, in a state of

---

[235] Gillis S, et al.' "Glucocorticoid induced inhibition of T cell growth factor production I. the effect on mitogen induced lymphocyte proliferation"; *J Immunol 123*: 1624-1630

[236] Gillis S., et al., "Glucocorticoid induced inhibition of T cell growth factor production. II. the effect on the in vitro generation of cytolytic T cells," *J Immunol* 123:1632–1638

[237] Kunz D., et al., 1996, "Molecular mechanism of dexamethasone inhibition of nitric oxide synthase expression in interleukin-1 stimulated mesangial cells: evidence for the involvement of transcriptional and post transcriptional regulation," *Proc Nat Aca Sci USA*; 93:255–259

[238] http://www.ncbi.nlm.nih.gov/pubmed/8899106 Brattsand R & Linden M; Cytokine modulation by glucocorticoids: mechanisms and actions in cellular studies. *Aliment Pharmacol Ther;* 1996;10 Suppl 2:81-90; discussion 91-2.

[239] Chambers, SK, et al., (2004), "An unexpected effect of glucocorticoids on stimulation of c-fms proto-oncogene expression in choriocarcinoma cells that express little glucocorticoid receptor," *Am J Obstet Gynecol*, 190(4):974–985

[240] http://www.ncbi.nlm.nih.gov/pubmed/6200936 Gallo R., et al, "Frequent detection and isolation of cytopathic retroviruses (HTLV-III) from patients with AIDS and at risk for AIDS"; *Science 1984* May 4;224(4648):500-3.

[241] Op Cit., Gillis 1979 a, 1979b

[242] Kremer, Op cit.

[243] http://www.jleukbio.org/content/58/2/225.long Cellular and molecular mechanisms of IFN gamma production by IL-2 an IL-12 in a human NK cell line

decompensated cell dis-symbiosis[244] (reduced vitality and mitochondria), and no longer show signs of programmed cell death. It is the leukemia cells and Th2 CD4+T cells that actually display HIV characteristics, e.g., increased RT production, increased budding of export particles for oxidized cell proteins as the already stressed Th1 cells likely undergo apoptosis under the stimulation of type I cytokines, and increased nitrous oxide production. Cancer cells respond to NO exposure, depending on the dosage, with either cell inhibition or subsequently with heightened counterregulation[245] (see the chapter on cell dis-symbiosis). So what Gallo did was not to isolate any virus but to finagle his cell cultures with knowledge gained during the Nixon War on Cancer to create two crucial HIV characteristics: the continuous production of reverse transcriptase and the apparent destruction of T4 cells by the retroviral HIV.[246,247]

The proteins obtained from the spun sediment from these cultures have never been identified as pure viral particles. In fact, it has been stated and will be shown to be mostly cell debris. The problem faced by virology researchers then and now is that not only are viral-like particles found in that sediment, so are a plethora of cellular proteins.[248,249] On the basis of reactivity with AIDS patient sera, only 20 percent of the proteins, which band at 1.16 gm/ml, are claimed to be HIV proteins by HIV/AIDS experts and, without proof, to be coded by HIV DNA.[250,251] The question then becomes quite obvious: if only 20 percent of the proteins are HIV, then what is the origin of the remaining 80

---

[244] Kremer, H, (2008), The Silent Revolution in Cancer and AIDS Medicine, Xlibris, pp 210-215

[245] Brüne, B. Mohr, S., Messmer, UK., (1996), "Protein thiol modification and apoptotic cell death as cGMP-independent nitric oxide (NO) signaling pathways," *Rev Physiol Biochem Pharmacol;* 127:1–30

[246] Popovic M., et al. "Detection, isolation and continuous production of cytopathic retroviruses (HTLV-III) from patients with AIDS and pre AIDS" *Science* 1984;224:497-500

[247] Gallo R, et al. "Frequent detection and isolation of cytopathic retrovirus (HTLV-III) from patients with AIDS and at risk for AIDS: 1984 *Science;*224:500-503

[248] Gluschankof P, Mondor 1, Gelderblom HR, Sattentau QJ. Cell membrane vesides are a major contaminant of gradient-enriched human immunodeficiency virus type-1 preparations. Virology 1997;230:1 25-1 33.

[249] Bess JW, Gorelick RJ, Bosche Wi, Henderson LE, Arthur LO. Microvesides are a source of contaminating cellular proteins found in purified HIV-1 preparations. Virology 1997;230:1 34-144.

[250] Henderson LE, Sowder R, Copeland TD. Direct identification of Class II Histocompatibility DR proteins in preparations of human T-cell lymphotropic virus type III. *J Virol* 1987;61:629-632.

[251] Hoxie JA, Fitzharris TP, Youngbar PR, et al. Nonrandom association of cellular antigens with HTLV-III-III virions. *Hum Immunol* 1987;18:39-52.

percent of the proteins in such particles and by what genes are they coded? Why are only 20 percent of the proteins viral and noncellular? Why not all of them, or was that simply a random number picked out of a hat?

Importantly, in 1988, the only EM study done[252] in which suitable controls were used and in which extensive blind examination of controls and test material was performed, "HIV particles" were found not only in 90 percent (18/20) of patients with persistent generalized lymphadenopathy attributed to HIV but also in 87 percent (13/15) of patients with "non-HIV lymphadenopathies." The authors of this study concluded that "viral particles in persistent generalized lymphadenopathy (PGL) lymph nodes are most likely HIV, but similar particles can be seen in reactive lymph nodes not associated with HIV infection. . . . The presence of such particles do not, by themselves indicate infection with HIV."

By now, it should be clear that the cultures from the original studies were grossly manipulated to obtain the desired indirect markers. The controls used from healthy patients did not produce viral markers; however, when cells from unhealthy patients (who, in fact, should have been the control sample in the original studies) are used, similar viral makers can be found. It should also be understood that the purification or isolation by density gradient centrifugation has never been achieved. Most of the material sedimenting at this density has been recognized as cytoskeletal proteins and proteins of the cell type used in the cell cultures.[253] To this day, there are no electron micrographs of purified material sedimenting at the specified density gradient. So finding RNA or proviral DNA, which bands at 1.16 gm/ml, does not constitute proof that this is HIV RNA. Thus far, the first four rules of viral isolation have been violated. Although reverse transcriptase has been identified, it is not a unique retroviral marker; and item number 6, the use of identical cultures from matched unhealthy controls, has not been the standard.

---

[252] O'Hara CJ, Groopmen JE, Federman M.(1988) "The Ultrastructural and Immunohistochemical Demonstration of Viral Particles in Lymph Nodes from Human Immunodeficiency Virus-Related Lymphadenopathy Syndromes" *Hum Pathol*;19:545.

[253] Op cit, http://www.virusmyth.com/aids/hiv/epreplypd.htm

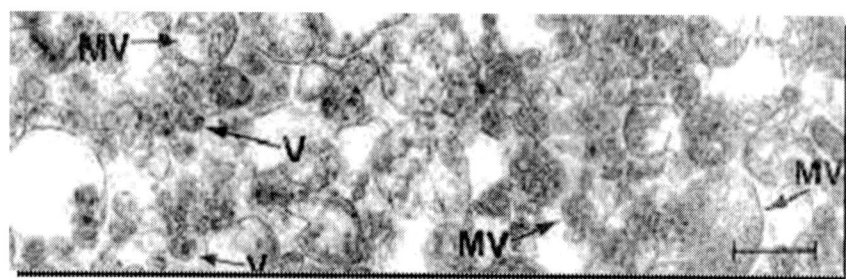

The first electron micrographs (EMs) of "purified HIV," published in the March 1997 issue of Virology, disclose "major contaminants." In the example above, note that the arrows labeled V point to the few particles that are "retrovirus like." The authors of these studies concede that their pictures reveal the vast majority of the material in the density gradient is cellular contamination.[254]

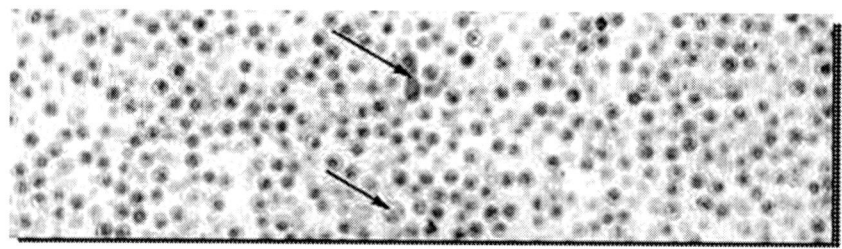

By contrast, this electron micrograph of the Friend virus shows, at a magnification of 19,500 times, an almost pure population of typical "type C" viruses (not yet called retrovirus in 1965). The arrows point at contaminating debris and microvesicles. The interpretation was that virus purification was satisfactory and that contamination rate was extremely low.[255]

When Luc Montagnier, who was award the Nobel Prize for his work on HIV, was interviewed by Djamel Tahi in 1997 for the magazine Continuum, Montagnier, although claiming that these indirect markers were sufficient evidence to declare a new virus, when asked by Tahi: "Why no purification?" he responded, "I repeat, we did not purify?" Which he had to say as they were also not able to publish an electron micrographs of the purified material sedimenting at 1.16 gm/ml in the sucrose gel. Neither was Gallo able to produce such photographs. At a 1994 meeting held in Washington sponsored by the National Institute of Drug Abuse, Gallo admitted, "We have never found HIV

---

[254] http://www.virusmyth.com/aids/index/hivpictures.htm
[255] Ibid

DNA in the tumor cells of KS.... In fact we have never found HIV DNA in T cells."[256] No matter.

Montagnier was asked by Tahi, "Why do the EM [electron micrographs] photographs published by you [in 1983] come from the culture and not the purification?" To which he honestly replied, "There was so little production of virus it was impossible to see what might be in a concentrate of the virus from the gradient. There was not enough virus to do that." Gallo also published EM photos without evidence of purification. A letter was found in the National Archives from Matthew A. Gonda, PhD, Head, Electron Microscopy of the National Cancer Institute, dated March 28, 1984, to Dr. Mika Popovic (one of the lead researchers in Gallo's lab) with a cc to Gallo:

"Dear Mika:

I am sending you 4 extra copies of results requested by Betsy Read. She said Dr. Gallo wanted these micrographs for publication because they contained HTLV (HTLV I, HTLV II, HTLV III which is HIV) particles. If this assumption is based on the cultures being antigen positive, I would like to point out that the "particles" in micrograph 0905 are in debris of a degenerated cell. No other extracellular "virus-like particles" were observed free between cells anywhere in the pellet. The small extracellular vesicles in 0904 are at least 50 percent smaller than HTLV mature particles seen in type I, II, or III. Again these vesicles can be found in any pellet. I do not believe any of the particles photographed are HTLV I, II, or III."[257]

Nevertheless, the second and third of the four Science articles of 1984 from Gallo's lab, with Gallo being the lead author on the second paper, included four micrographs of HTLV-III credited to Gonda. In the following text, Gallo claimed that all the particles were of the correct shape and size for HTLV-III, although if one examines these images, it can clearly be seen that this is more AIDSworld fantasy.

Since no particles were isolated, there is no evidence that any HIV particles have been analyzed and characterized for their physical, chemical, or biological properties. Since there is no proof that steps 1–5 were adhered to, there is a

---

[256] Lauritsen JL. NIDA meeting calls for research into the poppers-Kaposi's sarcoma connection. In: Duesberg PH, eds. AIDS: Virus- or Drug Induced. London: Kluwer Academic Publishers, 1995: 325-330.

[257] Roberts, J., "Fear of the Invisible" 2008-2009, Impact Investigative Media Productions, Bristol, U.K. p.275

decided lack of evidence that these indirect markers are a property only of putatively infected tissues. An even bigger issue is that there were no control cultures of similarly ill patients who had diseases other than AIDS—a violation of one of the most basic research design principles. Given these facts, there is indeed scant evidence that neither Gallo nor Montagnier isolated a unique infectious (exogenous) virus HIV. So in AIDSpeak, when they isolate, they really mean that they have found one or more indirect markers: reverse transcriptase, "virus like" particles, and some uncharacterized proteins (p24 has been selected) most likely to be cellular debris in the supernatant and/or the pellet found at 1.16 gm/ml in the sucrose gradient post-high-speed centrifugation of cellular material that includes rapidly dividing cancer cells or human cord blood cells that have been stimulated with mitogens, phytohemagglutinin and IL-2, and, in the case of Gallo, hydrocortisone.

Gallo and Montagnier were only able to cite indirect phenomena: reverse transcriptase, ultrathin electron micrographs, banding of a composite protein mixture at a given density, which, according to the established rules of virology, are not acceptable evidence for the existence of a virus or retrovirus. This is because these indirect anomalies can be obtained in the absence of any viral entity under certain cell conditions.[258,259,260,261] HIV has never been isolated or "purified" as complete intact viral particles. Needless to say, there is scant scientific evidence supporting the claim that what is commonly called HIV is, in fact, even a virus. What are being called HIV characteristics will be shown to be nothing more than decay products of the type 2 cytokine shift of stressed immune and cancer cells in response to glutathione depletion. This becomes even more important as these researchers were aware that the detection of RT and retroviral genetic sequences and release of retroviral particles depends on the metabolic state of the cells because the mere act of co-cultivation alone may lead to release of endogenous retroviral particles,[262] extracts, even from normal unstimulated cells, when added to the cultures

---

[258] Papadopulos-Eleopulos E, Turner VF, Papadimitriou JM. Is a positive Western Blot proof of HIV infection? BioTechnol 1993;1 1:696-702.

[259] Papadopulos-Eleopulos E, Turner VF, Papadimitriou JM. Has Gallo proved the role of HIV in AIDS? Emergency Med (Australia) 1993;5:71-74.

[260] Papadopulos E, Johnson C. Is HIV the cause of AIDS? Interview. Continuum 1997;5:8-19.

[261] Lanka S. HIV - Reality or artefact? Continuum 1995;3/1:4-9.

[262] Hirsch MS, Phillips SM, Solnik C. Activation of Leukemia Viruses by Graft-Versus-Host and Mixed Lymphocyte Reactions In Vitro. *Proc Natl Acad Sci U S A* 1972;69:1069-1072.

The Slow Death of the AIDS/Cancer Paradigm
and the Apocrypha of the Eukaryotic Cell

may increase endogenous retroviral expression.[263] They were aware that the appearance of "endogenous retrovirus" can be accelerated; and the yield increased a millionfold by stimulating the cultures with mitogens,[264] mutagen, chemical carcinogens, and radiation.[265,266] They also knew that in the presence of antioxidants, no "HIV" phenomena can be observed.[267,268,269] In a study entitled "Combined treatment with 3-aminobenzamide and N-acetylcysteine inhibits HIV replication in U937 infected cells" presented in July 1996 at the International AIDS Conference, researchers from Rome demonstrated using a combination of these antioxidants in vitro that they were able to alter the cellular redox balance and thereby modulate the expression of HIV. This was a significant discovery that confirmed the earlier research on the consistent finding of the reduction in master antioxidant glutathione levels in HIV positive and AIDS patients. It offered a way out of the quagmire and the possibility of a greater understanding of the metabolic chain reaction that has come to be known as AIDS. The alterations in the cellular metabolic processes that have been identified as the underlying defects in HIV positive and AIDS patients will be explored in later chapters. It can be shorthanded as thiol exhaustion → type 2 cytokine switch → NO inhibition → type 2 cell dis-symbiosis → HIV/AIDS, cancer, wasting syndrome, myopathy, encephalopathy and polyneuropathy, enteropathy, etc., in AIDS risk groups.[270]

Again and again, research has indicated that patients are suffering an energy imbalance that has manifested as a type 2 counterregulation of the immune system. However, only in AIDSworld can an obvious energy imbalance get dumbed down to a series of indirect markers that are called a virus.

---

[263] Toyoshima K, Vogt PK. Enhancement and Inhibition of Avian Sarcoma Viruses by Polycations and Polyanions. *Virol* 1969;38:414-426.

[264] Aaronson SA, Todaro GJ, Scholnick EM. Induction of murine C-type viruses from clonal lines of virus-free BALB/3T3 cells. *Science* 1971;174:157-159.

[265] Minassian A, Merges M, Garrity R, et al. Induction of a SMRV-like retrovirus from a human T-cell line after treatment with the mutagen ethyl-methyl-sulfonate. *J Acquir Immun Defic Syndr* 1993;6(No 6):738.

[266] Papadopulos-Eleopulos E, Turner VF, Papdimitriou JM. Is a Positive Western Blot Proof of HIV Infection? *Bio/Technology* 1993;11(June):696-707.

[267] Papadopulos-Eleopulos E, Turner VF, Papdimitriou JM. Oxidative Stress, HIV and AIDS. *Res Immunol* 1992;143:145-148.

[268] Papadopulos-Eleopulos E. Reappraisal of AIDS: Is the oxidation caused by the risk factors the primary cause? *Med Hypotheses* 1988;25:151-162.

[269] Papadopulos-Eleopulos E, Turner VF, Papdimitriou JM, et al. A critical analysis of the HIV-T4-cell-AIDS hypothesis. *Genetica* 1994;95:5-24.

[270] Kremer, H Op cit, p 345

CHAPTER 3

When an HIV Antibody Test Is Not an HIV Antibody Test

In 2006 the CDC began to recommend an "HIV test" for every American aged 13–64,[271] claiming that "human immunodeficiency virus (HIV) infection and acquired immunodeficiency syndrome (AIDS) remain leading causes of illness and death in the United States."[272] But if one examines the top ten leading causes of death in the United States for the period in question,[273] AIDS doesn't make the top ten. It doesn't even make the top twenty.[274] Suicide is listed as number ten, and there are 38,097 deaths recorded for this cause, with the implication that AIDS deaths must be less than 38,000/year. From the CDC, "an estimated 15,529 people with AIDS diagnosis died in 2010," but they don't know how many actually died of AIDS because "the deaths of persons with AIDS can be due to any cause—that is, the death may or may not be related to AIDS."[275] Yet in AIDSworld, this acknowledged low-level mortality, which is not even certain, is being presented as an "epidemic"; and therefore, something must be done. That something is to create an HIV test dragnet in the general population. But unfortunately there is no direct test to measure the unmeasurable. In the case of HIV, the test is not a direct test for the presence of a virus but an indirect assessment of the level of antibodies formed by an

---

[271] http://www.cdc.gov/mmwr/preview/mmwrhtml/rr5514a1.htm *MMRW* 2006),/55(RR14);1-17 Recommendations for HIV Testing of Adults, Adolescents, and Pregnant women in health care settings
[272] Ibid
[273] http://www.cdc.gov/nchs/fastats/deaths.htm Deaths and Mortality, data for 2010
[274] http://www.worldlifeexpectancy.com/united-states-life-expectancy
[275] http://www.cdc.gov/hiv/statistics/basics/ataglance.html HIV in the United States: At a Glance 7.25.14

The Slow Death of the AIDS/Cancer Paradigm and the Apocrypha of the Eukaryotic Cell

individual against proteins and glycoproteins that are said to be unique to the virus,[276] but there is a caveat. As discussed in the previous chapters, HIV is an idea; but a unique-entity HIV has never been isolated, purified, and characterized as an intact viral particle. The virus has never been analyzed for the physical, chemical, or biological properties that make it unique. The assertion that proteins found in AIDS patients are more common than in healthy controls is a specious argument. It is well understood that many HIV positive patients have been exposed to a higher levels of oxidative stressors that are known to lead to an increased level of cell death[277,278] and turnover and/or are genetically predisposed to have higher antibody levels,[279] and as a result, this increased rate of antibody production makes this population more likely to test positive. This has been the silent strategy for targeting populations of African origin. It is now claimed that black men are eight times more likely to be positive than white men with the same risk factors and fewer recorded sex partners and that black women are fifteen to twenty times more likely to be positive than white women with the same risk factors.

However, having elevated antibodies is not necessarily an indication that one is slated to develop a future disease, especially a disease that primarily effects the cell-mediated immunity system. For example, Reinhard Kurth, from the Paul Ehrlich Institute in Germany, and his colleagues reported that 70 percent of "HIV positive patients," compared to only 3 percent of blood donors, had antibodies that reacted with the retrovirus HTDV/HERV-K, an endogenous retrovirus present in all of us.[280] Using AIDSworld reasoning, does that mean that these patients have HTDV/HERV-K disease as well?

Before the AIDS era, a controlled experiment was construed as evaluating and comparing the results from experimental samples with control samples. The controls are practically identical to the experimental sample except for the one aspect whose effect is being tested. In the case of AIDS and in AIDSworld, ethically following this standard scientific protocol has been quietly altered to highlight exaggerated responses that may not exist. For example, much of

---

[276] Schupbach, J. et al, "Serological Analysis of a subgroup of human T-lymphotropic retroviruses (HTLV_III) associated with AIDS"; May 4, 1984 *Science* 224: pp. 503-505

[277] Pizarro, JG., et al., (2009), "Oxidative stress-induced DNA damage and cell cycle regulation in B65 dopaminergic cell line," *Free Rad Res;* 43(10): 985–994

[278] Cadenas, E., Davies, KJA., (2000), "Mitochondrial free radical generation, oxidative stress, and aging"; *Free Rad Bio Med;* 29(3-4): 222-230

[279] See attachment 7 Dixon (apr 14 draft)

[280] Papadopulos-Eleopulos, E., et al., (1996) "The Isolation of HIV—has it really been achieved? The case against" *Continuum;* 4(3) http://www.virusmyth.com/aids/hiv/epreplypd.htm

the AIDS literature defines *control* as either cells from healthy individuals or healthy individuals. However, in the real world where real science is done, a real control would be to use cells from people who are equally ill but with diseases other than AIDS or people who are equally ill with diseases other than AIDS in comparison to AIDS patients. Using cells from healthy people as a control is simply scientific malfeasance. Until those studies are presented as evidence, there is little justifiable scientific data validating the premise that what is currently referred to as HIV is, in fact, a virus and scant evidence that HIV proteins are indeed from a unique virus. One of the few AIDS studies in which an appropriate control was used found that while 90 percent of HIV positive patients with generalized lymphadenopathy had "HIV particles" by EM, so did 87 percent of controls who had persistent generalized lymphadenopathy not associated with HIV.[281] Another study was able to compile a list of over seventy entities that have been shown to cross-react with the HIV antibody test.[282] This is a veritable trap for the clinician who is expected to make what for the patient might be the most important decision in his life based on flawed evidence. All the noisy public relations gorilla chest pounding of the AIDS industry will not make false evidence true or redeem a physician who tells a patient who may have hepatitis or CMV or herpes simplex I or II, all common viral infections found in AIDS patients to which the test may be positive or recently had a flu shot or is pregnant or have nothing at all, that he/she has a deadly disease.

The overarching question, of course, is if there was no real isolation or purification, how is it possible to have a test that claims that it has a sensitivity and a specificity of 99.9 percent? The short answer is that it is not possible. Sensitivity measures how often a test is positive when you already know what you are testing for is present. Specificity expresses how often a test is positive when a patient does not have the condition. In AIDSworld, sensitivity and specificity have nothing to do with measuring the test against the "gold standard" of an isolated virus but refer to reported measures of performance and accuracy in relationship to other HIV tests on the market. In this *marketing* context, the meaning of sensitivity indicates how often a new test says a sample is positive when one already on the market says it is positive while specificity indicates how often this same test says a sample is negative when another test says it is negative. It is simply not possible to know the sensitivity and specificity of a test without measuring it against an independent, free, and purified particle. No HIV test on the market claims this. Thus, the clinician must understand that

---

[281] O, Harra, CJ, et al., (1988), "The ultrastructural and Immunohistochemical demonstration of viral particles in lymph nodes from human immunodeficiency virus-related lymphadenopathy syndromes," *Hum Pathol;* 19:545

[282] Johnson, Christine, (1996), "Whose antibodies are they anyway," *Continuum;* 4(3)

The Slow Death of the AIDS/Cancer Paradigm
and the Apocrypha of the Eukaryotic Cell

there is no test on the market that can conclude with any scientific certainty by employing one of these HIV tests that any patient is infected with HIV. If the clinician is unfamiliar with the metabolic processes that can result from the proton deficit with which these patients may present and be unaware of the appropriate laboratory measures available, this can present as an enormous diagnostic dilemma.

A great deal of AIDSworld uncertainty arises because information coming from the CDC and the FDA can be conflicting. The CDC and the FDA operate under different legal mandates. The CDC is a branch of the U.S. Public Health Service, and the Public Health Service operates under the auspices of the Department of Defense. As a public health agency, the CDC has a broad platform on which it can proclaim public health emergencies. They can and do stretch the truth. The FDA acts as an oversight agency for private corporations who operate under the Uniform Commercial Code, contract law, and the doctrine of informed consent. This presents a great confusion, and this is why the CDC can claim the accuracy of these tests as 99.9 percent while at the same time the package inserts, approved by the FDA, of most of the antibody tests have a disclaimer similar to this: "AIDS and AIDS-related conditions are clinical syndromes and their diagnosis can only be established clinically. EIA [enzyme immunoassay] testing cannot be used to diagnose AIDS, even if the recommended investigation of reactive specimens suggests that the antibodies to HIV are present. . . . **The risk of an asymptomatic person with a repeatedly reactive serum sample developing AIDS or an AIDS-related condition is not known.**"[283] (emphasis added) If, indeed, these tests have a sensitivity and specificity of 99.9 percent, there is no logical reason why this disclaimer should be inserted unless, as will be outlined, the companies who manufacture these tests understand something about the lack of purification of the HI virus, which they are choosing to share with neither the physician nor the patient and which the CDC completely and dishonestly ignores. One would expect that companies that manufacture tests of such high accuracy would have 99.9 percent trust in their product. This is not the case.

Thirteen years after the Gallo papers were published in *Science*, two separate research groups, one from the U.S. National Cancer Institute[284]

---

[283] Lucey, DR., et al., (1992), "Comparison by race of total serum IgG, IgA, and IgM with CD4+T cell counts in North American persons infected with immunodeficiency virus type 1," *J Acquir Immune Defic Syndr;* 5(4):325–32

[284] Bess, JW, et al, "Microvesicles are a source of contaminating cellular proteins found in purified HIV-1 preparations," Feb. 9, 1997 *Virology* 230: pp. 134-144

and the other from a French/German consortium[285] (figure 1 and figure 2), attempted to isolate and purify HIV-1 by the techniques of Gallo. Both groups discovered that Gallo could not possibly have isolated and neither could they by following the Gallo protocols. What both groups found were microvesicles, viral-like particles, containing proteins, DNA, and RNA extruded from the cancer cells and lymphocytes used in the study. The NCI paper (figure 1) clearly states that "identification and quantitation of cellular proteins associated with HIV-1 particles are complicated by the presence of nonvirion associated cellular proteins that copurify with virions. Many cellular proteins are associated with nonviral particles that bud from the surface of cells called microvesicles.[286] Microvesicles band in sucrose gradients in a range of densities that includes the same density as retroviruses. . . . We identify and partially characterize microvesicles from human T cell lines and PBL [peripheral blood lymphocytes] that constitute a significant source of cellular proteins found in purified preparations of immunodeficiency viruses, including HIV-1."[287] Only in AIDSworld, where most of the isolate is cellular debris and is admittedly from cellular proteins, can one find the implication of contamination of the spun specimen and the word *purified* in the same sentence.

---

[285] Gluschankof, P., et al, "Cell membrane vesicles are a major contaminant of gradient enriched human immunodeficiency virus type-1 preparations," Jan. 13, 1997 *Virology;* 230: pp. 125–133

[286] Other researchers have called these "virus like particles"

[287] Bess, Op cit.

The Slow Death of the AIDS/Cancer Paradigm
and the Apocrypha of the Eukaryotic Cell

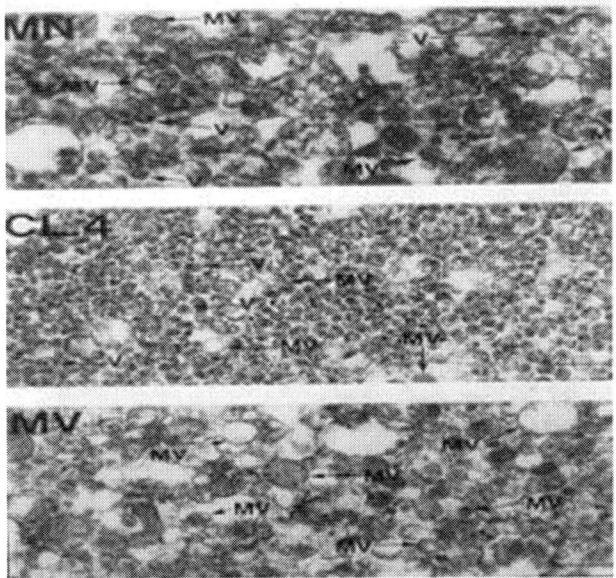

Fig. 1

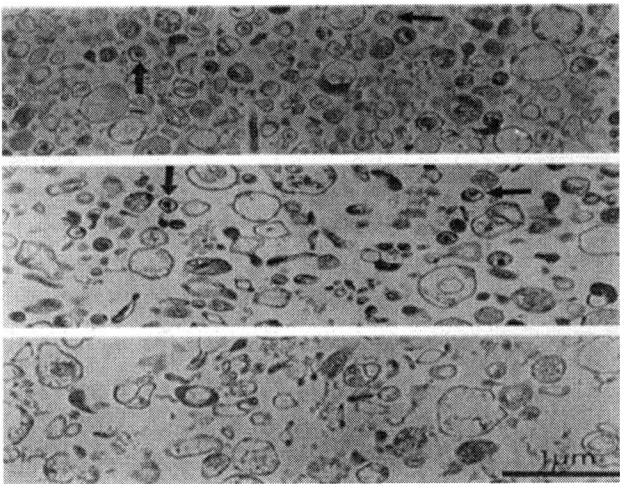

Fig. 2

Figure 1 slides are from the NCI, fig. 2 from the European consortium. The bars in the lower-right corner represent 1μm. There is nothing in either of these slides that is purified. While there are arrows pointing to particles that they claim are HIV, there is no proof offered that this is the case. Further, the particles identified as HIV in both groups are two to two and a half times the diameter that virologist claim for retroviruses.

The French/German paper (figure 2) acknowledged that *"none of the studies demonstrating the association of molecules of human origin with HIV or other retroviruses by biochemical or serological means has the purity of the virus preparation been verified.* (emphasis added) *We analyzed gradient enriched virus preparations and found that there is contamination with an excess of nonviral membrane vesicles of cellular origin. . . . HIV particles are a minority population, comprising about 25 to 50 percent of the vesicles in both infected preparations."*[288] However, if one examines carefully these published micrographs (figure 1 and figure 2), one can see that the evidence that HIV particles constitute 20 percent to 50 percent of this mixture is a pure hyperbole. Further, the particles identified as HIV are more than twice the normal retroviral size! These debris fields are the proteins used to make the HIV antibody tests, ergo, the package disclaimers.

Because of the abundance of contaminating material consistently found in these "isolating" experiments, every clinician must be aware that, to date, because of this contamination, there is no practical test for screening that indicates, with any medical or scientific accuracy, whether a person has the HIV virus and is infectious. In essence, if and until isolation and identification occurs, all HIV antibody tests should be construed as false-positive tests. If a test could be produced, a direct reliable method for determining the infection status of an individual would be to culture the virus from the blood or other body tissue. On the first Montagnier paper, to the following Gallo papers, to these two papers from the NCI and the European consortium, none of which have demonstrated the ability to isolate, rest the entire HIV/AIDS paradigm. Although the community of virologists has participated in this AIDSworld group delusion, convincing themselves and the world they have isolated a virus, their own literature (and the 1997 Montagnier interview) make it quite clear that in spite of the double talk and disingenuousness and the talk of contamination and purification in the same sentence, they are really not true believers of their own hype. It is unfortunate that most of the people who do this research are not clinicians and do not have to face the consequences of these experimental procedures that could not pass an undergraduate cell biology laboratory course and continue to support a broken theory that has done so much international harm.

Given this lack of purification, the most that can be said for any HIV test is that it is an assumption—but not direct proof—that the bands identified on the tests are from a unique HIV virus. That assumption is giving the test more credit than it deserves because the only way to distinguish between real reactions and cross-reactions is to use HIV isolation. As has been demonstrated,

---

[288] Gluschankof, P., et al, "Cell membrane vesicles are a major contaminant of gradient enriched human immunodeficiency virus type-1 preparations," Jan. 13, 1997 *Virology;* 230: pp. 125–133

The Slow Death of the AIDS/Cancer Paradigm
and the Apocrypha of the Eukaryotic Cell

all claims of HIV isolation are based on a set of indirect phenomena detected in tissue culture as have been described, none of which are isolation and none of which are specific for retroviruses. However, there is a much bigger issue: if HIV/AIDS has been defined as a problem of cell-mediated immunity, but the humoral immunity is known to be intact, why spend so much time on a test that tells you what you already know while ignoring what you do not know about the metabolic aberrations in the cell mediated immune system? This issue will be addressed in future chapters.

Because of the lack of purification the HIV, antibodies are nonspecific. The scientific literature reveals numerous studies demonstrating false-positive HIV-antibody reactions on the enzyme-linked immunosorbent assay (ELISA) and western blot (WB). A false-positive reaction means that antibodies to other germs, or naturally circulating antibodies in persons, coincidentally bind to the purported HIV proteins in test kits. HIV antibody tests have been found to be positive in Amazonian Indians who had no contact with the outside world, in dogs at the U. California Davis Veterinary School, and in mice of certain autoimmune strains. Fifty percent of 144 dogs tested were found to have antibodies to one or more HIV recombinant proteins.[289] The authors assumed that the dogs were not infected with HIV, but this is more evidence of the antibody cross-reactivity. The tests have been shown to cross-react with at least 70 other (human) factors[290] including flu, hepatitis and tetanus vaccines, acute viral infections, other retroviruses, autoimmune conditions, antimitochondria, pregnancy, antinuclear antibodies, among others.

Commonly used tests to detect HIV antibodies are of two general types, and both depend on a scaled decision variable. In the type of test used most, called enzyme-linked immunoassay (EIA or ELISA), the test result is one of a continuum of numerical values of optical density, as generated by a machine. As the main representative of the second type, regarded as more conclusive but more expensive and difficult, the western blot test (WB) produces several bands along a strip that vary in visual intensity according to the degree of reaction of various proteins. These bands are interpreted visually by a technician with a subjective positivity criterion; then positive judgments about various bands and various combinations of bands are taken as more or less indicative of HIV. The selection of a positivity criterion for the EIA test, a particular numerical value of optical density, is made by its manufacturer. Some data suggest the intent to

---

[289] Sandstrom HV, et al, "Studies with canine sera that contain antibodies which recognize human immunodeficiency virus structural proteins"; *Cancer Res* 1990:50: pp. 5628-5630
[290] http://www.virusmyth.com/aids/hiv/cjtestfp.htm

select the criterion that best discriminates between positive and negative cases, but there appear to be no published rationales for the criteria chosen.

The EIA tests were originally developed to screen donated blood, and their positivity criteria were set in that context. But when clinicians began to use these tests for the routine testing and diagnosis of patients, their positivity criteria remained unchanged. While the cost of a false-positive decision that leads to the unnecessary disposal of uncontaminated blood is negligible, the cost of a false-positive decision that leads to an improper diagnosis and additional testing of uninfected individuals is much greater. The cost of the fear, alarm, and social and psychological injuries that typically lead to costly treatment with highly toxic drugs often resulting in preventable errors and complications that lead to iatrogenic injuries and death is incalculable.

Figure 3 is a reproduction of a polyacrylamide gel electrophoresis—the HIV western blot test. Lane A is noninfected, and lanes B and C are "infected." What is visibly obvious on this electrophoresis is that all three lanes have all the same proteins. The difference between the bands on A and the B and C bands is quantitative only. Essentially, this can be interpreted to indicate that everyone has HIV proteins, simply in different ratios.[291] The infected cultures originate from AIDS patients who are highly oxidized to begin with (type 2 cell dis-symbiosis). Further, these proteins forming the darker lines are from cell cultures that have been mixed with cancer cells and have been chemically manipulated with mitogens and type 1 cytokines. Although the labels seem to distinguish actin and the MHC protein HLA-DR as non-viral, nevertheless, these two proteins are still a part of the western blot as is p24, another nonspecific protein, which has become the *sine qua non* of HIV identifiers.

---

[291] Giraldo, R., (1989/9), "Everybody reacts positive on the ELISA test for HIV," *Continuum*

The Slow Death of the AIDS/Cancer Paradigm and the Apocrypha of the Eukaryotic Cell

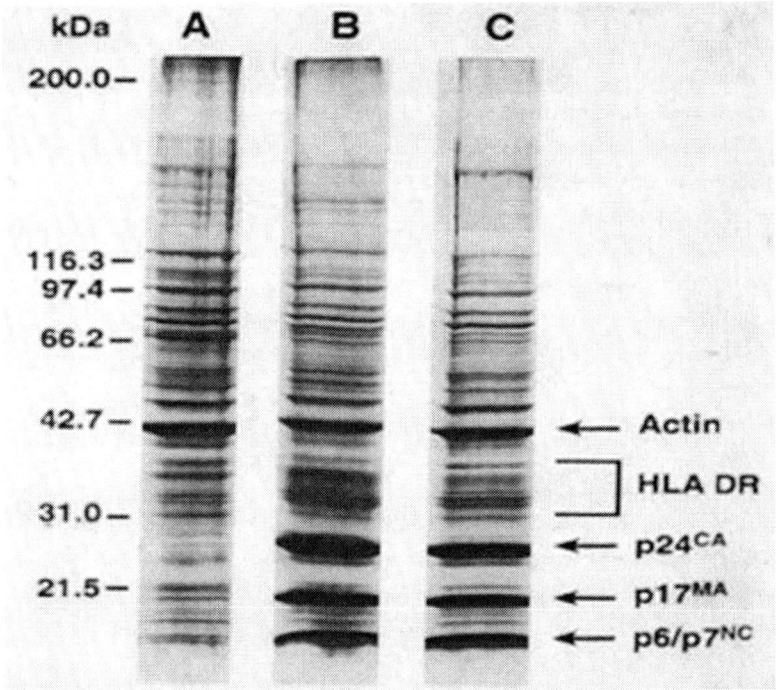

Fig. 3

The Perth group out of Australia asked the senior author the manner in which they were able to prove that the strong bands were HIV proteins. His reply avoided any mention of proof and simply informed them that the labels were added at the suggestion of the editor to better orientate the reader! Independent data demonstrate that the proteins labeled p24 and p18 have been found in a wide variety of uninfected human tissues using AIDS sera and monoclonal antibodies to the so-called HIV proteins. Where are the rest of the so-called HIV proteins in this purified virus? Where are p41 and p65 and p120 and p160? In other words, these data are better explained by HIV proteins being not viral but cellular. In fact, there is a significant body of independent data proving that all the HIV proteins are cellular or nonspecific.[292,293]

In the United States, theoretically, a diagnosis of HIV positivity can be done only after the same blood of a person has reacted positive on an ELISA three

---

[292] Bess, JW., et al., (1997), "Microvesicles are a source of contaminating cellular proteins found in purified HIV-1 preparations," *Virology;* 230: 134–144

[293] Papadopoulos, E., Turner, V., (2000), "HIV testing and surveillance," presentation presidential AIDS advisory panel meeting http://www.virusmyth.com/aids/hiv/eppretoria.htm

or four times on two consecutive days and one time on the western blot test,[294] although it must be stressed that these procedures are not consistently followed and there is evidence to support the contention of both racial and risk group bias in the reading of these tests.[295] For example, recently the CDC[296] claims that black men are eight times more likely than white men and black women are fifteen to twenty times more likely than white women, despite registering fewer sexual partners, to be HIV positive.[297] They completely ignore that the HIV test is, in fact, only a measure of antibody levels that have an arbitrary cut-off point and those people who are genetically predisposed to have a higher rate of production of antibodies to a given stimulus will be caught in the HIV antibody dragnet. The fact that it has been demonstrated that people of African ancestry have higher IGg antibody[298] levels than those of European ancestry has been discounted by the CDC who have historically consistently followed the precepts of the Rockefeller Foundation's Science of Man molecular biology agenda that continues to demonstrate malicious intent toward the African American community in both overt and subtle ways.[299]

If HIV is an infectious disease, it is the first infectious disease that requires the repetition of the same antibody test four times in order to know if those antibodies are present or not. If the ELISA test were 99.9 percent specific for HIV as claimed, there should be no need to repeat the test three or four times on the same blood specimen before declaring a positive result and then confirming with a western blot. This does not happen with any other well-known infectious disease; however, this was the standard from the iconic study by Colonel Donald Burke from the Walter Reed Army Institute, which has been used as definitive proof of the specificity of the western blot.[300]

---

[294] It should be noted that the most recent *MMWR* revised surveillance case definition for HIV infection—United States 2014 has all but abandoned any rational diagnostic criteria (e.g. eliminates the requirement of HIV infection in the child's biologic mother to define a case of HIV infection in a child < 18 months), etc.

[295] http://askdeblasiowhy.com/index.php?option=com_content&view=article&id=101

[296] http://www.cdc.gov/hiv/risk/racialethnic/aa/index.html

[297] Michael, Terry, (2013), "HIV an its amazing ability to tell whether you are white or black, and to cause heart attacks," http://www.terrymichael.net/Htm_InteriorPages/HIV_AIDS_Special_Report_RaceAndHeartAttacks.html

[298] Lucey, DR., et al., (1992), "Comparison by race of total serum IgG, IgA, and IgM with CD4+T cell counts in North American persons infected with immunodeficiency virus type 1," *J Acquir Immune Defic Syndr;* 5(4):325–32

[299] Cooper, LA., et al., (2012), "The Association of clinician's implicit attitudes about race with medical visit communication and patient ratings of interpersonal care," *JPHA;* 102(4): 979–987

[300] Burke, DS., et al., (1988), "Measurement of the false positive rate in screening program for human immunodeficiency virus infections," *NEJM,* 319:961-964

During an eighteen-month period, Burke, et al., tested 1.2 million applicants for U.S. military service. Burke's testing was consistent with a progression through two ELISAs and two western blots. The HIV seroprevalence was found to be 1.48/1,000. The study then retrospectively investigated a highly selected sample of this population in which the seroprevalence was one-tenth that of the 1.2 million. This group comprised 135,187 persons aged 17–18 years who resided in rural areas where the cumulative incidence of AIDS was low. This group should have been no different from healthy blood donors and regard all HIV positives as false positives, but the premise of the study was the opposite by assuming that there were true positives among healthy rural American youth. Wishing to evaluate the false-positive rate and specificity of the western blot, Burke needed to define HIV infection. This was done by performing a series of four more antibody tests on sera from the 15 out of 135,187 applicants who had already been found twice ELISA and twice western blot positive. Two of the extra tests were other western blots and two were similar tests. Any individual who was positive in all four extra tests, thereby making a total of eight positive antibody tests, was deemed HIV infected. Those who failed any of the extra four tests were deemed non-HIV infected. Of the 15, one failed to complete the panel; and thus, Burke conceded only one, not fifteen, false positives. From these data, Burke calculated the specificity of the HIV western blot to be in excess of 99.9 percent.[301] Disregarding the obvious flaws in this study, repeating the antibody test eight or more times is still not proof of a viral infection. It simply proves that something is wrong with the chosen test.

The epidemiological data from HIV tests collated on a wide variety of social groups between which the F(HIV) (frequency of a positive HIV test) varies enormously by nearly three orders of magnitude. Repeat blood donors test as low as 1 positive in 100,000. Gay men (MSM) test highest at 40 percent or even more. Injecting drug users (IDU) sometimes test as high as or close to the levels in MSM. Other groups fall between those extremes in a way that marks the level of F(HIV) as a nonspecific marker of the degree of challenged health or actual illness in the sampled population. As a non-specific indicator of physiological stress, it is inadequate for identifying those patients who have an abnormality in their cell-mediated immune function which, of course, is the fundamental diagnostic issue. This is a major clinical challenge as there are also patients

---

[301] Turner, V., (1996), "Do HIV antibody tests prove HIV infection? http://www.virusmyth.com/aids/hiv/vttests.htm

who are HIV negative yet have all the characteristics of AIDS patients.[302] These patients are defined as having CD4+ T lymphocytopenia, another misnomer, which again does not address the pathology of the cell-mediated immune system. Thus, the HIV test may be helpful in the clinical setting, but it is not diagnostic. It also cannot epidemiologically be used to reflect the mode of transmission of any of the known sexually transmitted diseases,[303] which have completely different epidemiological parameters. More than anything, it gives no explanation for the findings: anergy, the failure of an *in vitro* response of lymphocytes to mitogen stimulation and the immune shift in CD4+T cells from type 1 to type 2 with increased antibody levels, which are the hallmarks of the AID syndrome.

Several demographic studies have supported the notion of the non-transmissibility of this entity.[304] These studies help to explain the variation of the frequency of positivity between social groups and with age, sex, and population density.[305] These variations have been demonstrated to be incompatible with the behavior of a sexually transmitted infection. As an example, it was found that patients who are in hospital because of illnesses unrelated to HIV have a level of F(HIV) that is often ten times that of such generally healthy populations as military cohorts and even a hundred times greater than the level among repeat blood donors.[306] This also underscores the necessity of running matched controls of equally ill non-AIDS patients in AIDS studies—a practice that has been conspicuously absent over the years.

Physicians often use nonspecific indicators of physiological stress such as the ESR (erythrocyte sedimentation reaction), the C-reactive protein and pro-inflammatory cytokines,[307] to assess the health status of a patient. As an example, an elevated ESR, which is an indirect measure of generalized inflammation, is

---

[302] Smith, DK., et al., (1993), "Unexplained opportunistic infections and CD4+ T lymphocytopenia without HIV infection. An investigation of cases in the United States. The Centers for Disease Control Idiopathic CD4+ T lymphocytopenia task force," *NEJM*, 11(328): 373–379

[303] Bauer, HH., (2006), "Demographic characteristics of HIV: III. Why does HIV discriminate by race?," *J Scientific Explor;* 20(2): 255-288

[304] Padian, NS., et al., (1997), "Heterosexual transmission of human immune deficiency virus (HIV) in Northern California: Results from a 10 year study," *Am J Epidemiol;* 146(4): 350–357

[305] Bauer, Op cit.

[306] Bauer, Op cit.

[307] http://www.plosone.org/article/infopercent3Adoipercent2F10.1371percent2Fjournal.pone.0059107 Distinctive Cytokines as Biomarkers Predicting Fatal Outcome of Severe Staphylococcus aureus Bacteremia in Mice

caused by the dielectric effect of proteins in the surrounding plasma, especially fibrinogen, immunoglobulins, and other acute-phase reaction proteins, and their increased levels in some disease states. As a result, the red blood cells stick to one another and form stacks called rouleaux. Values exceeding 100 mm/hr have been shown to have a 90 percent positive predictive value for serious underlying pathology including infection, collagen vascular disease, or metastatic tumors.[308] Thus, like the HIV antibody test, an elevated ESR also predicts a number of unrelated diseases. However, there is no ESR syndrome disease; and it would be an absurdity to define, for example, congestive heart failure as ESR syndrome.

Nevertheless, clinicians should be aware that these tests are not diagnostic but ancillary and require an underlying evaluation of the patient's general health status and their cell-mediated immunity status as reflected in their DTH skin test, cysteine, glutathione, and other antioxidant and metabolic levels. This is consistent with how the manufacturers of HIV tests describe their product use. For example, the insert for the Abbott Laboratories HIVAB HIV-1/ HIV-2 (rDNA) EIA warns, "At present there is **no recognized standard** for establishing the presence or absence of antibodies to HIV-1 and HIV-2 in human blood.... False positive results can be expected with any test kit. Falsely elevated results have been observed due to non-specific interactions."[309]

From the beginning of the AIDS era, HIV tests were designed to support the assumption of immune deficiency caused by a virus in high-risk populations. HIV tests were never designed or approved as a direct measure of an infectious agent. The tests are notoriously inaccurate, especially in what are considered to be low-risk populations.[310] The frequency at which these tests are positive in defined groups varies in a manner that reflects the general health of that group. For example, military personnel have a lower rate of positivity in general testing than do Job Corps applicants and medical patients being treated for reasons unconnected to HIV or AIDS. Despite this fact, they test positive more often than do healthy people even when the medical condition is psychiatric. These variations mark a positive HIV test as indicating nothing specific to HIV but to something nonspecific about health in general such as the degree of physiologic or oxidative stress[311]. Much more will be discussed on the issue of immune deficiency as the result of an overload of oxidative stressors.

An application from the Cambridge Biotech Corporation to the FDA for the approval of a western blot test kit includes this disclaimer: "Although

---

[308] Brigden (Russell attachment 21)
[309] Abbott AXSYM© System. May, 1998
[310] Barry 1986 (Russell attachment 22)
[311] Papadopolus 1992 (Russell attachment 23)

a positive result may indicate infection with HIV-1, a diagnosis of Acquired Immunodeficiency Syndrome (AIDS) can be made only if an individual meets the case definition of AIDS established by the Centers for Disease Control."[312]

HIV WESTERN BLOT STRIP*		AFR	AUS	FDA	RCX	CDC 1	CDC 2	CON	GER	UK	FRA	MAC
ENV	p160 p120 p41	ANY 2	ANY 1	ANY 1	ANY 1	p160/ p120 AND p41	p160/ p120 OR p41	p160/ p120 OR p41	ANY 1	ANY 1	ALL 3	3 WEAK BANDS OR ANY STRONG BAND
POL	p68 p53 p32	ANY 3 GAG OR POL	p32 AND	ANY 1 AND		p32 AND	OR	ANY 1 GAG OR POL	p32 AND	ANY 1 OR		
GAG	p55 p39 p24 p18		p24	ANY 1		p24	p24		p24	ANY 1		

Fig. 4

An obvious anomaly on the WB is the absence of a designation for reverse transcriptase, which is said to have a molecular weight of 100,000 yet is nowhere to be found among the WB proteins.[314]

Figure 4 is a is a graphic of the western blot test (see figure 3) and the ten proteins used to make a diagnosis. Proteins (and glycoproteins) are delineated by *p* and a number indicating the molecular weight in kD. The kD numbers fall across from the area marked with *env, pol,* or *gag,* indicating the assumed location of the protein source on the viral genome.

The top of the diagram lists the various laboratories and/or countries around the globe as well as the various criteria used to diagnose from lab to

---

[312] http://www.fda.gov/downloads/BiologicsBloodVaccines/BloodBloodProducts/ApprovedProducts/LicensedProductsBLAs/BloodDonorScreening/InfectiousDisease/ucm094000.pdf
[313] http://www.theperthgroup.com/REJECTED/emergmedab.html
[314] http://www.sparks-of-light.org/263-Serology-HTLVIII-AIDS.pdf Schupbach J, et al, Serological analysis of a subgroup of human T lymphotropic retroviruses (HTLV-III) associated with AIDS, *Science* 1984;224:503-505

lab and country to country. Contrary to most diagnostic criteria for disease identification, there is a decided lack of standardization (e.g., the diagnostic criteria for diabetes are the same anywhere on planet earth). For example, in Africa, any two of the *env* proteins is considered a positive test while the requirements in Australia are much more stringent requiring one env and any three gag or pol proteins. That the diagnosis has different criteria based on geography may come as a surprise to many clinicians as this is certainly a unique diagnostic situation and one not well explained in the AIDS literature. An excuse is made for Africa where many countries lack public health budgets. As a result, the World Health Organization devised the Bangui definition in which no test is required, but the diagnosis is based on a series of nonspecific physical symptoms:[315,316]

Major signs
weight loss >= 10 percent of body weight
chronic diarrhea for more than 1 month
prolonged fever for more than 1 month (intermittent or constant)

Minor signs
persistent cough for more than 1 month
generalized pruritic dermatitis
etc.

You Can't Take These Numbers to Vegas: Why There Are Disclaimers in the HIV Antibody Tests

In vivo, it has been reported that what is being called HIV can only be found to be expressed in less than 1 in 10,000 of peripheral blood lymphocytes.[317] This is an infinitesimal amount considering that an adult human has a population of approximately 10^{11} naive T cells circulating in the peripheral lymphoid organs and blood.[318] From early in development, this population is generated and

---

[315] WHO case definitions for AIDS surveillance in adults and adolescents. Wkly Epidemiol Rec. 1994 Sep 16; 69(37): 273-5.

[316] WHO/CDC case definition for AIDS. Wkly Epidemiol Rec. 1986 Mar 7; 61(10): 69-76.

[317] Ou CY, Kwok S, et al., "DNA amplification for direct detection of HIV-1 in DNA of peripheral blood mononuclear cells" *Science* 1988 Jn. 15;239(4837): pp. 295-7

[318] Bains, I, et al., "Quantifying the development of the peripheral naive CD4+T cell pool in humans." *Blood* May 28, 2009; 113:22 pp 5480-5487

sustained by thymic export and division on the periphery and is estimated to comprise at least 10^8 different T cell receptor specificities.[319] The possibility of actually finding HIV becomes even less likely because what is being called HIV is not found in circulating Th1 CD4+T lymphocytes, but in naive Th0 and Th2 cells, which are found mainly in the bone marrow and to a lesser extent the lymph nodes.[320,321,322] That is correct. What researchers are calling HIV—the expression of RT and p24 under laboratory conditions—seems primarily to occur in the cells, which by definition are not "infected." The question then becomes what do these proteins actually represent?

A eukaryotic cell contains a billion or so protein molecules, and there are thought to be ten thousand different types of proteins in an individual vertebrate cell. Yet proteins are only 15 percent of the cell by dry weight.[323] Water molecules make up 99 percent of the molecules of the cell by number and 70 percent by weight. Only **1 percent** of the cell is composed of other molecules by dry weight 30 percent—proteins, 15 percent; RNA, 6 percent; ions and small molecules, 4 percent; polysaccharides, 2 percent; phospholipids, 2 percent; and DNA, 1 percent by weight.[324] From the numbers of cells identified and the content of these cells, what has been described as HIV proteins (or HIV RNA or HIV pro-viral DNA) have a much greater statistical probability of being cytoskeletal and/or upregulated stress proteins related to the (a) infectious conditions (and consequent apoptotic events) of the cells from patients with one or more AIDS-defining diseases or (b) the extruded oxidized proteins from the type 2 dis-symbiotic immortalized cancer cell line used in the original Gallo experiment.

The cytoskeleton is the main organizing structure of the cell and the scaffolding upon which the cell builds its infrastructure and carries out its functions. The cytoskeleton of eukaryotic cells consists of three main types of protein structures: microtubules, intermediate filaments, and actin filaments (microfilaments). Cytoskeletal filaments both generate and resist mechanical

---

[319] Arstilla, TP, et al, "A direct estimate of the human alphabeta T cell receptor diversity" *Science*. 1999 Oct 29;286(5441):958-61.

[320] Abbas A, Murphy K, Sher A. "Functional diversity of helper T lymphocytes." *Nature* 1996; 383: 787–793.

[321] Chehimi J, Frank I, Ma X, Trinchieri G. "Differential regulation of IL-10 and role of T-helper cells." In: Abstr. 408. Second National Conference on Human Retroviruses, Infectious Disease Society of America. Alexandria, Va.; 1995.

[322] Maggi E, Mazzetti M, Ravina A, et al. "Ability of HIV to promote a Th1 to Th2 shift and to replicate preferentially in Th2 and Th0 cells." Science, 1995; 265: 244–248.

[323] Popp, FA., Beloussov, L, editors (2003), Integrative Biophysics, Biophotonics, Kluwer Academic Publishers, Boston, Mass. p 180

[324] Alberts, B., et al, *Molecular Biology of the Cell;* Garland 3rd ed. 1994

loads, and they are largely responsible for the cell's ability to resist shape distortion.[325] In addition to the mechanical function, the cytoskeleton and especially microtubules generate a quasi-coherent electromagnetic field, which can both store energy and transmit it over distances.[326] They are highly electrically polar and possess nonlinear properties that may convert random thermal energy to quasi-coherent.

Intermediate filaments consist of a family of fiber-like vimentin and keratin proteins with molecular weights of 57kD and 52kD, respectively. The structural subunits of the microtubules are protofilaments composed of tubulin heterodimers consisting of α-tubulin and β-tubulin. Each tubulin monomer has a mass of about 55 kD.[327] Microtubules are located in strong static electric fields originating from mitochondria, and during mitosis, they form the structure called the mitotic spindle. Motor proteins transport along these intercellular and intracellular microtubular highways (see below).

Actin filaments have a double-helix structure. Individual units of actin filaments are globular proteins (G-actins, roughly 42 kD proteins), which polymerize to form filaments (F-actins). Bess[328] identifies gp41 as actin while Pinter found that gp160 and gp120 are tetramers and trimers of gp41[329] Actin is the most abundant intercellular protein in eukaryotic cells and in non-muscles cells makes up 1 to 5 percent of cellular protein.[330] Even Montagnier considered the p45 protein may be due to contamination by cellular actin.[331]

---

[325] Ingber, DE, "Tensigrity I. Cell structure and hierarchical systems in biology"; J *Cell Science;* April 1, 2003 116, 1157-1173

[326] Cifra, M, Doctoral Thesis, "Study of electromagnetic oscillations of yeast cells in Khz and GHz region," Prague, Jully 2009

[327] Cifra, Ibid

[328] Bess JW, et al, op cit

[329] Pinter A., et al, "Oligomeric structure of gp41, the transmembrane protein of human immunodeficiency virus type 1"; J Virol June 1989;63(6) pp. 2674–2679

[330] http://www.ncbi.nlm.nih.gov/books/NBK21493/

[331] Barré-Sinoussi, et al., (1983), "Isolation of a T-lymphotrophic retrovirus from a patient at risk for acquired immune deficiency syndrome (AIDS)," *Science;* 220(4599): 868–871

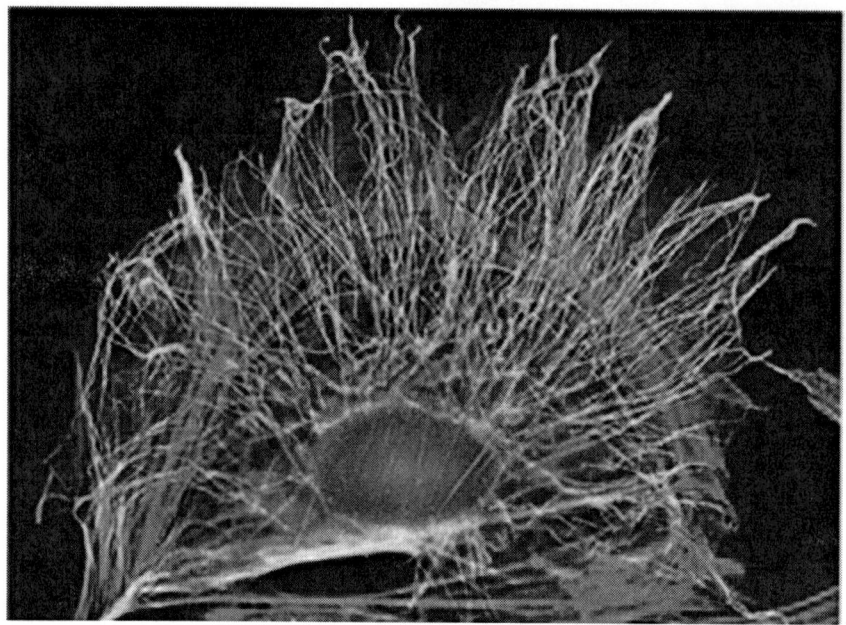
Cytoskeleton

The internal cytosol highways created by the cytoskeletal proteins allows the transport of organelles, macromolecules, membranes, or chromosomes within the cytoplasm. To assist in this transport are three known motor proteins: myosin, dynein, and kinesin. Dynein and kinesin move along the microtubules with energy supplied by ATP. As in muscle cells, in other eukaryotic cells, myosin is associated with actin microfilaments.

Motor protein dynein moves toward the cell center (negative end of the microtubule), and kinesin moves toward the cell periphery (plus end of the microtubule).

The Slow Death of the AIDS/Cancer Paradigm and the Apocrypha of the Eukaryotic Cell

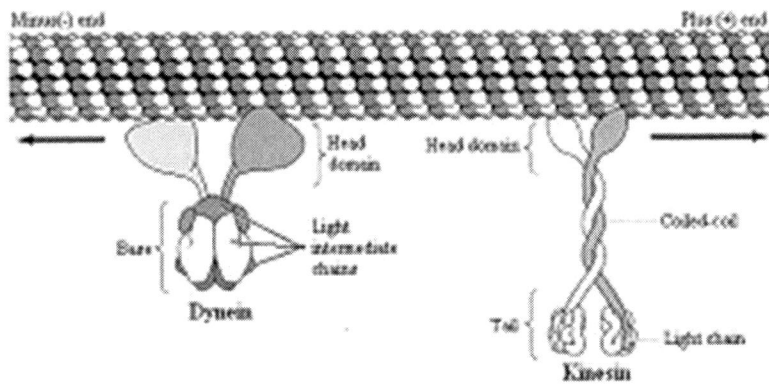

332

Dynein is composed of multiple chains including two 74 kDa intermediate chains, which are believed to anchor the dynein to its cargo and four 53–59 kDa intermediate chains and several light chains, which are less understood. Kinesin is also a large protein also composed of subunits: two heavy chains of 110–135 kDa and two light chains of 60–70 kDa.

At least fifteen myosin proteins have been identified, but only three have been well studied. Myosin II is associated with actin in the cytoskeleton. Myosin II is a large molecule of about 500 kD but has two light chains of about 20 kD each.[333,334] The organization and stiffness of the cytoskeleton are determined in large part by the forces generated by actin and myosin II.[335] The actin-myosin II interaction in smooth muscle and nonmuscle cells is regulated by the phosphorylation of serine 19 of the 20 kDa light chain of myosin II.[336] Already in 1987 it was shown that people who had "anti-HIV antibodies" had high IgG natural autoantibody titres to actin, DNA, tubulin, thyroglobulin, albumin, and myosin.[337]

---

[332] http://kc.njnu.edu.cn/swxbx/shuangyu/6.htm

[333] Ibid

[334] Fazal F, et al., "Inhibiting myosin light chain kinase induces apoptosis in vitro and in vivo" July 2005 *Mol Cell Bio;* 25(14): pp.6259-6266

[335] Elson, EL, 1988 "Cellular mechanics as an indicator of cytoskeletal structure and function," *Annu Rev Biophys. Biophys Chem;* 17:397-430

[336] Adelstein, RS 1983 "Regulation of contractile proteins by phosphorylation" *J Clin Investig;* 72:1863-1866

[337] Matsiota P, et al., "Detection of natural autoantibodies in serum of anti-hiv positive individuals" 1987 *Ann Inst Pasteur/Immunol;* 138: pp. 223-233

It is likely that microtubules play a direct role in the propagation of action potentials through the conductance of electric current.[338] Calcium has been shown to be critical for the propagation of action potentials. When calcium is removed from the extracellular solution, action potentials are immediately abolished.[339] Cytosolic calcium is also a key regulatory factor and perhaps the most widely used means of controlling cellular function.[340] Calcium is generally bound to calcium-binding proteins one of which has a molecular weight of 68,000. It is a major component of the human lymphocyte plasma membrane and is located on the cytoplasmic face of the plasma membrane.[341]

Finally, p32 has been identified as HLA-DR an MHC class II (HLA-human leukocyte antigen-D related and MHC-major histocompatibility complex) cell surface receptor encoded by the leucocyte antigen complex on chromosome 6. HLA-DR is involved in several autoimmune conditions, disease susceptibility, and disease resistance. It is upregulated in response to signaling. In the instance of an infection, the peptide (antigen) is bound into a DR molecule and presented to a few T-cell receptors found on T helper cells. These cells then bind to antigens on the surface of B cells, stimulating B cell proliferation.[342,343] The MHC HLA-DR5 is more commonly expressed in people of African and Mediterranean ancestry.

In a 1997 Djamel Tahi conducted an interview with Luc Montagnier where he asked Montagnier:

"*DT: At the density of retroviruses, 1.16, there are a lot of particles, but only 20 percent of them appertain to HIV. Why are 80 percent of the proteins not viral and the others are? How can one make out the difference?*

LM: There are two explanations. For the one part, at this density you have what one calls microvesicles of cellular origin, which have approximately the same size as the virus, and then the virus itself, in budding, brings cellular proteins. So effectively, these proteins are not viral. They are cellular in origin. So how to make out the difference? Frankly,

---

[338] Gardiner J., et al, "The microtubule cytoskeleton acts as a key downstream effector of neurotransmitter signaling."; Synapse. 2011 Mar;65(3):249-56. doi: 10.1002/syn.20841.

[339] Tasaki, I (1988) "A macromolecular approach to excitation phenomena: mechanical and thermal changes in nerve during excitation"; *Physiol Chem and Phys and Med, NMR* 20:251-268

[340] Rosado, JA et al., "Topical Review: the actin cytoskeleton in store mediated calcium entry," 2000, *J Phys; 562.2:* 221–229

[341] Owens, RJ., et al, "Cellular distribution of p68, a new calcium binding protein from lymphocytes"; 1984 *Embro J; 3(5):* 945-952

[342] Gluschankof, P, op cit.

[343] Bess, JW, op cit.

with this technique, one can't do it precisely. What we can do is to purify the virus to the maximum with successive gradients, and you always stumble on the same proteins."

And this is the rub as the trusting but gullible physician is expected to believe that HIV antibody tests have a sensitivity and specificity of 99.9 percent.

Only in AIDSworld does 20 percent trump 80 percent and where cytoskeletal proteins become viral proteins and where taking impure proteins from this cell mix and allowing them to react with antibodies from the blood serum of oxidatively stressed patients constitutes a positive diagnosis. So in AIDspeak, the HIV antibody test is not an HIV antibody test but an autoantibody test in ill patients who have catabolic stress, which leads to increased daily cell turnover or in people who are genetically predisposed to make more antibodies. The HIV antibody tests claimed to have a 99.9 percent specificity by the CDC, as stated by the test package inserts approved by the FDA, can never be used to diagnose because what pass as HIV proteins have a very low statistical probability of existing and even if existing have a low probability of being identified over the vastly larger number of cytoskeletal proteins sedimenting at 1.16 gm/ml in the sucrose gradient. What will be demonstrated in future chapters is the most that this test indicates is that the patient likely has a type 2 immune cell dominance with a consequent increase in antibody production, which may or may not, given the history and lifestyle of the individual, be predictive of future disease. It tells the clinician nothing about the state of the patient's cell-mediated immunity, which, of course, is the key issue for deciding whether or not therapeutic intervention is necessary in both those patients who have a positive HIV test and those who present with idiopathic CD4+T cell lymphocytopenia.

CHAPTER 4

When Viral Load Is Not Viral Load

The legal doctrine of informed consent has two distinct components: (1) the patient's right to determine what happens to his or her body and (2) the physician's duty to provide the patient with sufficient information to make an educated decision regarding any condition or proposed therapy.[344] Therein lies the rub. When the orthodoxy intentionally chooses to misrepresent or repress knowable information of vital interest to both the physician and his/her patient, and the patient suffers as a result. Who is at fault? The physician takes an oath to do no harm while the drug companies take an oath to make profit at any cost. Those goals are ethically and morally irreconcilable.

There are two ways by which the pharmaceutical industry accomplishes their profit goal that directly impacts the cost and quality of patient care. One is through the revolving door among pharmaceutical executives cycling into senior government bureaucratic positions, pushing through regulatory changes that directly impact their company's or industry's profits, and then returning to the private sector to cash in on those changes.[345,346] The other is by subsidizing research and direct monetary support to medical schools, hospitals, and physicians under various guises. As an example, when leading academic physicians serve as board members of major pharmaceutical corporations, taking money directly not only for their board participation but also for direct funding to their respective institutions, the first oath to do no harm is likely subsumed to the expediency of the profit motive. Perhaps if the Bayh-Dole

---

[344] Canterbury v Spence, 464 F .2d 772 (D.C. Cir. 1972)
[345] http://www.opensecrets.org/revolving/
[346] http://www.redicecreations.com/specialreports/monsanto.html

Act,[347] which was signed into law by Ronald Reagan (at about the same time as the AIDS crisis was developing) had never been passed, there would never have been an AIDS crisis. Unfortunately, the law allowed researchers and institutions to patent discoveries that had previously remained in the public domain because they were financed with public money. The law now allowed researchers such as Robert Gallo and his fraudulent patent on the HIV antibody test[348] to parasite off the largesse of the American taxpayer. Ultimately, the standard of care under this "privatized" system becomes corrupted, dangerous products and procedures are introduced to the market, while knowledge of not only their deleterious effects but their lack of clinical effectiveness is hidden from public scrutiny.[349] Physicians are rewarded by attending drug-company-sponsored conferences where they receive credits for passive indoctrination about how to sell (prescribe) the newest drugs or use an unproven test to make a false diagnosis. The patient suffers for lack of sufficient information to make an educated decision,[350] and iatrogenic morbidity and mortality numbers continue to spike.

As an example of medical disinformation that can be easily found on the government website AIDS.gov[351] is the description of *viral load*. This site advises the reader that "when healthcare providers discuss your 'viral load,' they are talking about the level of HIV in your blood." Is that a scientifically valid assertion? Has that patient been given reliable information on which to make a decision about whether or not to begin antiretroviral drugs (ARVs), or is that more AIDSpeak disinformation? Does the viral load actually have some relationship to complete infectious viral particles in the bloodstream, or is the test a measure of some other metabolic process that is being ignored in favor of pumping healthy HIV false-positive people full of experimental drugs with demonstrated negative outcomes? More importantly, because the theory posits that it is the level of HIV that causes AID, the decrease in CD4+T cells, is there indeed a causal relationship between the viral load and a reduction in circulating CD4+T cells? What AIDS.gov is not saying is that the test to detect the viral load, the polymerase chain reaction (PCR), detects gene fragments of

---

[347] Angell, M., (2004), "The truth about drug companies," *NY Rev Books;* http://www.nybooks.com/articles/archives/2004/jul/15/the-truth-about-the-drug-companies/ downloaded 13 April 2015

[348] Bauer, H, (2010), "HIV tests are not HIV tests," *J Am Phys Surg;* 15(1): 5–9

[349] http://www.bloomberg.com/news/2014-04-07/takeda-actos-jury-awards-6-billion-in-punitive-damages.html

[350] Anderson, TS., (2014), "Academic Medical center leadership on pharmaceutical company board of directors," *JAMA;* 311(13): 1353–1355

[351] http://www.aids.gov/hiv-aids-basics/just-diagnosed-with-hiv-aids/understand-your-test-results/viral-load/ 26 July 2014

unknown origin. Since the human genome is replete with retroid elements,[352] many isogenic to defined HIV genomic segments,[353] there is no universe in which this test can be construed as a reliable measure of the "level of HIV in your blood."

Mark Craddock, an Australian mathematician, has observed that *"one of the most disturbing aspects of what passes for AIDS research these days, is the separation between what researchers actually find, what they tell the press conference and what the media tells the public. To assume that these are identical or even similar would be pure folly."*[354] Unfortunately, clinicians have the responsibility to avoid becoming part of any intentional deception that allows egregious harm to patients. The deadly combination of Big Pharma money, the Epidemic Intelligence Service, and their public relations megaphones, willful ignorance, and arrogance born of insecurity and cowardice has created a system in which iatrogenic errors are the third leading cause of death in the United States.[355] The HIV/AIDS theory is fraught with obvious inconsistencies and urges medical intervention when none is required, especially the so-called "viral load" measure. Although it is widely known that natural-occurring polyphenols are protease inhibitors,[356] the latest AIDSpeak gimmick used to introduce the widespread use of a class of chemical and patented protease inhibitors was advanced by David Ho, [357] *Time* magazine's Man of the Year for 1996, and X. Wei, et al.,[358] in two papers published in *Nature* in 1995.

Ho and Wei were attempting to measure the rate at which both HIV and T cells are produced in infected people. The idea seemed deceptively simple, but it completely ignored several pertinent issues including low glutathione levels in T helper cells and the existence of operationally distinct subsets of CD4+T cells. By 1995 it was already clear that there is both a functional dichotomy

---

[352] McClure, MA., (1992), "Sequence analysis of eukaryotic retroid proteins," *Math & Computer Modeling;* 16(6-7), 121–136

[353] Duesberg, PH., (1989), "Human immunodeficiency virus and acquired immunodeficiency syndrome: Correlation but not causation," *PNAS USA;* 86: 755–764

[354] Craddock, M., "HIV: Science by press conference," 1996 P.H. Duesberg (ed.) AIDS: Virus or Drug Induced? 127–130

[355] http://jama.jamanetwork.com/article.aspx?articleid=192908 "Is US Health really the best in the world?"

[356] Cuccioloni, M., et al., (2009), "Natural occurring polyphenols as a template for drug design," *Chem Biol Drug Des;* 74(1): 1–15

[357] Ho, DD., et al, (Jan, 12 1995), "Rapid turnover of plasma virions and CD4 lymphocytes in HIV-1 infection," *Nature;* 373(6510): 123–126

[358] Wei, X., et al., (Jan 12, 1995), "Viral dynamics in human immunodeficiency virus type 1 infection," *Nature;* 373(6510):117–122

in T helper cells as well as a differential response to cytokine stimuli. Th1 cells are generally associated with cell-mediated immunity. This subset has the ability to upregulate the inducible nitric oxide synthase (iNOS) enzyme in response to intercellular pathogens. The Th2 cell subset is associated with humoral immunity and the production of antibodies. This subset has the constitutively expressed NOS but does not make use of iNOS for intracellular killing of foreign microbes with an NO gas attack. Since these pioneering discoveries by Mosmann[359] and Coffman in 1986, the number of Th subsets has grown to include Th9, Th17, Th22, regulatory T cells and T follicular helper cells.[360,361,362] What is important to the AIDS crisis and the fallacy of the Ho and Wei hypothesis is that it is the glutathione levels in antigen-presenting cells that modulates the expression of type 1 versus type 2 response patterns [363,364] and not the reputed HI virus. However, when Ho and Wei published their theoretical mathematical model, the knowledge of the existence of the heterogeneity of CD4+T cells was well established and widely accepted as the theoretical model of cellular/humoral immune cell dichotomy, and multiple papers by AIDS researchers had observed the depleted glutathione levels in T helper cells; yet the Ho/Wei modeling ignored the most basic functioning of the objects they were counting.

For that reason alone, the mathematical model was unreliable to make any rational clinical decision. The model also made multiple erroneous assumptions: (1) that viral load (bits of floating unidentifiable genetic material) was an accurate estimator of true complete viral particles, (2) that viral load could predict the rise and fall of the CD4+T cell count, (3) that these particles had the ability to infect and destroy CD4+T lymphocytes, and (4) that the CD4+T cell lymphocytes are a homogenous population and are destroyed equally (as opposed to leaving the circulation under stress conditions as had

---

[359] Mosmann TR, Cherwinski H, Bond MW, Giedlin MA, Coffman RL. Two types of murine helper T cell clone. I. Definition according to profiles of lymphokine activities and secreted proteins. J Immunol. 1986;136:2348–2357. [PubMed]

[360] Deenick, EK, Ma, CS., et al. (2011), "Regulation of T follicular helper cell formation and function by antigen presenting cells" *Curr Opin Immunol:* 23:111-118

[361] Ma, CS, Deenick, EK., et al, (2012), "The origins, function, and regulation of T follicular helper cells," *J Exp Med;* 209: 1241–1253

[362] Tangye, SG., Ma, CS., (2013), "The good, the bad and the ugly TFH cells in human health and disease," *Nat Rev Immunol;* 13: 412–426

[363] Peterson, JD., et al, (1998), "glutathione levels in antigen presenting cells modulate Th1 versus Th2 response patterns," *Proc Natl Acad Sci USA;* 95:3071–3076

[364] Lucey, DR., et al., (1996), "Type 1 and type 2 cytokine dysregulation in human infectious, neoplastic, and inflammatory diseases," *Clin Micro Rev;* 9(4): 532–562

been demonstrated by Fauci,[365,366] but what he conveniently forgot in his zeal to promote the AIDSworld view). It ignored the fact that HIV was not a cytocidal virus.[367] In the world of science, these would have been hugely unacceptable anomalies, and the model would never have found its way onto the pages of a journal that claims a high reputation in the scientific world. But in AIDSworld, one finds that the rules change to meet the expediency of the model. Moreover, the mathematical model ignored this little detail: that it had been demonstrated that even what were considered to be complete viral particles, after escaping from the cellular environment lacked the prerequisite knobs or spikes needed to latch onto and enter a new cell, making the *in vivo* process of infection highly improbable if not impossible.[368] For any mathematical model to have a reliable predictive value, it cannot pick and choose which variables to input. However, there are even more improbabilities.

Ho used the emerging field of genetic amplification techniques[369] to advance what he called his "kitchen sink theory" of the new HIV pathophysiology. In the kitchen sink model, it urged the physician to "hit early, hit hard" with ARVs (antiretroviral drugs) because the model predicted that from the beginning of contact with the virus it was rapidly replicating, making billions of copies daily and somehow (mechanism not specified) causing billions more T cells to die than were being produced. This was postulated without evidence of actual T cell kinetics in AIDS, non-AIDS well people, and equally ill non-AIDS patients. In the end, they claimed that more immune cells are lost from the system than are replaced, causing AID, the decline in CD4+T cells. Probably the most important issue ignored is the fact that at the earliest point in time of an "HIV seroconversion," there is a profound depletion of glutathione in T4 helper cells,[370,371] leading to a change in cytokine profile from type 1 to type

---

[365] Fauci, AS, Dale, DC., (1974), "The effect of in vivo hydrocortisone on subpopulations of human lymphocytes" *J Clin Invest;* 53:240–246

[366] Fauci, AS., Dale, DC, (1975), "The effect of hydrocortisone on the kinetics of normal human lymphocytes," *Blood;* 46: 235–243

[367] Duesberg, PH., (1987), "Retroviruses as carcinogens and pathogens: expectations and reality," *Can Res;* 47:1199–1220

[368] Hausmann, E.H.S., Gelderblom, H.R., Clapham, P.R. et al. 1987. Detection of HIV envelope specific antibodies by immunoelectron microscopy and correlation with antibody titer and virus neutralizing activity. J. Virol. Meth. 16:125-137.

[369] http://www.karymullis.com/pcr.shtml

[370] Buhl, R., et al. (1989) "Systemic glutathione deficiency in suptom free HIV seropositive individuals," *Lancet;* 2:1294-1297

[371] Eck, HP, et al, (1989), "Low concentrations of acid globule thiol (cysteine) in the blood plasma of HIV-1 infected patients," *Biol Chem Hippe Seyler;* 370:101-108

2.[372] (see chapter 9, "The Binary Strategy of Human Immune Defense"). Any intracellular virus that attacks these cells can only be eliminated by upregulation of inducible nitric oxide synthase and the production of NO gas. This only occurs in type 1 cells.[373] If there were HI viruses attacking glutathione-depleted Th1 lymphocytes, they would still be killed by other type 1 cells as a result of apoptosis or necrosis of the Th1 cell under attack. Therefore, the idea that the HI virus would become resistant in a few days[374] is more AIDSworld fantasy as neither the glutathione-depleted Th1 cells (normal half-life of one or two days) nor the infectious "virus" could survive the NO gas attack. As a result of the Th2 cell dominance early in the process and the fact that Th2 cells do not produce NO gas but stimulate antibody production in the B cells, they cannot eliminate the "virus." However, another issue ignored is that whether the T cells are programmed for a type 1 cytokine profile and NO gas production or a type 2 cytokine profile and NO gas inhibition is not determined by "HI viruses" but by glutathione content in antigen-presenting dendritic cells, macrophages, and B cells.[375,376] Unfortunately, for patients that submit to physicians, following the recommended "hit early, hit hard" ARV protocols promotes the further depletion of glutathione and loss of function and vitality of the mitochondria.[377]

Although HIV had been variously classified as a D retrovirus, then a C retrovirus, its last classification was as a "lentavirus" or slow virus. The theory of HIV/AIDS from the early days was that it would take eight to ten or more years for the syndrome to occur after the initial infection; and without nutritional and antioxidant replacement therapy, this had been the observed clinical experience, with many patients, especially those who eschewed AZT, remaining "long-term survivors."[378] The incidence of AIDS among antibody positive

---

[372] Lucey, D.R., et al, (1996), "Type 1 and type 2 cytokine dysregulation in human infectious, neoplastic, and inflammatory diseases," *Clin Micro Rev;* 9(4): 532-562

[373] Lincoln, J, et al., (ed. 1997), "Nitric Oxide in health and disease," Cambridge Univ. Press, Cambridge, U.K.

[374] Ho, DD., et al., (1995), "Rapid turnover of plasma virons and CD4 lymphocytes in HIV-1 infection," *Nature;* 373:123-126

[375] Peterson, JD., et al., (1998), "Glutathione levels in antigen presenting cells modulate Th1 versus Th2 response patterns," *Proc Natl Acad Sci USA,* 95:3071-3076

[376] Kremer, H, (2008), "The Silent Revolution in Cancer and AIDS Medicine," Xlibris

[377] Brinkman, K, et al., (1998), "Adverse effects of reverse transcriptase inhibitors: mitochondrial toxicity as common pathway," *AIDS,* 12: 1735-1744

[378] Shah, I., Nadiger, M., (2013), "Long term non progressors (LTNP) with vertically infected HIV children—a report from western India," *Indian J Med Res;* 137(1):210-212

persons varies from 0 percent to 10 percent depending on factors defined by lifestyle, health, and country of residence.[379]

Using traditional laboratory techniques as previously described, researchers were barely able to find HIV in CD4+T cells.[380,381] There was no free virus in most and very little in some persons with AIDS or in asymptomatic carriers.[382,383] Virus titers ranged from 0 to 10 infectious particle units per milliliter of blood.[384,385] What was being called HIV could only be expressed under laboratory conditions in 1 of every 10^4 cell.[386] Further, no provirus is detectable in blood cells of 70 percent to 100 percent of symptomatic or asymptomatic antibody positive persons if tested by direct hybridization of cellular DNA with cloned proviral DNA.[387,388,389]

In spite of what was already demonstrated about the elusive virus and the clinical progression from diagnosis to disease manifestation, the AIDS/drug industry embraced the Ho mathematical model that predicted that full-blown AIDS would develop in twenty to sixty days of infection;[390] and suddenly, the past twelve years of clinical medicine were obliterated. The slow virus was now officially an almost speed-of-light virus that while stubbornly refusing to multiply spontaneously *in vivo or in vitro* was made to alter its behavior with the new AIDSworld math. This immediately changed the clinical mandate from

---

[379] Anderson, RM. & May, RM, "Epidemiological parameters of HIV Transmission," *Nature* (9 June 1988) 333:514-519

[380] Harper, ME., et al., (1986), "Detection of lymphocytes expressing human T-lymphotropic virus type III in lymph nodes and peripheral blood from infected individuals by *in situ* hybridization," *Proc Natl Acad Sci USA;* 83:772-776

[381] Embretson, J., et al., "Analysis of human immunodeficiency virus infected tissues by amplification and *in situ* hybridization reveals latent and permissive infections at single cell resolution," *Proc Natl Acad Sci USA;* 90: 357-361

[382] http://www.allmystery.de/dateien/10435,1297581967, HIV_Isolation_aus_erkrankten_Personen.pdf Albert, J. et al., (1987) *J.Med.Virol.* 23, 67-73.

[383] Falk, L.A., Paul, D., Landay, A., & Kessler, H. (1987) N.Engl.J.Med. 316, 1547-1548.

[384] Ibid

[385] Albert, J., Op Cit

[386] http://www.virusmyth.com/aids/hiv/pdpnas89.htm Duesberg, PH, "Human Immunodeficiency virus and acquired immunodeficiency syndrome: Correlation but not causation";*Proc. Natl. Acad. Sci.* USA Vol.86, pp. 755-764, February 1989

[387] Richman, D., McCutchan, J., & Spector, S. (1987) J.Infect.Dis. 156, 823-827

[388] Shaw, G.M., Hahn, B.H., Arya, S.K., Groopman, J.E., Gallo, R.C., & Wong-Staal, F. (1984) Science 226, 1165-1167.

[389] Shaw, G.M., Harper, M.E., Hahn, B.H., Epstein, L.G., Gajdusek, D.C., Price, R.W., Navia, B.A., Petito, C.K., O'Hara, C.J., Cho, E.-S., Oleske, J.M., Wong-Staal, F., & Gallo, R.C. (1985) Science 227, 177-182.

[390] Craddock, M., (1995), "Analysis of the Ho & Shaw Papers," http://www.virusmyth.com/aids/hiv/mcreplyho.htm

The Slow Death of the AIDS/Cancer Paradigm
and the Apocrypha of the Eukaryotic Cell

something unheard of in the thousands of years of the practice of clinical medicine; that is to treat the disease when it arises and use prevention as a first measure. Now clinicians were urged to treat the numbers (whatever they meant) even when the patient is clinically well without consideration of the health history or further investigation of potential metabolic imbalances related to cell-mediated immunity. This new mathematical model predicted, against twelve years of clinical evidence, that once diagnosed HIV positive, the onset of full-blown AIDS would occur rapidly—within weeks. This model, although it made no clinical sense and was shown by the previous twelve years of clinical experience and by other mathematicians to be mathematically improbable[391] (it was called by critics Ho's intelligence-deficiency virus theory), was used to introduce a new class of expensive and very profitable mitochondrial toxic drugs, protease inhibitors, and a new expensive technology, quantitative competitive polymerase chain reaction (QC-PCR), to the expanding AIDS market.[392]

QC-PCR

The idea behind QC-PCR is to amplify target DNA (or RNA) with some DNA (or RNA), which acts as a control and is used to estimate the size of the unknown target. So if there is x amount of the target present, which is the unknown, you add y amount of the control and amplify the two together. After n PCR cycles, you end up with xn target DNA and yn control DNA. The assumption is that $xn/yn = x/y$ for all n. Because you can now measure xn/yn and you know y, then x can be figured.[393] The critical assumption is that these two ratios are always equal because any tiny difference will be enormously magnified over forty-five cycles of measurement because the numbers rise logarithmically for each measurement cycle.[394]

Ho's theory was etched out when he introduced this mathematical model using the new technology of genetic amplification, which had been introduced to the market by Nobelist Kary Mullis. Mullis is also one of the scientists who has

---

[391] Craddock, M., "HIV: Science by press conference," AIDS:Virus or Drug Induced? 1996, P.H. Duesberg (ed.): pp. 127-130

[392] Ho's paper used a slightly different technique, the branched DNA PCR http://www.virusmyth.com/aids/hiv/chjtests5.htm

[393] Craddock, M., Op Cit

[394] Piatak, M, et al., (1993), "High levels of HIV-1 in plasma during all stages of infection determined by quantitative competitive PCR," *Science*; 259:1749-1754

questioned the AIDS paradigm.[395] He has expressed doubt that his invention is capable of doing what Ho claims—measuring HIV in the bloodstream—and has warned that the amplification technique is highly efficient in that it will amplify whatever genetic fragment is in the sample regardless of where the RNA came from: HIV or a contaminant. Therefore, a very fundamental issue becomes, how is it possible to determine which part of the amplified material could be HIV and which part the contaminant(s), especially if there is no gold standard by which one can detect HIV? To date, no one has produced a single piece of evidence that the RNA fragments in blood plasma shown by this method presented in log scales actually originated from "HIV-RNA" as (1) there has been no isolation of a complete genome and (2) there is the isogenic retroid problem.[396]

Genetics is an evolving field, and some of its most cherished dogmas have led to conclusions that are not only illogical but hard to substantiate. This is especially the case in the realm of HIV genetic theory. The viral load model was a fallacious attempt to establish HIV as the cause of AID, the acquired immune deficiency, defined as the decrease in CD4+T cells from the bloodstream. What AIDS researchers have chosen to ignore is the emerging evidence of the functions of nonprotein-coding RNA (ncRNA). Because these bits of genetic material have the ability to store and transmit information, they have been recognized as important inter- and intracellular regulatory molecules.[397,398] Thus, finding bits of RNA in the bloodstream is not a rare event associated with a supposed infectious agent but a part of normal cell metabolism and homeostasis. However, other important aspects about the relationship between viral load and infectious virus particles and viral load and CD4+T cells counter viral load hypothesis. In other studies, it was found that many patients who had detectable viral loads had no evidence of virus by culture as there was a reported lack of correlation between viral load and infectious viral particles, as measured by co-culture.[399,400] Another study that directly challenges the

---

[395] Mullis, K., (1998), "The medical establishment vs. the truth," *Penthouse* Book Excerpt http://www.virusmyth.com/aids/hiv/kmdancing.htm

[396] Bannert, N., Kurth, R., (2004), "Retroelements and the human genome: new perspectives on an old relation," *PNAS;* 101: no. suppl 2: 14572-14579

[397] Dinger, E., et al., (2008), "RNAs as extracellular signaling molecules," *J Mol Endocrin;* 40:151-159

[398] Mattick, JS., (2004), "The hidden genetic program of complex organisms," *Scientific Am;* pp 51-67

[399] Sheppard, W., et al, (1993), "Viral burden and HIV disease," *Nature;* 364:291-292

[400] Bagasra, O., et al., (1992), "Detection of human immunodeficiency virus type 1 provirus in mononuclear cells by in situ polymerase chain reaction," *NEJM;* 305: 1425-1431

The Slow Death of the AIDS/Cancer Paradigm
and the Apocrypha of the Eukaryotic Cell

HIV causes AID theory was published in *JAMA* in 2006.[401] The research by Rodriguez, et al., demonstrated that changes in viral load were only able to explain ~4 percent of the changes in the CD4+T cell count in the patients observed. Specifically, the study found the coefficient of determination between viral load and CD4+ decline was only 4 percent. Mathematically, this means that the viral load (HIV genetic particles in the bloodstream by the theory) is not able to explain AID, 96 percent of the variation in CD4+T cell levels,[402] with the implication that other causal relationships, which have been ignored, need to be explored. Yet AIDSworld physicians absurdly continue to rely on a test that has a 4 percent probability of accuracy.

In another study that used co-culture (which is not isolation) that compared viral load results with detection of what they called HIV, 53 percent of HIV positive AIDS patients with detectable levels of viral load, many topping two hundred thousand and three hundred thousand, had *zero* co-cultured HIV.[403] As a result, the FDA has not approved PCR for HIV screening or diagnostic purposes; but even though it is not predictive of CD4+T cell number fluctuations, it is claimed to be useful as a marker for disease progression and physicians are urged to begin medicating patients based on this unreliable and meaningless test.

I have shortened the various linguistic conundrums from AIDSworld by calling the language changes AIDSpeak and thus far have attempted to translate from AIDSpeak into English the meaning of *virus, isolation,* and *antibody test*. This last area of exploration in this exercise on the deconstruction of linguistic rules or lack thereof will be in the area of HIV genetics. There is still much controversy in this area as genetic determinists, although having been proved incorrect in their predictions about the behavior of the genome in its relationship to protein production and RNA information transfer, its hierarchical status within the cell, and directionality of information flow, they unfortunately still hold sway over this discipline with concessions to virological interpretations of the mechanics of the central genome. This is not an attempt to rewrite the rules of genetics. The facts will ultimately stand on their own. It is the conclusions drawn from the facts that are open to reinterpretation.

---

[401] Rodriguez, B., et al, (2006), "Predictive value of plasma HIV RNA level on rate of CD4 T cell decline in untreated HIV infection," *JAMA;* 296: 1523-1525

[402] Culshaw, R.,

[403] Piatak, M, et al., "High levels of HIV-1 in plasma during all stages of infection determined by quantitive competitive-PCR," *Science,* 1993;259: 1749-1754

For most of the twentieth century, genes were considered to be stable entities arranged in an orderly linear pattern on chromosomes.[404] In the late 1940s, Barbara McClintock challenged this dogma when she demonstrated through her work on maize the unsettling idea that genes could be unstable. This instability was called genetic transposition, and it was in response to external stressors. She used X-rays to show that certain DNA fragments can be activated to transpose (jump) from one position on a chromosome to another. She hypothesized that transposition provides a means to rapidly reorganize genes in response to environmental cues. What she discovered was not merely something new, but it was an insight that turned conventional thinking upside down. Gene mutations were known and accepted, so it was not completely the idea of genetic instability, but the surprise was the idea that genes could move from place to place thousands of times more frequently than the rate at which mutations were known to occur.

McClintock finally won a Nobel Prize for her work in 1983; however, her work has yet to be fully understood especially by virologists who continue to interpret these transposable elements as viral and viral remnants even though it has been recently postulated that RNA may have been the initial genetic material.[405] The issue on which there is still not consensus is the question of why genes jump from place to place. McClintock's position was that when segments of DNA moved, they did so for specific reasons in response to external cues. Because of their demonstrated ability to regulate the functioning of other pieces of DNA in maize, which she used for her experiments, she coined the phrase *controlling elements* to describe these segments. She postulated that similar controlling elements might be responsible for choreographing the orderly changes in patterns of gene expression that underlie the development of a fertilized seed/egg into an adult in plants and animals. Indeed, recently, John Mattick—director of the Garvan Institute of Medical Research in Sydney, Australia—has argued that noncoding DNA is transcribed into the numerous ncRNAs that create the additional layers of developmental complexity required for the evolution of eukaryotes.[406] It seems that noncoding DNA increases with increasing complexity.[407] According to the latest estimate, ~80 percent of

---

[404] Morgan, TH (1922) Croonian lecture: On the mechanism of heredity, *Proc R Soc Lond, B* 94(659):162-197

[405] De Duve, C, (1991) "Blueprint for a cell: the nature and origin of life"; Neil Patterson Publishers, Burlington, N.C.

[406] Mattick, JS, (2004), "RNA regulation: a new genetics?" *Nat Rev Gen;* 5:316-323

[407] Mattick, Ibid

what has been referred to as junk DNA is dynamically transcribed mainly into noncoding RNAs.[408]

By the mid-1970s, researchers reported that reverse transcriptase had been found in a variety of cells, not just virus-infected cells, and that this was a repair process often found in embryonic and cancer cells.[409,410] The fact that the human placenta is full of what are called human endogenous retroviruses[411] or HERVs has still not brought wide support for McClintock's ideas. HERVs make up to 8 percent of the human genome[412] and are called endogenous retroviruses because they have genetic similarities to what have been labeled "exogenous retroviruses." Genetically, they consist of a long terminal repeat (LTR) followed by gag, pol, and env, which is flanked by another LTR. Segments of these genetic areas have the same coding as what has been called HIV DNA.[413] Further, the "specific genes" of HIVs are alternative reading frames of essential genes shared by all retroviruses.[414,415,416,417] Their apparent novelty is more likely to reflect new techniques of gene analysis than to represent HIV-specific retroviral functions.[418] Analogous genes have been found in other retroviruses, including one bovine and at least three other human retroviruses

---

[408] Bernstein, BE, et al., (2012), "An integrated encyclopedia of DNA elements in the human genome," *Nature;* 489: 57-74

[409] Temin, HM, "Reverse transcription in the eukaryotic genome: retroviruses, pararetroviruses, retrotransposons and retrotranscripts" 1985 *Mol Biol Evol* 2:455-468

[410] Baltimore, D., "Retroviruses and retrotransposons: the role of reverse transcription in shaping the eucaryotic genome" 1985 *Cell;*40:481-482109341109

[411] http://www.ncbi.nlm.nih.gov/pmc/articles/PMC1187282/pdf/mp56000011.pdf Nelson, PN., et al, Demystified...human endogenous retroviruses"

[412] Schust, DJ, "Review: Human endogenos retroviruses and the placenta"; Nov. 2009 *Reproductive Sciences;* 16(11) pp. 1023-1033

[413] http://jvi.asm.org/content/86/20/11194.abstract Monde, K, et al., "Human Endogenous Retrovirus K Gag Coassembles with HIV-1 Gag and Reduces the Release Efficiency and Infectivity of HIV-1";*J. Virol.* October 2012 vol. 86 no. 20 11194-11208

[414] Institute of Medicine (1986) Confronting AIDS (N.A.S., Washington, D.C.).

[415] Institute of Medicine (1988) Confronting AIDS-Update 1988 (N.A.S., Washington D.C.).

[416] Duesberg, P.H. (1987) Cancer Res. 47, 1199-1220.

[417] Clavel, F. (1987) AIDS 1, 135-140.

[418] Duesberg, P., "Human immunodeficiency virus and acquired immunodeficiency syndrome: Correlation but not causation" *Proc. Natl. Acad. Sci.* USA.86, pp. 755-764, February 1989

that do not cause AIDS.[419,420,421] According to retroviral expert Peter Duesberg, because HIV and all other retroviruses are isogenic, the newly discovered genes cannot be HIV specific. Moreover, it is unlikely that these genes even control virus replication. *In vivo*, HIV lies chronically dormant, although the presumed suppressor genes are not expressed.[422] This, of course, becomes relevant to QC-PCR measurements as the technology measures not infectious virus units but fragments of genetic material that are assumed to belong to HIV.

Because of the money that has been thrown at the virus/cancer industry, the tendency has been to identify the transposable elements as parasitic molecules of DNA that have no purpose as such besides that of ensuring their own survival and reproduction.[423] As previously discussed, many of these elements are retrotranscribed from RNA into DNA with the enzyme reverse transcriptase and have a variety of names that fall under the common rubric of "retroids."[424] When virologists had the idea that they were going to find viruses that caused cancer, because they were both either unfamiliar with McClintock's work or did not know how to back out of their own fixed ideas about cancer transformation, they mistakenly claimed that these "oncoviruses" that came to be known as retroviruses were the cause of disease rather than the end result of metabolic stressors and altered cell metabolism attempting to find a new homeostatic level.

---

[419] Duesberg, P.H. (1987) Cancer Res. 47, 1199-1220.
[420] Weiss, R.A. (1988) Nature (London) 333, 497-498.
[421] Haseltine, W.A., & Wong-Staal, F. (1988) Sci.Am. 259 (4), 52-62.
[422] Duesberg, op cit. 1989
[423] http://www.ias.ac.in/womeninscience/Barbara.pdf
[424] Cordaux, R., Batzer, MA., (2009), "The Impact of retrotransposons on human genome evolution," *Nat Rev Genet;* 10(10): 691-703

The Slow Death of the AIDS/Cancer Paradigm and the Apocrypha of the Eukaryotic Cell

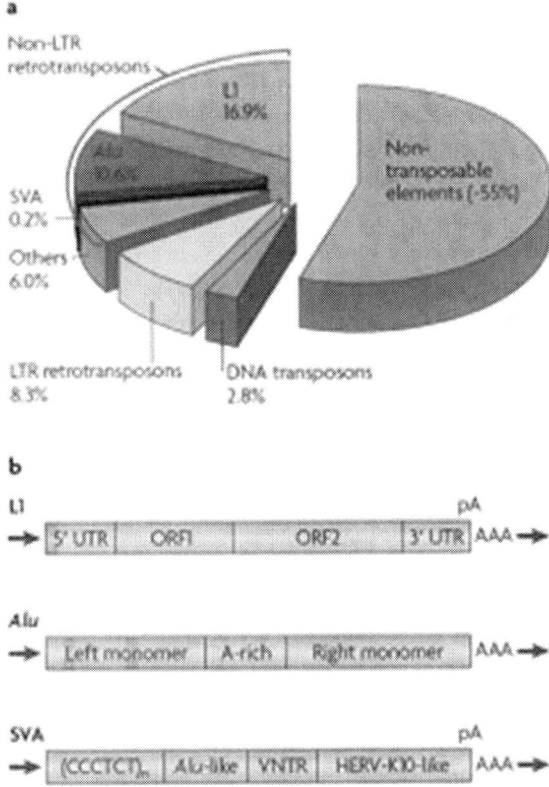

The transposable element content of the human genome[425]

Unfortunately, this focus on the molecular arithmetic has narrowed the focus of the debate away from the core cellular energetic processes. Ultimately, it is not the genome that determines the fate of the cells but rather the thermodynamic fluctuations of energy that precede gene mutations/alterations that are the material traits of such energy fluctuations. It is the thermodynamic shifts that alter both the molecular and informational structure of the cell network.[426]

It has been observed that "it is no accident that a mechanistic, market-obsessed culture should reify processes to things, for things, unlike processes,

---

[425] Cordaux, Batzer Ibid
[426] Waliszewski, P et al., "On the holistic approach in cellular and cancer biology: nonlinearity, complexity, and quasi-determinism of the dynamic cellular network"; 1988 *J of Surg Onc*;68:70-78

can readily be turned into commodities."[427] It follows that the genetic expression of various unusual proteins during cell metabolism is the effect, not the cause. As has been discussed in the previous chapters, the identification of shadow elements that are not always highly expressed under stable conditions of cell metabolism (e.g., RT, p24) used to claim the presence of retroid elements can be commonly found in the activated cells of very ill people and can be made to be expressed from cells in the course of laboratory experimentation as the result of the culture conditions of the experiment itself. In fact, the "infected" cells from AIDS patients caused no infection (expression of RT and p24) until they were activated by laboratory manipulations. This is not the pattern of an aggressive virus. The HIV researchers are only able to demonstrate "HIV characteristics" in stimulated cells[428] to which has been added strong oxidizing mitogens (PHA, Con A., etc.) and type 1 cytokine interleukin-2 (IL-2). IL-2 activates Type 1 cytokine interferon-γ (IFN-γ). IFN-γ stimulates cytotoxic nitric oxide (NO) production.[429] This sets in motion a cascade of cellular repair events, including the synthesis of reverse transcriptase, the enzyme for the synthesis of DNA from RNA.

In 2001, when the sequencing of the human genome was completed, the genetic determinist point of view suffered a crippling blow to the idea that our fate is determined solely by our genes. This incorrect assumption was largely due to attempts by geneticists to infer a priori that the same metabolic parameters observed in the simple prokaryotic cell could be assumed to be the same operational parameters of the much more complex eukaryotic cell. Unfortunately, this simplistic view has been rather premature. The eukaryotic cell operates at a much higher functional level. By use of this inappropriate operational model, genetic determinism held fast to several basic assumptions: that genes determine characters in a straightforward, additive way—one gene, one protein, and, by implication, one character trait. Environmental influence, if any, can be neatly sorted from the genetic; genes and genomes are stable and, except for rare, random mutations, are passed on unchanged to the next

---

[427] Ho, MW., (2003), Living with the Fluid Genome, "Institute of Science and Society, Penang, Malaysia p 39

[428] Klatzmann D., et al., "Selective tropism of lymphadenopathy associated virus (LAV) for helper-inducer T lymphocytes, *Science*; 225:59-63

[429] Totemeyer, S., et al., (2006), "IFN-gamma enhances production of nitric oxide from macrophages via a mechanism that depends on nucleotide oligomerization," *J Immunol;* 176(8): 4804-4810

generation; genes and genomes cannot be changed directly in response to the environment, and characteristics acquired in life are not inherited.[430]

Experimental data suggests that the relationship between genotype and phenotype in eukaryotic cells is nonbijective (i.e., a gene can contribute to the emergence of more than just one phenotypic trait or a phenotypic trait can be determined by the expression of several genes). This implies nonlinearity (i.e., lack of the proportional relationship between input and outcome), complexity (i.e., emergence of the hierarchical network of multiple cross-interacting elements that is sensitive to initial conditions, possesses multiple equilibria, organizes spontaneously into different morphological patterns, and is controlled in dispersed rather than centralized manner) and finally is quasi-deterministic (i.e., coexistence of deterministic and nondeterministic events) of the cellular network.[431] The energy required to animate this system arises from inputs into complex cascades of coupled cyclic processes—ATP/ADP, NADH/NAD, GSH/GSSH, the tricarboxylic acid cycle, etc.—and the various redox reactions that inform the system to up- or downregulate genetic expression appropriate to the state of the cell. These are not linear processes.

It was revealed that the human genome has only about 20,000 genes, twice as many as a fruit fly and only 10,000 more than a roundworm. As all humans the world over share 99.9 percent of their DNA, race then can only be defined as a social and cultural construct; until recently, it was unclear what 95 percent or the human DNA does and therefore has been cavalierly dubbed "junk" DNA. The coding regions for proteins occupy only ~1.1 percent of the human genome, and about 50 percent of the human genome are "proviral sequences" and transposable elements, many with reverse transcriptase.[432] There are an estimated 250,000 to 1 million proteins made by the 20,000 genes. The dog is 85 percent identical to a human in terms of genetic sequence.[433] According to Evan Eichler, a member of the genome research team at the University of Washington

---

[430] Ho, MW, "Living with the fluid genome" 2003, Institute of Science in Society, London, England p. 15

[431] Waliszewski, P., Op Cit.

[432] Ref. "Genome project" The Guardian Feb. 12, 2001; "Unexpected bits and pieces" Henry Gee, The Guardian Feb. 12, 2001; "Genome discovery shocks scientists: Genetic blueprint contains far fewer genes than thought – DNA's importance downplayed" Tom Abate, San Francisco Chronicle, Feb. 11, 2001; "Analysis of human genome discovers far fewer genes" Nicholas Wade, The New York Times, Feb. 12, 2001.

[433] Ho, MW, 2001 "The human genome map, the death of genetic determinism and beyond" *Isis Report*

in Seattle, the human and chimp sequences differ by only 1.2 percent in terms of single-nucleotide changes to the genetic code.[434]

The initial blow to genetic determinist logic was McClintock's work, which demonstrated that genes had mobile elements. However, it was the discovery of reverse transcriptase by Howard Temin and David Baltimore that began the process of rethinking the manner in which the genome functioned in relation to the holistic structure of the cellular network. Apparently, the base sequences of DNA can be read in more than one reading frame (shifted one or two bases from the usual) to give different triplets that code for entirely different proteins.[435] The same gene can be read at different starting points to give different transcripts that result in distinct proteins, and the message encoded in the gene can be changed after it is transcribed. The gene transcript can become "edited" by chemical modifications or by addition of bases to change the base sequence of the RNA transcript so that it is translated into a protein entirely different from the one encoded.[436] It turns out that the gene does not even determine the amino acid sequence of the protein encoded. Instead, the precise protein made depends on influences from the context—the state of the cell and the organism as a whole—propagating back to affect transcription at all stages.[437] Finally, some genes are represented in superfamilies of hundreds or thousands of similar sequences, all encoding slightly different versions of the same proteins.[438] Therefore, what AIDSworld claims as the rapid mutation of the HIV genome can more plausibly be understood to be the spontaneous RNA modifications in response to varying information inputs.

In light of these genetic possibilities, it becomes important to consider because of the way in which "HIV RNA" has been described, whether it is really an epiphenomenon of thermodynamic fluctuations (oxidative stress) rather than a unique entity. By 1985 it was already known that the envelope genes of what would eventually become HIV (LAV and HTLV-III) differed by more than 20 percent.[439] Gallo and his fellow researchers were claiming that the HIV genome has a "far greater variability" as "compared to HTLV" and, in fact, "the rate of genetic change for the AIDS virus is more than a millionfold greater than for most DNA genomes and may even be tenfold greater than for some

---

[434] http://news.nationalgeographic.com/news/2005/08/0831_050831_chimp_genes_2.html
[435] Ho, MW, Op Cit p. 41
[436] Ho, MW., Op Cit. p.44
[437] Ho, MW., Op Cit. p, 46
[438] Ho, MW., Op Cit. p 43
[439] Marx JL. A virus by any other name... Science 1985;227:1449-1451.

other RNA viruses including certain retroviruses and influenza A virus."[440] By 1988 it was acknowledged that "no two isolates are identical and that each isolate contains many variants."[441] Researchers at the Pasteur Institute in Paris were finding that "an asymptomatic patient can harbor at least 10^6 genetically distinct variants of HIV, and for AIDS patients, the figure is more than 10^8."[442,443] Another paper claimed that 99.9 percent of the HIV genomes may be defective and, by implication, not infectious.[444] By 1990, HIV researchers began to divide the HIV genome into subtypes A, B, C, etc.[445] They asserted that the basis for the system was that "...subtypes are approximately equidistant from one another in *env* {a 'star' phylogeny}; that the *env* phylogenetic tree is for the most part congruent with *gag* phylogenetic trees; and that two or more samples are required to define a sequence subtype"[446] Before subtyping, the HIV sequences were classified as either African or USA/European, with sequence differences of 20 percent to 30 percent between the two groups.[447]

There are several red flags that are raised from this discussion. To review, it has been found that there is only a 1.2 percent to 1.3 percent difference in the genomes of humans and chimpanzees and 15 percent between humans and canines. Humans have ~20,000 genes with 3 billion base pairs.[448] The HIV genome has been found to be of various sizes between 9,150 and 9,749 base pairs (every genome of a unique entity, in fact, should be of equal length) and yet has been claimed to have as much as a 30 percent sequence variability and still is stated to be the same entity that has the same function of disrupting the immune system no matter how its genomic structure may fluctuate! With this much variability in gene sequencing and subtypes, how is it possible to

---

[440] Hahn BH, Shaw GM, Taylor ME, et al. Genetic variation in HTLV-III/LAV over time in patients with AIDS or at risk for AIDS. Science 1986;232(June):1548-1553.
[441] Newmark P. Receding hopes of AIDS vaccines. Nature 1988;333:699.
[442] Vartian JP, Meyerhans A, Henry M, et al. High-resolution structure of an HIV-1 quasispecies: Identification of novel coding sequences. AIDS 1992;6:1095-1098.
[443] Wain-Hobson S. Virological mayhem. Nature 1995;373:102.
[444] Sheppard HW, Ascher MS, Krowka JF. Viral burden and HIV disease. Nature 1993;364:291.
[445] http://www.hiv.lanl.gov/content/sequence/HIV/COMPENDIUM/1996/PART-III/3.pdf, Genetic subtypes of HIV-1
[446] Myers G. Nucleic acids alignments and sequences. The human retroviruses and AIDS Compendium on Line: Web site: http://hiv-web.lanl.gov. USA: US Government, 1995: I-1-I-2.
[447] Blomberg J, Lawoko A, Pipkorn R, et al. A survey of synthetic HIV-1 peptides with natural and chimeric sequences for differential reactivity with Zimbabwean, Tanzanian and Swedish HIV-1-positive sera. AIDS 1993;7:759-767.
[448] The National Human Genome Research Institute: https://www.genome.gov/11006943 downloaded 12 April 2015

have any stability in the proteins coded for by these ever-changing genes? The proteins in the antibody tests have not changed over time although the genes coding for these proteins are claimed to have changed enormously. It has been acknowledged that 8 percent of the human genome can be identified as human endogenous retroviruses and that as much as 45 to 50 percent may be other retroid elements that are identified by a gag and pol region, yet the AIDS literature is mute on how they have identified what are uniquely "HIV" genomic elements as opposed to other retroid elements without ever having isolated a unique virus and without ever having characterized its proteins and genomic material. Claiming the PCR has any hope of specificity amid this complexity is nothing more than a pipe dream.

There are a number of reasons to question the use of the polymerase chain reaction for making decisions about clinical intervention. Certainly, not knowing the origin of the genetic fragments that are being amplified is near the top of the list, e.g., the PCR primers and probes are taken from HIV grown in tissue culture using a T4 cell leukemia cancer cell line, which Gallo claims is caused by HTLV-1, a retrovirus said to be similar to HIV. Even if the origin could be validated by the gold standard of an isolated virus, another problem is that not only does viral load overestimate what is called infectious virus by an average of factor of 60,000:1[449] to 100,000:1,[450] but this estimation is not consistently linear. Thus, there is no way to make an accurate estimate of infectious virus—if one could find infectious virus. What is referred to as the "efficiency" of PCR must be perfect, or else, any estimate obtained using PCR will be wrong.[451] The technique is complicated and not always reproducible. This is why the CDC acknowledges that the specificity and sensitivity of PCR are "unknown" and that "PCR is not recommended and is not licensed for routine diagnostic purposes."[452] By 1993 the CDC announced that the "PCR is not recommended nor approved for the purpose of routine diagnosis. . . . Neither the specificity [must be negative against the HIV test] nor the sensitivity [must be congruent with HIV positives] is known."[453]

---

[449] Piatak, M, et al., "High levels of HIV-1 in plasma during all stages of infection determined by quantitive competitive-PCR," *Science*, 1993;259: 1749-1754

[450] Raeymaekers, L, "Quantitative PCR: Theoretical Considerations with Practical Implications," *Anal Biochem* (1993), 214: 582-585

[451] Culshaw, RV., "Mathematical modeling of AIS progression: limitations, expectations, and future directions," *J Am Phy & Surg* winter 2006, 11(4): 101-105

[452] Maggiore, C., (2007), "What if everything you thought you knew about AIDS was wrong?," The American Foundation for AIDS Alternatives; Studio City California, p 37

[453] Johnson, C., (1996), "Viral load and the PCR—why they can't be used to prove HIV infection," *Continuum;* 4(4): 32-37

The Slow Death of the AIDS/Cancer Paradigm and the Apocrypha of the Eukaryotic Cell

The Ho kitchen sink hypothesis claimed that these billions of bits of genetic material of unknown origin represented infectious virus production and when counted by this method had some clinical relevance. The lack of correlation between viral load and infectious particles, as measured by co-culture, has been noted elsewhere.[454,455] A significant lack of correlation has also been demonstrated between CD4+T levels and viral load as noted in the *JAMA* study,[456] which found that changes in viral load were only able to explain no more than 4 to 6 percent of changes in the CD4+T cell count in the patients observed. In clinical practice, these findings have profound implications: if viral load is correlated neither with infectious virus nor CD4+ T cell levels, this means that the measurement constitutes insufficient evidence for T cell decline and other factors must be considered. It also calls into question the nature of the metabolic response to antiretroviral drugs (ARVs) and the so-called HIV resistance.

What is missing from the equation on the focus of CD4+T cell number over CD4+T cell functions has been an understanding of the meaning of severely reduced glutathione levels consistently found in pre-AIDS and AIDS patients.[457,458] In the coming chapters, the role of glutathione (GSH) as a sensor for the redox milieu for the number of T helper cells (type 1 or type 2 immune cells) as effectors of the balance of the redox milieu; for the amounts of RNA in the blood plasma as indicator for the repair of DNA and the role of antiretroviral therapy as a stressor of the counter-regulation via the GSH sensor; the immune cell effectors and the RNA-DNA software will be explored in greater detail. Here, I will briefly address the response of the viral load to the introduction of ARVs.

An important issue about the fall and subsequent rise of genetic fragments in the bloodstream, which are claimed to be from HIV, after the patient is given ARVs (HAART) must be addressed, especially as one will encounter some whiner from AIDSworld triumphantly glued to the falling PCR numbers post

---

[454] Sheppard W, Ascher M, Krowka J. "Viral burden and HIV disease." Nature, 1993; 364: 291–292.

[455] Bagasra O, Hauptman S, Lischner H, Sachs M, Pomerantz R. "Detection of human immunodeficiency virus type 1 provirus in mononuclear cells by in situ polymerase chain reaction." N Engl J Med, 1992; 326: 1385–1391.

[456] Rodriguez B, Sethi A, Cheruvu V, et al. "Predictive value of plasma HIV RNA level on rate of CD4 T-cell decline in untreated HIV infection." JAMA, 2006; 296: 1523–1525.

[457] Buhl, R. et al., "Systemic glutathione deficiency in symptom free HIV seropositive individuals" *Lancet* 1989; 2: 1294-1297

[458] De Rosa, SC., et al., "N-acetylcysteine replenishes glutathione in HIV infection." *Eur J Clin Invest*. 2000 Oct;30(10):915-29.

the introduction of ARVs but never understanding its true clinical relevance. One of the AIDSworld magic tricks is the introduction of patients to highly active retroviral therapy (HAART) based on elevated PCR levels. From a PCR test perspective, after the initiation of HAART, the numbers may initially fall but after a time begin to rise again. Accordingly, the AIDS theorists claim that the drugs are initially killing the virus, causing the fall in PCR numbers, but that the virus then develops a resistance to the drugs and breaks free from suppression. This is the cause of the rise of viral load after the introduction of HAART therapy and of the patient's ultimate decline. However, as plausible as this might sound, it has no firm basis in cell physiology.

"HIV positives" from the earliest have been observed to have a systemic glutathione deficiency of immune and nonimmune cells. This deficiency is crucial to understanding the pathological process as it triggers a cascade of downstream events (type 1 to type 2 cytokine expression, etc.), which can stimulate the formation of polyamines and the repair and regeneration of DNA.[459,460] Arginine is processed by macrophages in response to the cytokines to which these cells are exposed. Th 1 type cytokines induce NO synthase II, which metabolizes arginine into nitrites.[461] On the other hand, the cells responsive to Th 2 type cytokines produce arginase, which converts arginine into polyamines and proline.[462] NO (type 1 cytokines) has been described to exert cytostatic effects on cellular proliferation while polyamines (type 2 cytokines) are required components of cellular proliferation.[463]

HAART therapy has multiple deleterious consequences. The drugs in the HAART regimen, both nucleoside reverse transcriptase inhibitors (NRTI)[464]

---

[459] Wang C, et al. (November 2003). "Defining the molecular requirements for the selective delivery of polyamine conjugates into cells containing active polyamine transporters." *J. Med. Chem.* 46 (24): 5129–38.

[460] Satriano, J., (2004), "Arginine pathways and the inflammatory response: interregulation of nitric oxide and polyamines: review article," *Amino Acids;* 26(4): 321–329

[461] Yeramian, A., et al., (2006), "Arginine transport via cationic amino acid transporter 2 plays a critical regulatory role in classical or alternative activation of macrophages," *J Immunol;* pp.5918–5924

[462] Yeramain, Ibid

[463] Satriano, J, et al., (1999), "Regulation of intracellular polyamine biosynthesis and transport by NO and cytokines TNF-α and IFN-γ," *Am J Physiol;* 276(4 Pt 1): C892-899

[464] Glesby, MJ, (2001), "Overview of mitochondrial toxicity of nucleoside reverse transcriptase inhibitors," *International AIDS Soc. USA;* pp 42-46

and protease inhibitors,[465] are not only mitochondrial toxic[466] but also act as pro-oxidative[467] substances that aggravate the already GSH deficit. This treatment protocol can therefore intensify the type 2 cytokine profile and DNA synthesis by use of RNA from blood plasma as building blocks for synthesis. If it is assumed that the PCR can measure the RNA level in blood plasma, then the decreased levels of RNA after the introduction of HAART therapy is not because there is an inhibition of any "HI viruses" but because of increased recycling of RNA in an attempted repair process under an altered redox milieu of the stress of the drugs themselves. As these drugs intensify the glutathione deficiency, this triggers an increase in glycolytic biosynthesis activities in which RNA is used so that the RNA decrease in the blood plasma is not the inhibition of HI viruses but the aggravation of the underlying metabolic pathology. Under conditions in which cells are proliferating, glycolytic enzymes are upregulated as a result of changing redox conditions and/or oxygen tension. By this process, there is an increased need for recycled RNA. This concept is supported by the finding of increased values of niacin levels in the serum of HIV positives. Niacin levels were higher among HIV-infected subjects both on average and in proportion with above-normal levels. Furthermore, higher niacin levels were highly correlated with lower CD4+ T cell counts. The significance of this inverse relationship is not clear[468] from an AIDSworld point of view. However, niacin is a component of the coenzyme NAD that is enzymatically split for DNA repair.[469] In HIV positives and AIDS patients, the increased niacin level is associated with the progression of clinical symptoms and the decline in RNA values in serum.[470] That nucleotides released by intracellular degradation are

---

[465] Apostolova, N., et al., (2011), "Mitochondrial interference by anti-HIV drugs: mechanisms beyond Pol-γ inhibition," *Trends Pharmacol Sci;* 32(12):715-725

[466] Apostolova, N., et al., (2011), "Mitochondrial toxicity in HAART: an overview of in vitro evidence," *Curr Pharm Des;* 17(20): 2130-2144

[467] Mondal, D., et al., (2004), "HAART drugs induce oxidative stress in human endothelial cells and increase endothelial recruitment of mononuclear cells: exacerbation by inflammatory cytokines and amelioration by antioxidants," *Cardiovasc Toxicol;* 4(3): 287-302

[468] Skurnick, JH., et al., (1996), "Micronutrient profiles in HIV-1 infected heterosexual adults," *J Acquir Immune Defic syndr Hum Retrovirol;* 1;12(1): 75-83

[469] Mazurek, S., et al., (1997), "The role of phosphometabolites in cell proliferation, energy metabolism and tumour therapy," *J Bioenerget Biomembr;* 29(4): 315-330

[470] Murry, MF., (1999), "Niacin as a potential AIDS preventive factor," *Med Hypotheses;* 53(5):375-379

salvaged and reused has been demonstrated in several studies.[471,472] Therefore, the decrease in viral load (RNA in plasma) is in response to the increased oxidative stress/mitochondrial toxicity of HAART and not to the imagined decrease in the "HI virus." The use of recycled genetic material is consistent with Bauer's principle of stable nonequilibrium in that "all the work that may be performed by living systems is done only at the expense of structural energy [of its excited elements]—that is, by forces generated by a living system itself."[473] Further, Bauer's principle of augmentation of external work performance" observes that during the performance of external work, a living system loses its structural energy, thus sliding toward equilibrium. In an attempt to survive the onslaught of additional oxidative stressors, the cell metabolic systems make a decision based on the redox milieu and cytokine profile: to die by apoptosis necrosis or to continue living at a lower energetic state.

ARVs attack mitochondria on two levels: (1) by decreasing the ability of the ETC to transport electrons[474] and (2) by attacking the ability of mtDNA to replicate.[475] Once that lower energetic state is reached and the living system begins to lose its structural energy, it may no longer be able to incorporate recycled genetic material because of disruptions to nucleic acid synthesis and secondary RNA/DNA defects (as the result of HAART) that lead to the deficient transformation of RNA and leads to a backlog of genetic fragments in blood plasma.[476] It is not any putative HIV resistance to the drugs, but it is the drugs that are altering in a harmful way, the very basic life force of cell metabolism—the function of the mitochondria. These findings support the fact of a type 2 cell dis-symbiosis[477] as the result of toxic and pharmacotoxic prooxidative glutathione deficiency with a primary inhibition of the mitochondrial respiratory chain is leading to DNA defects. Thus, the fall and rise of the PCR post introduction of ARVs is the consequence of the toxicity of these drugs

---

[471] Grimble, G.K., (1994), "Dietary nucleotides and gut mucosal defense," *Gut;* supplement 1:S46-S51

[472] Kulkarni, A.D., et al., (1986), "Influence of dietary nucleotide restriction on bacterial sepsis and phagocytic cell function in mice," *Arch Surg;* 121(2):169-172

[473] Bauer, ES, *Theoretical Biology;* Reprint of the 1935 edition with a preface, a biographical and critical essay, Akadémiai Kiadó, Budapest 1982

[474] Yerroum, M, et al, (2000), "Cytochrome c oxidase deficiency in the muscle of patients with zidovudine myopathy is segmental and affects both mitochondrial DNA- and nuclear DNA-encoded subunits," *Acta Neuropath;* 100(1): 82-86

[475] Mukhopadhyay, A., et al., (2002), "In vitro evidence of inhibition of mitochondrial protease processing by HIV-1 protease inhibitors in yeast: a possible contribution to lipodystrophy syndrome," *Mitochondrion;* 1(6): 511-518

[476] Kremer, Op Cit. p 368

[477] Kremer, Op cit., p 369

on the already-stressed mitochondria, and the manifestation of the fall and rise of genetic elements in the bloodstream is the evolutionary biologically programmed metabolic response to this stress load. It is not because the HI virus has become "resistant."

The "hit them early and hard" that was a natural consequence of Ho's fuzzy math kitchen sink hypothesis has led to the practice of aggressively giving drugs to patients who are not ill and who may never become ill and ignoring known physiologically reversible parameters in favor of drug only therapy. The kitchen sink concept has advanced an endless cycle of counting things rather than exploring cellular metabolic functions that are naturally more complex but knowable outside of the AIDS paradigm. The questions about how those functions have been altered under a particular set of oxidative stressors at a particular time in history to a particular group of "high risk" individuals are a little more arcane and don't have quite the pizazz (or economic rewards) as a singular identifiable target whose existence can only be surmised by indirect markers imagined in the fertile minds of HIV researchers to have originated from a virus, that can only be made manifest with the use of high tech laboratory alchemy and methodology that has come to dominate and obscure this field. It is the basic core of medical practice that of necessity asks and answers the appropriate questions, posits theories that have predictive value and plots a course of action and has the humility to change action if the course is proven wrong.

Another clue that undermines the idea of billions of T cell turnover in the kitchen sink hypothesis is the nonshortening length of the T cell telomeres, which theoretically would shorten under this much cell division and destruction. It has been observed that with every division, a part of the telomere is lost. The telomeres are constructed by the enzyme telomerase, which regulates the transcription of an RNA template in a DNA sequence (reverse transcriptase),[478,479] which was misconstrued by Montagnier, Gallo, and other AIDS researchers to arise from an HI virus.

Researchers at the Netherlands Red Cross Blood Transfusion Service and the Academic Medical Center of Amsterdam University have measured the wear on the telomeres of chromosomes in T-4 immune cells of "HIV positive" patients:[480] *"If T-4 immune cells have a rapid turnover and thus a high proliferation rate during an HIV infection this must be reflected in an accelerated loss in the length of the telomeric terminal restriction fragments (TRF). Telomeres are the extreme ends of*

---

[478] Temin, HM, Baltimore, D., (1972), "RNA-directed DNA synthesis and RNA tumor viruses," *Adv Virus Res;* 17:129-186

[479] Boeke, JD, (1996), "DNA repair: A little help for my ends," *Nature;* 383:579-581

[480] Kremer, Op cit., p 372

chromosomes that consist of TTAGGG repeats [linear sequences of the pyrimidine base, thymine (T) and the purine bases, adenine (A) and guanosine (G), ~10kb long in humans. Some findings have led to the belief that the telomeric length can be used as a marker of the replicative history of cells and can indicate the accelerated deterioration or increased cell history of cells and can indicate the accelerated deterioration or increased cell division rates. Firstly, body cell telomeres shorten with increasing age [roughly 30 to 50 base pairs (bp) per year] and after in vitro *cultivation. Secondly, telomeric length* in vitro *lymph cells and fibroblasts dictates the division capacity. Thirdly, just like tumor cells and germ cells, the telomeric length in cultivated cells that continuously divide and are immortal is maintained by the enzyme telomerase. These cells display an elevated telomerase activity, while body cells show limited or no telomerase activity. . . . Longitudinal analysis of samples of lymph cells showed no accelerated loss of TRF length during the [alleged] HIV infection phase before the clinical diagnosis of AIDS. Other research teams have also observed no loss of TRF length of T-4 immune cells of HIV infected individuals. . . . Consequently, telomeric length is not impaired in HIV infection. . . . There is no evidence of increased turnover in T-4 immune cells and thus the reduction in numbers of T-4 immune cells as a consequence of continued HIV induced cell destruction. . . . The depletion in regeneration driven by a rapid turnover in T-4 cells no longer seems a plausible cause for the loss of T-4 immune cells."*[481,482]

It would be inappropriate to leave this chapter on HIV genetics without addressing the issue of cloning because AIDS researchers have begun to claim that cloning (joining together in the laboratory diffuse segments of genetic material by a process called template switching, a property of RT,[483] and claiming that it is the HIV genome) is isolation. In the cloning procedure, defined genetic material, DNA or RNA, is introduced into cells; and the cells then are able to produce the "virus" from which the genetic material originated. However, the genetic material introduced has to have already been proven to be the genome of a specific virus. As has been consistently stressed here, all cells contain retroviral elements as a normal part of their genome, which can be made to be expressed in cell culture under certain laboratory conditions. Both the cells in the culture from which the original particle were obtained and the transfected cells may release identical or similar retroviral particles

---

[481] Rosenberg, YJ, et al, (1998), "HIV-induced decline in blood CD4/CD8 ratios: Viral killing or altered lymphocyte trafficking?," *Immunol Today;* 19(1): 10-17

[482] Wolthers, KC., et al., (1998), "T-cell telomere length in HIV-1 infection: no evidence for increased CD4+T cell turnover," *Science;* 274:1543-1547

[483] Guangxiang Luo and John Taylor. 1990. Template Switching by Reverse Transcriptase during DNA Synthesis. J Virol 64, 4321-4328. Goodrich D.W. and Duesberg P.H. 1990. Retroviral recombination during reverse transcription. *PNAS* 87: 2052-2056.

even if there is no cloning.[484] Therefore, for cloning, the virus must be isolated twice: the first time to obtain the viral genome and the second time to prove that the particles released by the cell after the introduction of the viral genome are identical to those from which the genome was originally obtained. In AIDSworld, the first isolation has been short-circuited, which is why there is a database with ~100,000 different HIVs on file.[485]

Cloning is not now and has never been isolation. Cloning is multiplication of viral process that has nothing to do with structural identification. It is unclear where the pieces of DNA or RNA come from because the thing to be cloned has never been identified as a part of HIV. No structural criteria with which one can exactly identify genuine biological entities are used in the case of HIV—no analysis of the form and size of an isolated virus, the kind and composition of its proteins, and its genetic substance.[486]

It can be understood that it is normal that genetic material, whether natural or multiplied, when placed in cell cultures is able to enter into the chromosomes of those cells and may even eventually produce proteins. The idea of vaccination with "naked DNA" is based on these known mechanisms. To add a DNA clone to cells and later to prove its presence and probable activity is simply standard experimental technique in biology, but it is not proof for the existence of HIV. If there is no HIV isolation, there can be no HIV cloning.

In AIDSpeak, the words used do not necessarily mean what is commonly understood. In AIDSpeak, a viral load is simply unidentifiable floating genomic objects and not really a viral load. A clone is another laboratory artifact produced by a process called template switching and not a viral genome. This is why the tests for viral load are neither licensed nor recommended by the FDA to diagnose HIV infection, and this is why any clinician who continues to rely on these tests to institute ARV therapy is committing malpractice. As these drugs will continue to attack the cells' energy centers—the mitochondria—practicing physicians must of necessity develop some modicum of understanding of how acquired mitochondrial diseases originally progress and how they can be nontoxically treated.

---

[484] Papadopulos-Eleopulos, E., et al., (1996), "The Isolation of HIV—has it really been achieved? The case against," *Continuum;* 4(3):
[485] http://www.oxfordjournals.org/nar/database/summary/76 downloaded 10 April 2014 "HIV sequence database"
[486] Lanka, S., "Lanka replies to Duesberg (II)," *Continuum* Feb./March 1997

CHAPTER 5

Volatile Nitrites, Folic Acid Inhibitors, and AZT— a Lethal Combination

Revolutions sometimes begin with a bang, and so it was for a group of targeted individuals who had been pushed to the limit by years of police and civilian harassment. In the early hours of June 28, 1969, several customers at the Stonewall Inn, a popular gay bar in Greenwich Village, took a stand and confronted the police. As rumor spread throughout the city about the demonstration, the customers of the inn were soon joined by other gay men and women who started throwing objects at the police and began shouting "gay power."[487] This spontaneous outbreak of collective resistance was a landmark event in the gay community as many had for years been taunted and persecuted by both law enforcement and private citizens. That event continues to be celebrated annually as Gay Pride Day.

However, it also marked the beginning of a decade in which a subset of homosexual and bisexual men began an experiment in behavioral changes that presaged a massive increase in sexual promiscuity and an explosive growth in pharmaceutical and recreational drug use, including the nitrites: amyl, alkyl, isobutyl and isopropyl.[488] The metabolic consequences of this combination of factors sparked an epidemic of environmentally induced cellular energy deficiency that clinically presented as classic type 2 cell dis-symbiosis— opportunistic infections and Kaposi's sarcoma. These changing sexual and

---

[487] http://www.civilrights.org/archives/2009/06/449-stonewall.html
[488] Root-Bernstein, R.S. "Non HIV immunosuppressive factors in AIDS: A multifactorial, synergistic theory of AIDS etiology"; *Res Immunol,* Paris 1990;141:815-838

social habits were combined with other drugs (barbiturates, amphetamines, cocaine, heroin, ethyl chloride, LSD, PCP, Quaaludes, alcohol, etc.)[489] including the erratic and inappropriate use of immune-suppressing antibiotics such as trimethoprim/sulfamethoxazole (T/S), and other lifestyle habits that almost guaranteed an inevitable health catastrophe. In this subgroup, it was more of a gay frenzy rather than a gay pride.

T/S, which is still widely used both prophylactically and therapeutically for AIDS patients, not only acts as a double folate and DNA synthesis inhibitor but also produces as an intermediate product, hydroxylamine, which produces an N-nitroso metabolite that has to be detoxified with glutathione. The principal function of folate coenzymes is to accept or donate one-carbon units in key metabolic pathways. Adequate folate levels are essential for cell division and homeostasis. It plays an essential role in folate coenzymes required for nucleic acid synthesis, methionine regeneration, and shuttling, oxidation, and reduction of one-carbon units required for normal metabolism and regulation.[490,491] The rate-limiting step for the synthesis of DNA is the conversion of uracil (deoxyuridine monophosphate) to thymine (deoxythymidine monophosphate). This step requires tetrahydrofolate as a cofactor. Other critical pathways dependent on folate as a one-carbon source include RNA and protein methylation as well as the aforementioned DNA synthesis and maintenance. Folate can be a limiting factor in all these reactions.[492]

Added to the long list of toxins that were being freely ingested by this population was the tragic iatrogenic introduction of the drug AZT[493] (Zidovudine, Retrovir), which not only further lowered the glutathione concentration in these patients[494] but also attacked the mitochondrial[495] oxidative phosphorylation

---

[489] Haverkos, H.W., R Pinsky, R Drotman & D.J. Bregman, 1985. Disease Manifestation among Homosexual Men with Acquired Immunodeficiency Syndrome: A Possible Role of Nitrites in Kaposi's Sarcoma. Sexually Transmitted Diseases 12: 4.

[490] Wagner, C., (1995), Biochemical role of folate in cellular metabolism, In: Folate in Health and Disease (Bailey, L.B., ed.) pp. 23-42, Marcel Dekker, New York, N.Y.

[491] Baily, LB., Gregory III, JF, (1999), "Folate metabolism and requirements," *J Nutr;* 129(4): 779-782

[492] Crider, KS., et al., (2012) "Folate and DNA methylation: A review of molecular mechanisms and the evidence for folate's role," *Adv Nutr;* 3: 21-38

[493] Chemical warfare on a civilian population

[494] Yamaguchi, T., (2002) "Azidothymidine causes functional and structural destruction of mitochondria, glutathione deficiency and HIV-1 promoter sensitization," *Eur J Biochem;* 269(11):2782-2788

[495] Benbrik, E., et al., (1997), "Cellular and mitochondrial toxicity of zidovudine (AZT), didanosine (ddI), and zalcitabine (ddC) on cultured human muscle cells," *J Neuro Sci;* 149(1):19-25

energy production system, ultimately killing thousands of mostly young men. The drug company responsible for the introduction of nitrites, T/S and AZT, was the British firm, Burroughs Wellcome. Burroughs Wellcome merged with Smith Kline and Beecham in 2000 and is now known as GlaxoSmithKline.

Nitrites NO_2

Amyl nitrite was marketed as a prescription drug in the United States in 1937 for acute relief of angina pectoris. The drug came to be called poppers because initially it was packaged in small glass ampules that were "popped" open to release fumes that were inhaled for relief of intermittent chest pain. It remained a prescription drug until September 1960 when the Food and Drug Administration (FDA) eliminated the prescription requirement. This was principally because after the introduction of nitroglycerin sublingual tablets, dermally applied ointments, and, later, transdermal patches. Amyl nitrite lost most of its market share in cardiac therapeutics.

During the 1960s, the drug made its way to U.S. soldiers fighting in Vietnam along with a variety of other drugs, including marijuana, heroin, opium, LSD, and amphetamines.[496] When the soldiers returned to the United States after their tour of duty in Vietnam, many continued their poppers habit. The FDA reinstated its ban on amyl nitrite without a prescription in 1969 following reports from soldiers and former soldiers in the United States of serious problems caused by the drug. These problems included skin burns, fainting, dizziness, breathing difficulties, and blood anomalies. The National Institute of Drug Abuse was also beginning to compile data that implicated amyl nitrite in increased emergency room admissions as a result of the side effects of the drug,[497] ranging from dyspnea and flushing to tachycardia and death. However, other nitrites, butyl and isobutyl, soon replaced the vacuum created by this prohibition; and because they did not fit the criteria of a food, drug, or cosmetic as specified by the Federal Food, Drug and Cosmetic Act, they have not been subject to government regulation. The United Kingdom, however, recognizes isobutyl and isopropyl nitrites as class 2 carcinogens, and they are controlled under the UK Dangerous Substances and Preparations (Safety) Regulations 2006.[498]

---

[496] Young, I., (1995), "The poppers story, the fall and rise of 'the gay drug'," *Steam;* 2(4)
[497] Reed, D., (1979), "The multi-million dollar mystery high," *Christopher Street;* 2:21-27
[498] http://www.emcdda.europa.eu/publications/drug-profiles/volatile (last accessed 23 April 2014) http://www.legislation.gov.uk/uksi/2006/2916/pdfs/uksi_20062916_en.pdf

While amyl nitrite was originally manufactured and marketed by the British firm Burroughs Wellcome to treat angina, as other drugs garnered a bigger market share, it was repositioned and marketed as a "room odorizer" in gay men's magazines. It became a staple of the gay scene and grew in popularity as word spread that it seemed to intensify sexual orgasm.[499] Although there was little research that suggested that amyl nitrite is an effective aphrodisiac, by the 1950s, it had gained a reputation in the British show business industry for enhancing sexual orgasm.[500] There were isolated reports of amyl nitrite use in the United States as early as the 1960s,[501] but it was not until the 1970s that reports of nitrite use for augmentation of sexual experiences along with descriptions of their aphrodisiac properties began to surface.[502,503] However, the popper craze really skyrocketed during the years 1974 to 1977. By 1979, when the first early cases of immune suppression were beginning to surface, over five million people in the United States were reportedly using these drugs more than once a week.[504]

By the late seventies,[505] it was being reported that the sale of nonprescription volatile nitrites had become a huge business. An estimated total of $50 million a year was made from the sales of more than one hundred thousand bottles a week in just one city. Further, it was claimed that, prior to 1978, male homosexuals indulged in the use of volatile nitrites more than any other group. Someone even produced a guide to homosexual lovemaking and asserted that the use of amyl nitrite has "passed into every corner of gay life."[506]

Because these nitrite drugs were found to reduce social and sexual inhibitions as well as heighten sexual arousal and facilitate relaxation of the anal sphincter, they were being touted and used primarily as sexual doping agents.[507,508]

---

[499] Labataille, L, (1975), "Amyl nitrite employed in homosexual relations," *Med Aspects Human Sexuality;* 9:122
[500] Young, Op Cit.
[501] Israelstam, S., et al, "Poppers, a new recreational drug craze"; *Can Psychiatr Assoc J*; 23:493-495, 1978
[502] Hollistter, LE, "The mystique of social drugs and sex" In: Sandler, M. et al. eds. *Sexual Behavior: Pharmacology and Biochemistry.* New York: Raven Press, 1975 pp.85-92
[503] Pearlman, JT & Adams, GL., "Amyl nitrite inhalation fad; *JAAMA* 212:160, 1970
[504] Mayer, KH., "Medical consequences of the inhalation of volatile nitrites: In: Ostrow, DG. et al., *Sexually transmitted diseases in homosexual men.* New York: Plenum Medical Book Co., 1983. pp.237-242
[505] Newell, GR., Mansell PWA., et al., (1985), "Volatile Nitrites, use and adverse effects relaed to the current epidemic of the acquired immune deficiency syndrome," *Am J Med;* 78: 811-816
[506] Sigell, Ibid
[507] Lubell, I. Correspondence with Burroughs Wellcome Co., 1964; U.S. FDA, 1967
[508] Israelstam et al., Op Cit.

However, poppers also induce a list of acute, dose-dependent, deleterious effects as well: abrupt drop in blood pressure (flushing) and tachycardia; heat loss and chills; skin irritation upon direct contact to lip, nose, penis, scrotum, and elsewhere; allergic reactions; tracheobronchitis with cough, fever, hemoptysis, and dyspnea; dizziness, headaches, and nausea; and disturbances in oxygen transport of the red blood cells, methemoglobinemia.[509,510,511] These drugs also can produce chronic depletion of T-cell ratios associated with severe immune dysfunction.

Even after the AIDS crisis began and there were strong epidemiological indications of the link between gay-related immune disease (GRID), as it was first called, and the chronic use of poppers, the gay press remained silent to the harmful effects of these potent toxins, which were often their main source of advertising revenue. Just as mainstream medical journals had long taken ads from cigarette companies, gay journals followed suit and put their advertising revenues ahead of their customers' welfare. One magazine, the Advocate, even ran a series of ads promoting poppers as a "blueprint for health."[512]

By 1978, which was approximately seven to ten years after the extreme use of this drug metastasized throughout the gay community, unusual medical symptoms began to appear in the cohort who were known to have had an increased exposure, namely, a "fast track" subset of homosexual men in large urban centers. These men were beginning to not only have the symptoms noted above but were beginning to present with significant immune imbalances expressed as opportunistic diseases—diseases not generally seen in well-nourished Western populations, mainly PCP and candidiasis, as well as with malignant cancers of vascular endothelial cells called Kaposi's sarcoma. The KS lesions were commonly found on the face, nose, and chest.

The CDC's first official notification of these various illnesses was posted in 1981 when a brief report was published regarding five cases of illness in homosexual men who suffered from an opportunistic lung infection. All the patients were nitrite abusers. All had pneumocystis carinii pneumonia, all had CMV, all exhibited immunosuppression.[513] "The patients did not know each other and had no known common contacts or knowledge of sexual partners who had had similar illnesses. Two of the 5 reported having frequent homosexual contacts with various partners. All 5 reported using inhalant drugs, and 1

---

[509] Jackson, CD, 1979 Volatile Nitrites, NTP working paper, National Center for Toxicological Research, Office of Scientific Intelligence
[510] http://www.medsafe.govt.nz/profs/datasheet/a/Amylnitriteinh.pdf
[511] http://archives.drugabuse.gov/pdf/monographs/83.pdf
[512] Young, I., Op Cit
[513] http://www.cdc.gov/mmwr/PDF/wk/mm4534.pdf

reported parenteral drug abuse. Three patients had profoundly depressed in vitro proliferative responses to mitogens and antigens. Lymphocyte studies were not performed on the other 2 patients."[514] Ignoring their long health history of drug abuse and lifestyle, the attending physicians claimed that these diseases were occurring in "previously healthy homosexual men."[515] One of the CDC "geniuses" responsible for avoiding this obvious health hazard was Dr. Harold Jaffe. Jaffe is a CDC-trained spy from the Epidemic Intelligence Service, a branch of the government that is wedded to the belief that every mysterious disease outbreak has an infectious origin. From early on, the CDC was committed to positioning HIV as (a) infectious and (b) as a sexually transmitted disease, evidence to the contrary notwithstanding.

To the gynecologist who is expertly trained in the recognition and treatment of sexually transmitted diseases (STDs), STDs have historically and wisely been confined to manifestations that occur in the reproductive organs. Somehow AIDSworld was now going to absurdly claim that a vascular cancer and a lung fungus, both far removed from the reproductive system, were somehow "sexually transmitted". Jaffe claimed that "nitrite use among gay men also tends to be associated with other behaviors. Men with a heavy use of nitrite inhalants often also are highly sexually active, and have other sexually transmitted diseases. So it's very hard in doing studies to be able to separate out all of these behaviors that are highly associated."[516] However, Jaffe's bias (and his ignorance of STDs) was focusing on the behaviors rather than the metabolic consequences of the entire constellation of behaviors of this subgroup. He was also rather cavalierly discounting the known immunosuppressive and carcinogenic potential of N-nitroso compounds, problems that had been reported in medical literature as early as 1956.[517] The astute clinician will immediately understand the fallaciousness of this rather insipid and tendentious argument. It can also be gleaned by these remarks that a case was being made, based on both bad epidemiology and bad science, to convince the world of a new sex-and-blood plague. Known cellular metabolic responses to the identifiable toxins that could have, even by 1984 standards, answered many of the AIDS conundrums were to be blatantly ignored.

---

[514] http://www.cdc.gov/mmwr/preview/mmwrhtml/june_5.htm
[515] Gottlieb, MS, et al., "Pneumocystis carinii pneumonia and mucosal candidiasis in previously healthy homosexual men: evidence of a new acquired cellular immunodeficiency"; *NEJM.* 1981 Dec 10;305(24):1425-31.132
[516] Bethell, T., (1996), "AIDS and Poppers" http://www.virusmyth.com/aids/hiv/tbpoppers.htm
[517] Magee, PN, Barnes, JM, (1956), "The production of malignant primary hepatic tumours in the rat by feeding dimethylnitrosamine," *Brit J Cancer;* 10: 114-122

A crucial and disastrous decision was made at this juncture. For almost a century, physicians had been steeped in the lessons of Pasteur and Koch and had all but ignored the theories of Antoine Béchamp,[518] who had posited that disease arose in the organism that already has some underlying damage and not the other way around. This is still the pressing issue in medicine that has never been dealt with sufficiently—which is more important: the milieu of the human organism or the organisms that take hold? Physicians have been taught that there is a microbe lurking behind every disease, including cancer. The bioterrain is an afterthought. When the first cases of AIDS were identified in 1981, poppers were briefly considered as an etiologic agent. Already both in vitro and in vivo studies, it was demonstrated that these drugs damaged the immune system and could lead to two types of anemia: methemoglobinemia[519] and hemolytic anemia.[520]

Red Cell Metabolism

Hemoglobin (Hgb), the redox-sensitive metalloprotein oxygen-carrying molecule in red blood cells, is continuously oxidized from the ferrous (Fe^{2+}) to the ferric (Fe^{3+}) form and reduced back again. The ferric form, termed methemoglobin (MetHb), is incapable of transporting oxygen. In the normal physiological state, the concentration of methemoglobin is less than 1 percent. Studies have shown that MetHb levels of 10 to 25 percent produce cyanosis, 35 to 45 percent produce mild symptoms (e.g. dyspnea), levels of 60 percent produce lethargy and coma, and levels of 70 percent or more are lethal.[521,522]

---

[518] http://www.mnwelldir.org/docs/history/biographies/Bechamp-or-Pasteur.pdf Bechamp or Pasteur? A lost chapter in this history of biology"

[519] Edwards, RJ, Ujma, J., (1995), "Extreme methaemoglobinaemia secondary to recreational use of amyl nitrite," *J Accident & Emerg Med;* 12:138-142

[520] Brandes, J.C., et al, (1989), "Amyl nitrite induced hemolytic anemia," *Am J Med;* 86(2):252-4

[521] Wintrobe, MM, Less, GR., Boggs, IR, et al, (1974), *Clinical Hematology,* 7th edition. Lea & Febiger, Philadelphia (1991)

[522] Forsyth, RJ., Moulden, A., (1991), "Methemoglobinemia after ingestion of amyl nitrite," *Archives of Diseases in Childhood;* 66: 152

Table 1 – Clinical Manifestations of Methemoglobinemia.

fMetHb (%)	Signs and Symptoms
< 3 (normal)	None
3 - 15	Frequently none
	Grayish skin
15 - 30	Cyanosis
	Chocolate-brown blood
30 - 50	Dyspnea
	Headache
	Fatigue, weakness
	Dizziness, syncope
	SpO_2 ~ 85%
50 - 70	Tachypnea
	Metabolic acidosis
	Cardiac arrhythmias
	Seizures
	CNS depression
	Coma
> 70	Death

CNS – central nervous system. [523]

The iron in the heme moiety of hemoglobin must be maintained in the reduced (ferrous) state in order to bind oxygen reversibly despite exposure to a variety of endogenous and exogenous oxidizing agents. The red blood cell (RBC) has several metabolic pathways to counter the actions of oxidizing agents and to reduce hemoglobin iron if it becomes oxidized. Cellular enzymes for preventing or reversing oxidative denaturation of hemoglobin in RBCs include methemoglobin reductase, superoxide dismutase, glutathione peroxidase, and catalase. Most of the physiologically important methemoglobin reduction occurs enzymatically but may be reduced nonenzymatically by certain

---

[523] Souza do Nascimento, T., et al., (2006), "Methemoglobinemia: from diagnosis to treatment," *Rev Bras Anestesiol;* 58(6): 651-664

compounds found in erythrocytes: ascorbic acid and glutathione. Glutathione is the principal nonenzymatic-reducing agent in RBCs and is the essential cofactor in the glutathione peroxidase reaction.

In the course of reactions protecting hemoglobin from oxidation, GSH (reduced) is oxidized to GSSG—two GSH molecules joined by a disulfide linkage. GSSG rapidly exits the erythrocyte; therefore, for a continuous supply of GSH to be maintained, glutathione reductase catalyzes the reduction of GSSG by NADPH (a product of the pentose phosphate shunt). The production of both glutathione and NADPH are dependent on folic acid levels.[524]

The erythrocyte membrane is the platform for thiol-based circulatory signaling, and it requires sufficient free thiol for maintenance. Hypoxic erythrocytes have a greater loss of reduction potential, and this loss impairs the ability of RBCs to recycle either oxidized glutathione or adenine dinucleotide phosphate (NADPH). As a result, these RBCs lose the ability to defend membrane thiols from oxidative attack.

Hemoglobin conformation controls glycolytic flux through the hexose monophosphate shunt, the sole source of NADPH in RBCs. NADPH acts as a co-factor in the reduction of oxidized glutathione (GSSG) to GSH. When there is sustained hypoxia, ROS cascades may exceed antioxidant capacity, leaving biochemical changes consistent with hypoxia-induced oxidative stress leading to changes in hemoglobin conformation that controls coupled glucose and thiol metabolism of erythrocyte vascular-based signaling.[525]

Ninety percent of the glucose entering RBCs is metabolized by the anaerobic glycolytic pathway, which produces three important products: NADH, a cofactor in the methemoglobin reductase reaction; ATP; and 2,3,-diphosphoglycerate (2,3 DPG), a regulator of hemoglobin function.

---

[524] Fan, J., (2014), "Quantitative flux analysis reveals folate dependent NADPH production," *Nature;* 510(7504): 298-302

[525] Rogers, SC., Said, A., et al., (2009), "Hypoxia limits antioxidant capacity in red blood cells by altering glycolytic pathway dominance," *FASEB J;* 23: 3159-3170

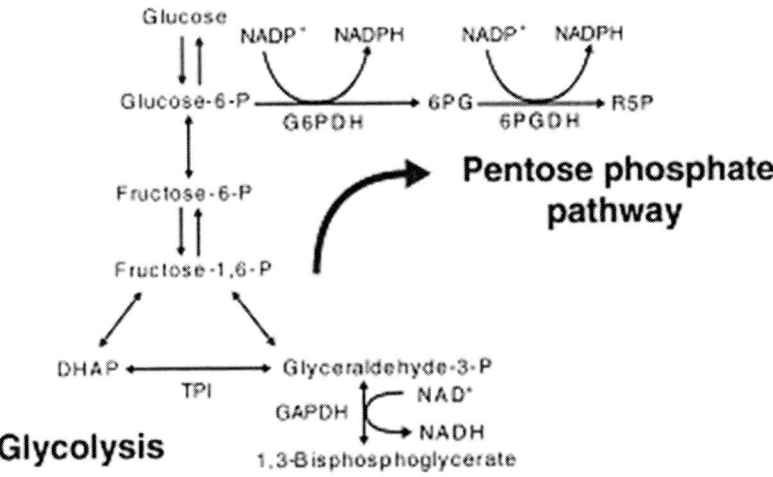

A simplified diagram of the link between glycolysis and the pentose phosphate pathway. The pentose phosphate pathway is linked to glycolysis through glucose 6-phosphate; if it is oxidized, it enters the pentose phosphate pathway whereas if it is isomerized to fructose-6-phosphate, it continues through glycolysis.

Another crucial question about the consequences to oxygen transfer and energy metabolism as a result of prolonged exposure to nitrites was left insufficiently explored in the virus quest. The issue in need of serious investigation was this: what happens to OXPHOS energy production in the mitochondria after long-term reduction in GSH levels contributes to a prolonged decrease in the level of oxygen substrate available for oxidative ATP formation?[526] The issue was partially addressed by the CDC, but both the epidemiological and clinical research studies were manipulated in such a way as to obscure the answer.

The CDC chose to rule out poppers as an etiologic agent in AIDS pathology, citing two reasons. They asserted that there were some AIDS patients who claimed to deny the use of poppers. However, the CDC chose to limit the question about use to a previous two-year time span, ignoring the previous years when the drug may have been utilized as well as the possibility of bias and incorrect data input. Patients are not always willing to freely expose their deleterious lifestyle habits. This was a convenient way of ignoring not only the complete panoply of important and acknowledged risk factors to which these patients were known to have been exposed but, importantly, the duration of exposure. This was also the beginning of the effort to solidify the idea that AIDS

---

[526] Rogers, SC., Said, A., et al., Ibid

was one disease rather than a syndrome with multiple causes, thus ipso facto the AIDS/poppers connection was denied as a causative factor. This assertion was also based on a dubious mouse study that the CDC conducted in 1982[527] that claimed they found "no evidence of immunotoxicity" from nitrite drugs. The National Institute for Occupational Safety and Health, which conducted the study, noted that during the experiment, the nitrite doses were reduced to subclinical levels after they found that the mice in the study were dying,[528] which, in most laboratories, would be considered a serious side effect, except at the CDC. Methemoglobinemia as well as some evidence of thymic atrophy was noted in some animals exposed. This study was rather disingenuous in that it employed a method of manipulation common to both drug companies and government laboratories who work with those companies. In order to obtain the desired results from drug and/or clinical trials, they not only control the dose (to subclinically relevant levels) but also control the length of exposure (which is inevitably less than mirrored in actual clinical use).[529] In this way, a claim can be made that the drug was not found to cause the anticipated harm—if one does not consider death by drug a harm as the CDC.

However, another series of studies done by Lee Soderberg[530,531] used three times the maximum dose employed by the National Institute for Occupational Safety and Health, which more closely mirrored levels in human ingestion. What he found in the study mice after only fourteen days of exposure was evidence of the same serious immune deficits in T cell-mediated immune responses as were presenting in the AIDS patients: decreased cytotoxic T lymphocyte activity and decreased responses to mitogenic and allogenic stimulation. Soderberg's studies noted the T-dependent antibody responses of nitrite-treated mice were reduced by 50 to 65 percent, cytotoxic T cell (CTL) induction was reduced by 40 percent, and the tumoricidal activity of peritoneal exudate macrophages was reduced by 40 percent. In a later experiment, inhalant exposure increased the tumor incidence from 21 percent of control mice to 75 percent of inhalant-

---

[527] http://www.cdc.gov/mmwr/preview/mmwrhtml/00000135.htm Epidemiologic notes and reports an evaluation of the immunotoxic potential of isobutyl nitrite

[528] Lauristen, J., (1994), "The Poppers-Kaposi's sarcoma connection, *New York Native*; 13 June

[529] Ioannidis, JP, (2005), "Why most published research findings are false," *PLoS Med*; http://www.plosmedicine.org/article/infopercent3Adoipercent2F10.1371percent2Fjournal.pmed.0020124

[530] Soderberg, L, (1995), "Acute exposure to inhaled isobutyl nitrite causes massive destruction of peripheral blood cells," NIDA Conference, "HIV and substance abuse" Poster P-20, Scottsdale, AZ.

[531] Soderberg L, (1994), "T cell functions are impaired by inhaled isobutyl nitrite through a T independent mechanism," *Toxicology Letter*; 70: 319-329

exposed mice. The rate of increase in mean tumor weight was nearly fourfold faster in nitrite-exposed mice.[532] Unlike the CDC study, death, disease, and metabolic abnormalities were considered relevant.

The cohort of immunosuppressed men began to appear in big-city emergency rooms just as the Nixon Virus Cancer Program had unsuccessfully sought for ten years to prove that cancer was a contagious disease that had a retroviral etiology. This fruitless search not only wasted billions of dollars, it directed research away from the basic science of the molecular, electrical, and quantum dynamics of cell physiology and the alteration in cancer energy metabolism from OXPHOS to glycolysis noted by Otto Warburg decades before. Rather than investigating the role that the long-term use of immune-suppressing drugs and toxic lifestyle had on altering cell metabolism and producing this syndrome, a decision was made to look for an infectious agent, even with the epidemiological knowledge that "the [original] patients did not know each other and had no known common contacts or knowledge of sexual partners who had had similar illnesses." The shared psychosocial issues that pertained to lifestyle choice and drug use patterns were, in fact, the real common denominators that the CDC conveniently chose to ignore in an effort to consolidate the single-disease hypothesis. By ignoring these controversial matters as the real precipitating and causative factors of this crisis, the keys to understanding the underlying metabolic changes and reversing them with appropriate therapy have been both medically and psychically obliterated.

Dr. Harry Haverkos of the Public Health Service noted that twice as many whites as blacks use poppers and twice as many get Kaposi's.[533] Furthermore, by 1990, there were no white women between the ages of eighteen and forty-five who were sexually linked to a man with Kaposi's sarcoma and who did not use poppers who presented with a case of the new "sexually transmitted disease" of Kaposi's. By ignoring the obvious critical effects that volatile nitrites can have on available oxygen and glutathione supplies and thus on redox metabolism, oxygen availability, and energy production, what the CDC was in the process of creating was the beginning of a thirty-year-and-counting disaster. The "experts" at the CDC ignored the sage advice of Paracelsus who noted more than five hundred years ago, "The poison is in the dose."

Early studies of Kaposi's sarcoma (KS), which was identified as a part of the AID syndrome (KS and OI), found that a majority of the people with KS had been anything but "previously healthy." A review of their health histories revealed that they held these things in common: a greater number of male

---

[532] Soderberg, Op cit.
[533] Bethell, Op Cit.

sex partners per year; exposure to feces during sex often because of an anal penetration by fisting; histories of syphilis and non-B hepatitis and other STDs; prior treatment for enteric parasites, and quite heavy usage of various illicit substances including volatile nitrites.[534,535]

Why was the long-term use of these nitrites so hazardous to health? In vivo, nitrites may be converted to N-nitroso compounds, which are known to be mutagens, teratogens, and strong carcinogens. Additionally, studies found nitrites to have strong immunosuppressive characteristics.[536] Hersh, et al.,[537] demonstrated that "isobutyl nitrite has nonspecific cytotoxic activity on various cells in vitro and could have immunosuppressive effects on tissues exposed in vivo during its recreational use. Their group speculated that these immunosuppressive effects, combined with the ability of nitrites to convert amines to nitrosamines, might be related to the development of opportunistic infections and Kaposi's sarcoma in homosexuals who used this agent. They noted that concern about nitrites had been mainly related to their carcinogenic potential. However, they also found that nitrites have other acute or subacute toxicities including the production of methemoglobinemia, Heinz body hemolytic anemia, splenomegaly, skin rash, and death after acute over-ingestion causing methemoglobinemia and hypokinetic anoxia."

A consistent finding of the original group of AIDS patients was the failure of lymphocytes to respond to mitogenic stimulation. The Hersh study also found that very low doses of isobutyl nitrite inhibited in vitro lymphocyte blastogenic responses to phytohemagglutinin, pokeweed mitogen, and concanavalin A.[538] In another study using human neutrophils, it was determined that nitric oxide caused a depletion of intracellular glutathione and that depletion of this molecule was accompanied by a rapid and simultaneous activation of the

---

[534] Jaffe, HW et al., "National case control study of Kaposi's sarcoma and pneumocystis carinii pneumonia in homosexual men: Part I. Epidemiologic results *Ann Intern Med 1983*;99:145-151

[535] Rogers, MF., et al, "National case control study of Kaposi's Sarcoma and *pneumocystis carinii* pneumonia in homosexual men: part 2, laboratory results" *Ann Intern Med* 1983;99(2):151-158

[536] Newell, GR., et al., "Nitrite Inhalants: Historical perspective," NIDA Res Monogr. 1988;83:1-14.

[537] Hersh, EM., et al., "Effect of Recreational Agent Isobutyl Nitrite on Human peripheral blood leukocytes and on *in vitro* interferon production"; March 1983 *Cancer Res;* 43:1365-1371

[538] Hersh Ibid

hexose monophosphate shunt.[539] In essence, the symptoms directly proven to be caused by excessive nitrite use were, in fact, the hallmarks of AIDS in the early patients: anergy, decreased CD4+T cell lymphocytes, and failure of lymphocytes to respond to mitogens in vitro.

Thus, a big question in medicine has been what positive role if any do nitrites or nitrite metabolites have in human physiology. Clearly, before the onslaught of the AIDS era, they had been useful in clinical practice. It has only been within the last three decades that this fundamental question in cardiocirculatory research been explored and answered. In the late 1970s and early 1980s, real evidence began to be produced that mammalian cells produce nitrates, which have been shown to be essential modulators and mediators of all cellular life on earth—including humans. Nitric oxide is part of the redox signaling system that controls the post-translational modification of proteins. The redox and phosphorylation modification systems have been conserved throughout evolution.[540] The impact of NO-mediated redox modification is felt dramatically not only in the cardiocirculatory system but the nervous system and, importantly to the AIDS story, the immune system.

How the AIDS industry has negligently ignored information about the role of nitric oxide in health and disease and has consistently denied, in favor of a viral etiology, the fundamental and life-preserving relationship between this small molecule and the cellular thiol pool has been the sad saga that has played out over the last three decades. It is the reciprocal nature of the delicate balance between NO and sulfur-containing molecules that drive the balance of cellular redox homeostasis. The mechanisms of this relationship will be explored in the next chapter.

Trimethoprim/Sulfamethoxazole

On many surgical floors in U.S. hospitals during the 1970s, it was noted that the consequence of long-term antibiotic therapy was often superinfection with fungal and viral agents. As a result, questions were raised and studies conducted on the effect of chronic antibiotic use on cell-mediated immunity. As suspected, the results of several of these studies indeed indicated a suppression

---

[539] Clancy, RM, et al., (1994), "Nitric oxide reacts with intracellular glutathione and activates the hexose monophosphate shunt in human neutrophils: evidence for s-nitrosoglutathione as a bioactive intermediary," *PNAS USA;* 91: 3680-3684

[540] Stamler, JS., (2001), "Nitrosylation: the protytypic redox-based signaling mechanism," *Cell;* 106: 675-683

of cell-mediated immunity with many of the antibiotics examined.[541] At the beginning of the AIDS crisis, it was also observed that "gay men were aware of their disease susceptibility long before AIDS emerged as a problem. . . . They made chronic use of antibiotics, some prophylactically and some to treat recurrent venereal and other infections. . . . It was not uncommon to take a few antibiotics and sniff an ampule or two of amyl nitrite on the way to the baths or bars for a round of anonymous sex. . . . In one study, over 40% of the men surveyed responded that they 'routinely' treated themselves with prescription antibiotics."[542,543]

One of the diseases most frequently observed in AIDS patients in the United States and Europe has been a fungus, pneumocystis (PCP now called Pneumocystis jiroveci). It is routinely treated acutely or prophylactically with the double folic acid blockers Bactrim, Septra, or Cotrim—not without consequences. These drugs are combinations of two antibiotics (trimethoprim and sulfamethoxazole, or TMP/SMX, T/S), both known folate inhibitors. Sulfonamides, as antimetabolites, compete in bacteria and human mitochondria with para-aminobenzoic acid (PABA) for incorporation into folic acid. Trimethoprim is an inhibitor of dihydrofolate reductase (DHFR), an essential enzyme that converts folic acid to the biologically active form of tetrahydrofolate (THF). It acts as a carbon donor for construction of amino acids and DNA and the coenzymes NAD(P)H, FAD (flavin adenine dinucleotide), and FMN (flavin mononucleotide). Folate inhibitors, including trimethoprim, are purposely designed to have multiple deleterious effects on cell metabolism and division: disruption of certain amino acids as well as disruption of certain coenzymes and DNA synthesis.

Germane to the AIDS story is the role of NADPH in the pentose monophosphate shunt whose main purpose is to regenerate NADPH from $NADP^+$ via an oxidation/reduction reaction. NADPH is then used to reduce the disulfide form of glutathione to the sulfhydryl form. Glutathione reductase catalyzes the reduction of glutathione disulfide (GSSG) to the sulfhydryl form glutathione (GSH). Glutathione reductase utilizes an FAD prosthetic group and NADPH to reduce one mole of GSSG to two moles of GSH.

---

[541] Munster, AM et al., (1977) "The effect of antibiotics on cellmediated immunity," *Surgery;* 81(6):692695

[542] Piffer, LL, et al., (1987), "Borderline immunodeficiency in male homosexuals: is life style contributory?" *South Med J;* 80(6):687-691, 697

[543] Root-Bernstein, RS., (1993), The tragic cost of premature consensus, The Free Press, New York

The Slow Death of the AIDS/Cancer Paradigm and the Apocrypha of the Eukaryotic Cell

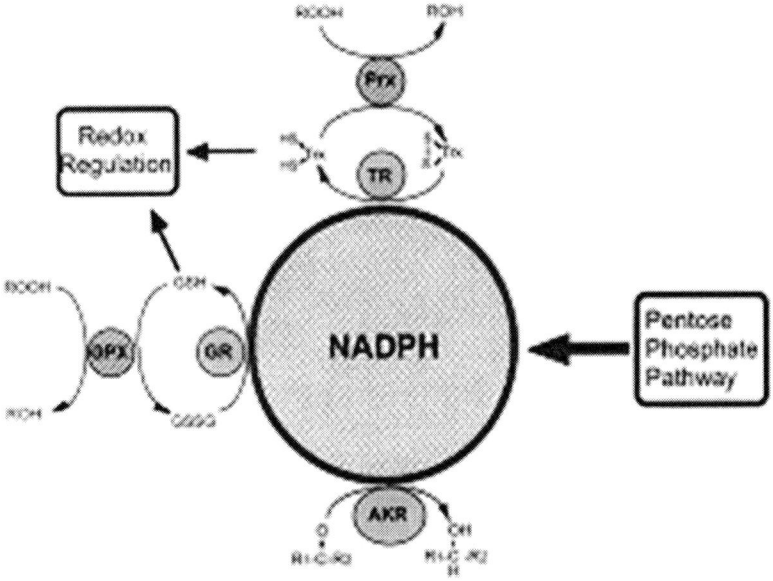

Fig. 1

Instead of attempting to alleviate the metabolic imbalances in these patients, AIDSworld enthusiasts pushed these people over an iatrogenic cliff to drown in a sea of toxicity. As glutathione deficiency has been a known problem in both HIV positive and AIDS patients, and as these antibiotics have the potential for aggravating that deficiency, that they continue to be recommended and used in this clinical context without a recognition of the need for glutathione and/or folate replacement therapy is more than disturbing. It has been noted that "AIDS patients may not tolerate or respond to Bactrim in the same manner as non-AIDS patients. The incidence of side effects, particularly rash, fever, leukopenia and elevated aminotransferase [transaminase] values, with Bactrim therapy in AIDS patients who are being treated for Pneumocystis carinii pneumonia has been reported to be greatly increased compared with the incidence normally associated with the use of Bactrim in non-AIDS patients."[544]

---

[544] Hardy DW, et al. (1992) "A controlled trial of trimethoprim-sulfamethoxazole or aerosolized pentamidine for secondary prophylaxis of Pneumocystis carinii pneumonia in patients with the acquired immunodeficiency syndrome." *N Engl J Med*; 327: 1842–1848.

The blocking effects of trimethoprim are complex. It disrupts the metabolism of amino acids, one of which is the transformation of the amino acid serine to glycine, which supplies one of the three building blocks of glutathione. Glycine also acts in the recovery of the essential amino acid methionine from homocysteine.[545] Elevated levels of homocysteine have been associated with atherosclerosis, but they can also stimulate inducible nitric oxide synthase expression in macrophages,[546] thereby increasing the oxidative stress load in cells, which are already experiencing a deficit of the glutathione-reducing molecule. Additionally, activated folic acid (methyltetrahydrofolic acid) also mediates the methylation of biogenic amines (dopamine, adrenaline, noradrenaline, serotonin, melatonin),[547,548] which have crucial roles in the stabilization of the nervous system including sleep/wake cycles and the fight-or-flight response patterns. Consequently, trimethoprim has multiple effects consistent with the complexity of pathways affected by folic acid. Not only can it effect the maturation function (DNA synthesis) and detoxification (glutathione deficit) of immune cells but also may disrupt the biosynthesis of the coenzymes of the respiratory chain of the mitochondria as mitochondria in all human cells originate from proteobacteria.[549] Unfortunately, to date, Hoffman Laroche, now the main producer of Bactrim and Septra, have not addressed this serious and important clinical issue with appropriate mitochondrial studies.[550]

Additive to the biological stressor effects of these drugs is the metabolic degradation product of sulfamethoxazole: hydroxylamine. Under physiological conditions, hydroxylamine can be oxidized spontaneously to nitroso compounds. These compounds are more highly reactive and more toxic than

---

[545] Barra, Lise, et al., (2006), "Interrelations between glycine betaine catabolism and methionine biosynthesis in *Sinorhizobium meliloti* Strain 102F34," *J Bact;* 188(20): 7195-7204

[546] Woo, CW., et al., (2003), "Homocysteine stimulates inducible nitric oxide synthase expression in macrophages: antagonizing effect of ginkgolides and bilobalide," *Mol Cell Biochem;* 243(1-2):37–47

[547] Lambie, DF, Johnson, RH., (1985), "Drugs and folate metabolism," *Drugs;* 30:145–155

[548] Banerjee, SP, Snyder, SH, (1973), "Methyltetrahydrofolic acid mediated N and O methylation of biogenic amines," *Science;* 182(4107): 74-75

[549] Gray, MW., et al, (1999), "Mitochondrial Evolution," *Science;* 283: 1476-1481

[550] Kremer, H, (2008), "The Silent Revolution in Cancer and AIDS Medicine," Xlibris p 294

hydroxamines[551,552] and have to be detoxified by glutathione.[553] Unfortunately, the glutathione deficit can lead to increasing levels of oxidative and nitrosative stress and to inhibition of cytochrome c oxidase in the respiratory chain.[554] This can cause irreversible inhibition of the respiratory chain, uncoupling, mitochondrial membrane permeability, and/or cell death (type 1 overregulation of cell dis-symbiosis) or to cell transformation as glycolytic tumor cells (type 2 counterregulation of cell dis-symbiosis).

Trimethoprim/sulfamethoxazole perfectly illustrates the concepts of the nonlinearity and complexity of the network. While the pharmaceutical industry continues to push the concept of "selective bonding," as demonstrated by the numerous metabolic functions of folic acid and its derivatives and the deleterious consequences of its "selective inhibition" of DHFR on multiple cell systems, it becomes incumbent on the clinician to understand the consequences of blocking a number of crucial metabolic functions, including both the detoxification process and DNA and protein synthesis, as well as neurohormone and energy production. The nocuous side effects of these drugs are not, in fact, "side effects" but effects. Importantly, the mitochondria still has many characteristics of the ancient proteobacteria from which it is descended, and until the pharmaceutical companies begin to do appropriate studies to answer questions about how their products' effect this organelle, extreme caution is advised. This is not to deny a drug's potential use. It is a word of caution that the patient's disposition must be considered and metabolic status must be compensated before considering these drugs for either short- or long-term chemotherapy.

By 1981, at the beginning of the AIDS era, a research team was already disclosing evidence that pathological transformation of nuclear DNA was appearing in patients who had been treated with customary doses and duration of co-trimoxazole for urinary tract infection. A 1981 report concluded that "the present study shows that trimethoprim-sulfamethoxazole [co-trimoxazole], like other folic antagonists [for instance, methotrexate for the treatment of

---

[551] Cribb, AE., Spielberg, SP., (1992), "Sulfamethoxazole is metabolized to the hydroxylamine in humans," *Clin Pharmacol Ther;* 51(5): 522-526

[552] Sanderson, JP.,(2008) "Nonenzymatic Formation of a Novel Hydroxylated Sulfamethoxazole Derivative in Human Liver Microsomes: Implications for Bioanalysis of Sulfamethoxazole Metabolites," *Drug Metab Disposition;* 36(12): 2424-2428

[553] Tsikas, D., (1995), "Formation of S-nitroso compounds from sodium nitroprusside, nitric oxide or nitrite and reduced thiols: analysis by capillary isotachophoresis," *J Chromatog;* 699: 363-369

[554] Brown, GC., (2001), "Regulation of mitochondrial respiration by nitric oxide inhibition of cytochrome c oxidase," *Biochim Biophys Acta*; 1504(1): *46-57*

leukemia], damage human genetic material."[555] In spite of the clear warning, AIDSworld specialists were advising long-term prophylaxis for patients who were already immunologically and cytologically impaired.[556,557]

THE LESSONS LEARNED FROM AZATHIOPRINE WERE IGNORED BY THE ADHERENTS OF AZIDOTHYMIDINE: AZT AND THE CALLED-FOR HUMAN EXPERIMENTATION

Azathioprine is another Burroughs Wellcome immunosuppressive drug that came into widespread use during the 1960s and 1970s mainly to prevent organ transplant rejection. The drug was developed as a purine analog and an inhibitor of DNA synthesis. As a result, the drug targets rapidly proliferating cells, including bone marrow and T and B immune cells. It effectively dampens both the cell-mediated and humoral immune response. As a result of the use of this drug, a number of transplant patients developed what can be defined as transplantation AIDS: Kaposi's sarcomas, lymphomas, and opportunistic infections. A lesson that could have been learned about immune suppression and recovery, (but was known and ignored) from the use of this drug by AIDSworld adherents, was that patients often recovered when the drug was withdrawn, even from disseminated KS[558] and even while continuing on other immune-suppressive agents prescribed to inhibit the rejection response. Thus, the symptom presentations of the early AIDS patients were neither a sudden nor a unique clinical syndrome confined to a group of fast-track urban gay males. The identical disease constellations had been seen, treated, and written about in the medical literature as a clinical syndrome that did not require a viral explanation. But AIDSworld chose to ignore this relevant history. The HIV theory was easier to advance than taking a critical look at the dark side of the pharmaceutical industry and the complicity of the medical profession in the creation of iatrogenic disease. Thus, when patients started to present as severely immune suppressed as a result of the long-term use of multiple

---

[555] Sörensen, PJ, Jensen, MK., (1981), "Cytogenetic studies in patients treated with trimethoprim-sulfamethoxazole," *Mutat Res;* 89(1): 91-94

[556] Gottlieb, MS., et al., (1981), "Pneumocystis carnii pneumonia and mucosal candidiasis in previously healthy homosexual men. evidence of a new acquired immunodeficiency," *NEJM;* 305: 1425-1431

[557] De Wys, WD, et al., (1982), "Workshop on Kaposi-Sarcoma Meeting report," *Cancer Treatment Reports;* 66(6): 1387-1390

[558] Montagnino, G., et al., (1994), "Clinical features and course of Kaposi's sarcoma in kidney transplant patients: report of 13 cases," *Am J Nephrol;* 14(2): 121-126

environmental stressors, including pharmaceutical drugs, that were going to continue to be used in this patient population as part of the called for "human experimentation" rather than apply what had already been learned from recent transplantation history, a new viral theory was advanced. When no HIV could be found to be associated with KS[559] and the rate of KS began to rapidly decline with the disuse of poppers,[560,561] KS was still kept as an AIDS-defining disease; but instead of assessing the metabolic situation, a new viral agent was proposed here as well: HHV-8.[562] AIDSworld continues to confuse association with causation and epiphenomena with pro-phenomena.

When the FDA approved the addition of AZT for the treatment of AIDS patients as another Burroughs Wellcome drug to this already-lethal brew of nitroso compounds and folate inhibitors, it was the wish come true of the august Dr. Lewis Thomas, the then-director of the Memorial Sloan Kettering Cancer Center. In a lecture delivered at the first World AIDS Conference, Dr. Thomas clearly stated the direction of AIDS research, which continues to the present: "Whatever we learn about the mechanisms releasing Kaposi's sarcoma in AIDS will be useful information for the study of cancer in general, and whatever we can discover about the role of immunity in cancer will turn out to be a piece of applied science for the AIDS problem. . . .What is needed, of course, is a series of human experiments, planned and executed in order to answer the sort of question which automatically raises itself: what would happen if you were to remove the putative defense mechanism of cellular immunity in human beings?" Would this affect either the incidence or clinical course of cancer? As it happens, unplanned experiments have already been done. . . . It seems to me that there are two alternative explanations for the high incidence of cancer in AIDS patients, and the same alternatives exist for the patients with organ homografts treated with immune suppressive drugs. One is that the impairment of cellular immunity has allowed an oncogenic virus to invade and proliferate, and what we are seeing is a human cancer running wild. This would seem plausible enough for the AIDS patients with Kaposi's sarcoma if this were the only neoplasm, but these patients are developing other types of neoplasms as well, including the same lymphomas with special predilection for

---

[559] Papadapulos-Eleopulos, E., et al. (1992), "Kaposi's sarcoma and HIV," *Med Hypothesis;* 39: 22-29

[560] Lauritsen, J., (1989), "Poppers: The end of an era," *New York Native*

[561] Haverkos HW, (1990) "The changing incidence of Kaposi's sarcoma among patients with AIDS" *J Am Acad Dermatol;* 22:1250

[562] Moosa, MR., et al., (1998), "Detection and subtyping of human herpesvirus-8 in renal transplant patients before and after remission of Kaposi's sarcoma," *Transplantation;* 66(2): 214-218

invading the central nervous system, which are seen in the homograft patients. The second possible explanation, which I favor, is that the AIDS agent, whatever its nature, is not a cancer virus, but has as its sole action the suppression of cellular immunity. This action opens the way for a multitude of opportunistic pathogens and at the same time releases any clone of transformed, neoplastic cells that happen to turn up."[563,564]

Only in AIDSworld can the director of a major world medical institution make such a morally reprehensible desire calling for human experimentation and then a simultaneous idiotic statement about cellular immunity allowing oncogenic viruses to invade when, in fact, cellular immunity (T helper cells) can only recognize intracellular viruses once they have already invaded the cell. Lewis further stated, "The most remarkable feature of the phenomenon [in transplantation patients], apart from the cancers themselves, has been that a few of these spontaneous tumors have regressed when the immune suppressive drugs were discontinued. On a few occasions, malignant growths the size of a hen's egg or larger, some with already established lymph node metastases, some of them Kaposi's, have been reported to melt away after stopping the drugs."[565] Clearly, Thomas was aware of the relationship between immune-suppressing drugs and transplantation AIDS. The question is why look for an oncogenic virus when the process of drug withdrawal and reversal of cancer and OI had already been demonstrated in another population as a metabolic response without a viral etiology? Why avoid the obvious unless to do a series of human experiments?

Indeed this became a reality when the FDA rushed through in about seventeen weeks a shelved cancer drug that generally takes ten years to get through the approval process. It was a moribund product because it was found not to prevent but to cause cancer[566] and therefore was not authorized for human trials. The AIDS crisis allowed the drug to be repurposed, claiming that it was now a "reverse transcriptase inhibitor" that could target HIV reverse transcriptase, thereby inhibiting viral proliferation in cell cultures.[567] What

---

[563] Thomas, L, (1984), AIDS and the immune surveillance problem, In: Friedman-Kien AE, Laubenstein LJ (ed.)
[564] Kremer, op cit p 68
[565] Thomas, op ci.
[566] Adams, J, (1989) AIDS, The HIV Myth, St. Martin's Press, New York
[567] Mitsuya, H et al. (1985) "3'-Azido-3'-deoxythymidine (BW A509U): an antiviral agent that inhibits the infectivity and cytopathic effect if human T-lymphotropic virus type III/ lymphadenopathy-associated virus in vitro," *Proc. Natl. Acad. Sci. USA*; 82: 7096-7100

the approval of this drug did was to do the desired human experiment and add another chapter in this sad saga of AIDSworld iatrogenic poisoning and deaths. However, AIDSworld quickly and cynically used these tragic deaths to their benefit by promoting an updated version of the Bizet's opera *Carmen*, calling it *Philadelphia* and making Tom Hanks the dying lawyer. It was a good sob story that played well to the American audience by allowing Hollywood to put a human face on this self-inflicted health crisis.

It is of interest that AZT was first isolated from herring and salmon sperm cell extracts in 1961 and synthesized as 3'-azido-3'-deoxythymidine by the Michigan Cancer Foundation.[568] This raises an intriguing issue about the mechanism of fertilization and the role that this compound might play in the disappearance of paternal mitochondria during embryogenesis. The typical mammalian sperm midpiece contains approximately fifty to seventy-five mitochondria with one copy of mtDNA each.[569] The human oocyte contains about one hundred thousand mitochondria—a veritable energetic army. Although the entire sperm enters the oocyte, there is still paucity of research and little understanding as to the fate and the mechanism of disappearance of the of the paternal organelles.[570] Only the maternal mitochondrial genes are transferred to the developing embryo.[571] Research in the area of fertilization and embryogenesis has not answered this intriguing question, but AZT could be a link because although AZT is claimed to be a nucleoside analog reverse transcriptase inhibitor, it does much of its damage by way of its mitochondrial toxicity.[572]

Burroughs Wellcome, the National Cancer Institute, and Duke University claimed that AZT acts as a targeted DNA chain terminator for the HIV virus and that in vivo AZT was two thousand to twenty thousand times more inhibitory to HIV replication than to the nuclear DNA of uninfected cells.[573] Again, what was measured were the nonspecific markers that in AIDSworld are called

---

[568] Horwitz, JP, et al., (1964), "Nucleosides. V. The monomesylates of 1-(2,—deoxy-beta-D-Iyxofuranosyl) thymidine," *J Org Chem*; 29: 2076

[569] Bedford, JM, et al., (1994), "Distinctive features of the gametes and reproductive tracts of the Asian musk shrew, Suncus murinus," *Bio Reprod*; 50(4): 820-834

[570] Hecht, NB., et al., (1984), "Maternal inheritance of the mouse mitochondrial genome is not mediated by a loss or gross alteration of the paternal mitochondrial DNA or by methylation of the oocyte mitochondrial DNA," *Dev Biol*; 102(2):452-461

[571] Giles, RE., et al., (1980), "Maternal inheritance of human mitochondrial," *PNAS U.S.A.*; 77(11):6715-6719

[572] Samuels, DC., (2006), "Mitochondrial AZT metabolism," *IUBMB Life*; 58(7): 403-8

[573] Furman, PA., et al., (1986), "Phosphorylation of 3'-azido-3'-deoxythymidine and selective interaction of the 5'-triphosphate with human immunodeficiency virus reverse transcriptase', *Proc Nat Acad Sci USA*; 83: 8333-8337

HIV; and again, the result of this hyperbole was deadly, even by AIDSworld logic. Chiu and Duesberg[574] made the observation that "even if AZT were to inhibit HIV DNA synthesis, it could not 'selectively' inhibit HIV, as is claimed by the manufacturer [Furman et al., 1986]. Since HIV DNA measures only 10 kb and cell DNA measures 10^6 kb, and since both DNAs are made in vivo simultaneously inside the same cell, cell DNA provides a 10^5-fold bigger DNA target for AZT toxicity than does HIV DNA. Therefore, the 100 fold higher selectivity of AZT claimed for HIV DNA synthesis is immaterial." They further make the observation (if one does agree with HIV as a defined entity) that since what is called HIV can only be found in less than 0.1 percent of susceptible T cells,[575] (1) HIV has already been effectively neutralized and (2) and there is no correlation between the number of HIV infected cells and AIDS,[576] i.e., there are healthy HIV-positive persons who have thirty to forty times more HIV-infected cells than AIDS patients.[577]

AZT, like the antibody test, became a global marketing success even though researchers from Burroughs Wellcome and the NCI and any of the researchers who were involved in the production of this drug were disingenuous as to the actual mechanisms of AZT function in vivo. It was simply assumed that AZT as a hypothetical thymidine analog would be integrated into the DNA in the place of thymidine either by the RT or by one of the DNA polymerases. Theoretically, in the transcription of DNA into RNA, in the thymidine base, the OH group is replaced by an azido group, thereby, with this false insertion, terminating any further nucleotide additions. Therefore, the provirus genome would remain incomplete and stop producing. That is the theory. What is the reality?

AZT is a nucleoside monophosphate. DNA bases are nucleoside triphosphates. The researchers from Burroughs Wellcome, the NCI, and allied institutions somehow assumed that AZT monophosphate, like other nucleotides, would be triphosphorylated in vivo, thereby able to be incorporated into proviral DNA. What was discovered in the decade after the release of the drug by multiple researchers was that only about 1 percent of AZT is transformed to AZT-TP, making the prescribed doses of between 500 and 1,500 mg per day

---

[574] Chiu, DT, Duesberg, PH, (1996), "The toxicity of azidothymidine (AZT) on human and animal cells in culture at concentrations used for antiviral therapy," P.H. Duesberg (ed.). AIDS: Virus-or Drug Induced?, 143-149

[575] Duesberg, PH, (1992), "AIDS acquired by drug consumption and other noncontagious risk factors," *Pharm Therapeutics;* 55: 201-277

[576] Piatek, M, et al, (1993), "High levels of HIV-1 in plasma during all stages of infection determined by competitive PCR," *Science;* 259: 1749-1754

[577] Simmonds, P., et al., (1990) "Human immunodeficiency virus infected individuals contain provirus in small numbers of peripheral mononuclear cells and at low copy numbers," *J Vir;* 64: 864-872

insignificant for the task of inhibition of "HIV provirus DNA" or nuclear DNA as a "DNA terminator"[578] but powerful enough to cause multiple life-threatening side effects including bone marrow suppression[579] and muscle wasting.

That AZT was isolated from fish sperm was a possible clue to its action. An important prerequisite for a successful pregnancy is that the maternal immune system does not reject the fetus. At some point between fertilization and implantation, there is downregulation of Th1 cytokines in favor of Th2 profile.[580] Azidothymidine, as a nitrosative substance, may service to induce this shift; and since the azido groups of this molecule inhibit mitochondrial cytochrome oxidase,[581] not only could it shift the cytokine profile, it could simultaneously disable the paternal mitochondria. This is also why AZT may seem to have some beneficial effect in HIV patients—not because it is able to stop the replication of the "proviral HIV DNA" but because it can attack the cytochrome oxidase in the electron transport system of certain microbes,[582,583] effectively acting as an antibiotic. There is a deficit in research as to whether substances similar to azidothymidine are formed in human sperm cells, but there are indications that similar compounds may be found. Human sperm cells,[584] malignant cancer cells,[585,586] and proliferating microbes[587] contain high amounts of polyamines that are formed in the ornithine decarboxylation cycle. Ornithine decarboxylase inhibitors have been used to treat lethal protozoa

---

[578] Papadopulos-Eleopulos, E., et al.,(1999), "A Critical analysis of the pharmacology of AZT and its use in AIDS," *Cur Med Res & Opin;* 15 supplement

[579] Weinkove, R., et al., (2005), Zidovudine induced pure red cell aplasia presenting 4 years after therapy," *AIDS;* 19(17): 2046-2047

[580] Reinhard, G., et al., (1998), "Shifts in the TH1/TH2 balance during human pregnancy correlate with apoptotic changes," *Biochem Biophys Res Commun;* 245(3): 933-938

[581] Tyler, DD., (1992), The mitochondria in health and disease, VCH Publishers, New York

[582] Lewis, W., et al., (1995), "Mitochondrial toxicity of antiviral drugs," *Nat Med;* 1(5): 417-477

[583] Lewis, W, et al., (2003), "Mitochondrial toxicity of NRTI antiviral drugs: an integrated cellular perspective," *Nat Rev Drug Discov;* 2(10): 812-822

[584] Coffino, P, (2000), "Polyamines in spermiogenesis: not now, darling," *PNAS;* 97(9): 4421-4423

[585] Fozard, JR, Prakash, NJ, (1982), "Effects of dl-α-difluoromethylornithine, an irreversible inhibitor of ornithine decarboxylase, on the rat mammary tumour induced by 7,12-dimethylbenz[a]anthracene," *Naunyn-Schmiedeberg's Arch Pharmacol;* 320:72-77

[586] Davidson, NE., et al., (1999), "Clinical aspects of cell death in breast cancer the polyamine pathway as a new target for treatment," *Endocrine Related Ca;* 6: 69-73

[587] Kusano, T., (2008), "Polyamines: essential factors for growth and survival," *Planta;* 228: 367-381

infections[588] and AIDS-associated PCP.[589] Recently, the University of Minnesota has developed an ornithine decarboxylase inhibitor for cancer therapy.[590] While this may be of some usefulness because the upregulation of the ornithine decarboxylase enzyme is under the regulation of type 2 cytokines acting on L-arginine by the activation of arginase with a simultaneous counterfeedback inhibition on the increased production of NO by the suppression of inducible nitric oxide synthase,[591] it fails to take into account the full spectrum of the metabolic derangements of type 2 cell dis-symbiosis.

Lymphoid cells treated with AZT in vitro had a 60 percent decline in cellular glutathione concentration, loss of mtDNA integrity, and decreased energy production.[592] This is because AZT has two fundamentally negative impacts on mitochondria metabolism: the direct inhibition of enzymes of the respiratory chain[593] and inhibition of the enzymes (DNA polymerase) for the replication of mitochondria.[594] The azido group of azidothymidine N_3 has a triple nitrogen configuration, which is as reactive as nitrosative molecules—NO and its derivatives. As such, the azido group can oxidize metal ions such as those in cytochrome oxidase. It also has the ability to oxidize sulfhydryl groups in thiols (glutathione, cysteine) and thiol proteins (R-SH). This is one of the reasons that azide (N_3) has been used by researchers to inhibit the electron transfer from complex IV to molecular oxygen in the respiratory chain of the mitochondria.[595] However, by inactivating cellular respiration in the OXPHOS system, while being able to have antibacterial effects that target this system in bacteria, protozoa, and fungi, AZT also produces immunosuppressive

---

[588] Sjoerdsma, A., et al, (1984), "Successful treatment of lethal protozoal infections with the ornithine decarbosylase inhibitor, alpha-difluoromethylornithine," *Trans Assoc Am Phys;* 97:70

[589] Gilman, TM., et al., (1986), "Eflornithine treatment of Pneumocystic carinii pneumonia in AIDS," *JAMA;* 256(16): 2197-2198

[590] http://license.umn.edu/technologies/20110052_cancer-treatment-uses-ornithine-decarboxylase-inhibitor 1 August 2014

[591] Hesse, M., et al., (2001), "Differential regulation of nitric oxie synthase 2 and arginase 1 by type1/type2 cytokines in vivo: granulomatous pathology is shaped by the pattern of L-arginine metabolism," *J Imm;* 167(11): 6533-6544

[592] Yamaguchi, T., et al., (2002), "Azidothymidine causes functional and structural destruction of mitochondria, glutathione deficiency and HIV-1 promoter sensitization," *Eur J Biochem;* 269(11): 2782-2788

[593] Benbrik, E., et al., (1997), "Cellular and mitochondrial toxicity of zidovudine (AZT), didanosine (ddI) and zalcitabine (ddc) on cultured human muscle cells," *J Neuro Sci;* 149(1): 19-25

[594] Lewis, W., Dalakas, MC., (1995), "Mitochondrial toxicity of antiviral drugs," *Nat Med;* 1(5): 417-422

[595] Tyler, op. cit.

and carcinogenic effects in humans. Thus, AZT may be able to decrease the microbial stress load for a limited period. However, there is a heavy price to pay.

The immediate response to AZT, depending on dosage and disposition of the patient, can cause a sudden reduction in the ATP produced by blockage of cytochrome c oxidase, leading to apoptosis because of a decrease of the mitochondrial membrane potential and massive increase in Ca^{2+} cycling. If the ratio of ADP to ATP dips below the critical level of 0.2, necrosis ensues.[596]

The introduction of the chronic use of AZT exacerbated an already critically depleted glutathione and thiol pool leading to a balance shift in the type 2 counterregulated cellular dis-symbiosis:[597] decrease in O_2 uptake with a concomitant decrease in OXPHOS ATP synthesis, reduction of mtDNA per cell, increase in glycolysis, and lactate production.[598] Clinically, these patients now not only had a decrease in function of their cell-mediated immunity but also experienced a decrease in the maturation of their red blood cells as well as increased potential for tumorigenesis, degeneration of nerve and muscle cells, liver failure, and wasting syndrome.[599,600,601,602] It was not only the called-for human experimentation but an iatrogenic atomic bomb.

---

[596] Richter, C., (1996), "Nitric Oxide and its congeners in: Moncada S., Bagetta G. (eds.) Nitric oxide and the cell: Proliferation, differentiation an death," Portland Press Limited, London, UK

[597] Lucey, DR., et al., (1996), "Type 1 and Type 2 cytokine dysregulation in human infectious, neoplastic, and inflammatory diseases," *Clin Micro Rev;* 532-562

[598] Hobbs, GA., et al, (1995), "Cellular targets of 3'-azido-3'-deoxythymidine: an early (non-delayed) effect on oxidative phosphorylation," *Biochem Pharmacol;* 50(3):381-390

[599] Cherfas, J., (1989), "AZT still on trial," *Science;* 246(4932): 882

[600] Bach, MC., (1989), "Failure of zidovudine to maintain remission in patients with AIDS.," *NEJM;* 320(9): 594-5

[601] Pluda, JM, et al., (1990), "Development of non-Hodgkin lymphoma in a cohort of patients with severe human immunodeficiency virus (HIV) infection on long-term antiretroviral therapy," *Ann Intern Med;* 113(4):276-282

[602] Dalakas, MC., et al., (1990), "Mitochondrial Myopathy Caused by long term zidovudine therapy," *NEJM;* 322: 1098-1105

CHAPTER 6

Nitric Oxide: The Multifaceted Mighty Mouse of Molecules

At the period in history when poppers were becoming a staple of the gay sex scene, various researchers were beginning to uncover the mysteries of the small molecule, nitric oxide (NO), and its myriad metabolic functions. Had these discoveries been applied in the clinical setting, they would have helped to unravel the AIDS puzzle and avoid thirty years of nonstop nonsense. To date, AIDSworld has continued to ignore this crucial information. This research established the relationship and cellular homeostatic function between the reducing molecule, glutathione, and the oxidizing molecule, nitric oxide (and its congeners). It was discovered that not only was the free radical nitric oxide synthesized in a variety of different mammalian cell types but that this molecule controls and influences a number of critical physiological processes directly through its metabolites and with the counterregulatory action of the reducing agent glutathione.[603,604] NO functions both as a signaling molecule,[605] and as an energy molecule as it participates in the generation of ROS. It is the constant churning of ROS that give rise to the energy of electronic excitation (EEE).[606] It is the EEE that becomes part of the coherent energy in the space/time cell

---

[603] Harbrecht, BG, et al., (1997), "Glutathione regulates nitric oxide synthase in cultured hepatocytes," *Ann Surg;* 225(1): 76-87

[604] Clancy, R, et al., (1994), "Nitric oxide reacts with intercellular glutathione and activates the hexos monophosphate shunt in human neutrophils: evidence for S-nitrosoglutathione as a bioactive intermediary" *PNAS USA;* 91: 3680-3684

[605] Khan, AU, Wilson, T., (1995), "Reactive Oxygen as Second Messengers," *Chem Biol;* 2:437-445

[606] Voeikov, VL, (2006), "Reactive oxygen species—pathogens or sources of vital energy?," *J Alt Compl Med;* 12(2): 111-118

structure that is capable of doing work. NO also has antioxidant properties, not directly but in its ability to inhibit oxygen-initiated ROS chain reactions.[607] It can function as a cytotoxic gas in immune cells,[608] and it was found to control mitochondrial respiration.[609] Importantly, it is the differential regulation by NO feedback that determines the secretion of type 1 or type 2 cytokines that control whether L-arginine will be shuttled into either the nitric oxide synthase or arginase pathway, each having very distinct metabolic consequences.[610] Nitric oxide is the vital link in the mitochondria between energy production and the control of cell death or survival.[611]

NO has a high diffusion capacity and can move freely through cell membranes, acting as both a messenger molecule or a cytotoxic gas. It can interact with molecular oxygen, thiols, and reduced hemoproteins. The nature of the interaction depends on the microcellular environmental conditions under which NO is released and, importantly, the concentration of other bioreactants.[612] In the vascular system, NO has vasodilatory effects based on the activation of the ferrous enzyme[613] guanylate cyclase. In vascular smooth muscle, NO binds with iron in guanylate cyclase, activating the production of cyclic guanosine phosphate, thereby relaxing this muscle and thus lowering blood pressure.[614] In addition to helping to regulate vascular tone, the NO/cGMP signaling pathway inhibits platelet aggregation, neuronal transmission,

---

[607] Zhao, J., (2007), "Interplay among nitric oxide and reactive oxygen species," *Plant Sig Behav;* 2(6): 544-547

[608] Nathan, CF, Hibbs, JB, Jr., (1991), "Role of nitric oxide synthesis in macrophage antimicrobial activity," *Curr Opin Immunol;* 3(1):65-70

[609] Benamar, A., et al., (2008), "Nitrite-nitric oxide control of mitochondrial respiration at the frontier of anoxia," *Biochim Biophys Acta;* 1777(10): 1268-1275

[610] Yeramian, A., et al., (2006), Arginine via cationic amino acid transporter 2 plays a critical role in classical or alternative activation of macrophages," *J Immunol;* 176(10): 5918-5924

[611] Brüne, B., (2003), "Nitric oxide: NO apoptosis or turning it on?," *Cell Death Differen;* 10: 864-869

[612] Kelm, M., et al., (1997), "The nitric oxide-sueroxide assay: insights into the biological chemistry of the O_2/No-interaction," *J Biol Chem:* 272: 9922-9932

[613] Murad, F., et al., (1978), "Guanylate cyclase: Activation by azide, nitro compounds, nitric oxide, and hydroxyl radical and inhibition by hemoglobin and myoglobin" *Advances in Cyclic Nucleotide Res* 9: 145-158

[614] Gruetter, CA., et al., (1979), "Relaxation of bovine coronary artery and activation of coronary guanylate cyclase by nitric oxide, nitroprusside and a carcinogenic nitrosamine," *J Cycl Nucleotide Res;* 5;211-224

and cytostasis.[615,616] High levels of (NO) are involved in hypotension associated with endotoxic shock,[617] inflammatory-response-induced tissue injury,[618] mutagenesis,[619] and formation of carcinogenic N-nitrosamines.[620]

Under the influence of type 1 cytokines, activated macrophages oxidize L-arginine into nitrate and nitrite-forming (NO) gas as an intermediate product used to neutralize intracellular parasites.[621,622] Molecules of (NO) bind to sulfur-containing compounds to create nitrosothiols[623]—a function important to AIDS research as it was ultimately the exhaustion of the thiol pool by nitrosylation of the thiol proteins by a continuous and long-term supply of exogenous nitrite/(NO) (poppers) and endogenous (NO) production (i.e., in response to the innumerable chronic infections), which contributed to the initiating factors in the cellular process of dedifferentiation and counterregulations of the vascular endothelial cells and the immune cells respectively that presented clinically as Kaposi's sarcoma and opportunistic infections. When human plasma is exposed to (NO) or (NO2), a rapid loss of antioxidants (e.g., ascorbic acid, uric acid, and, most importantly, thiols) occurs.[624]

---

[615] Marletta, MA, et al., (1990), "Unraveling the biological significance of nitric oxide," *Biofactors;* 2(4): 219-225

[616] Moncada, S., et al., (1991), "Nitric oxide: physiology, pathophysiology, and pharmacology," *Pharmacol Rev;* 43(2): 109-142

[617] Kilbourn, RG., et al., (1990), "Reversal of endotoxin-mediated shock by NG-methyl-L-arginine, an inhibitor of nitric oxide synthesis," *Biochem Biopohys Res Commun;* 172(3): 1132-1138

[618] Mulligan, MS., et al., (1991), "Tissue injury caused by deposition of immune complexes is L-arginine dependent," *Proc Natl Acad Sci USA;* 88(14): 6338-6342

[619] Nguyen, T., Brunson D., Crespi, CL., et al., (1992), "DNA damage and mutation in human cells exposed to nitric oxide in vitro," *Proc Natl Acad Sci USA;* 89(7): 3030-3034

[620] Miwa, M., Stuehr, DJ, et al., (1987), "Nitrosation of amines by stimulated macrophages," *Carcinogenesis;* 8(7):955-958

[621] Hesse, M., et al., (2001), Differential regulation of nitric oxide synthase-2 and arginase 1 by type1/type 2 cytokines in vivo: granulomatous pathology is shaped by the pattern of L-arginine metabolism," *J Immunol;* 6533-6544

[622] Munder, M, et al., (1998), "Alternative metabolic states in murine macrophages reflected by nitric oxide synthase/arginase balance: competitive regulation by CD4+ T cells correlates with Th1/Th1 phenotype," *J immunol;* 5347-5354

[623] Ignarro, LJ., et al., (1981), "Mechanism of vascular smooth muscle relaxation by organic nitrates, nitrites, nitroprusside and nitric oxide: Evidence for the involvement of S-nitrosothiols as active intermediates," *J Pharmacal Experiment Therapeutics;* 218: 739-749

[624] Halliwell, ML., et al., (1992), "Interaction of Nitrogen dioxide with human plasma," *FEBS Lett;* 313: 62-66

Although compounds that release nitric oxide (NO) in vivo have been used in medical practice for well over one hundred years, it has only been in the last three decades that the extraordinary biological significance and versatility of this small molecule has begun to be appreciated, so much so that it was named Molecule of the Year in 1992.[625] The importance of (NO) in mammalian metabolism was underscored in 1998 when the Nobel Prize for Physiology and Medicine[626] was awarded to Robert Furchgott, Louis Ignarro, and Ferid Murad for the critical work they began in the 1980s, enabling a greater understanding of how this small diffusible paramagnetic molecule could play such an important role in biological signaling. In the 1990s, it was discovered that (NO) could reversibly inhibit mitochondrial respiration at the level of cytochrome oxidase. The more current research has determined that (NO) also plays a role in modulating mitochondrial events that are involved in cell death and transformation.[627]

Nitric oxide is one of the smallest molecules produced by mammalian cells and is composed of one atom of nitrogen and one atom of oxygen. Because it is an uncharged lipophilic molecule, it can diffuse across membranes freely. (NO) has an unpaired electron and is relatively unstable compared to other free radicals. Aside from its reaction with O_2, (NO) mainly reacts by electron gain to form the nitroxyl anion (NO-) and by electron loss to form (NO+), the nitrosonium ion.[628] It has a brief half-life, and shortly after it is produced, it can be oxidized into stable end products nitrite (NO2) and nitrate (NO3).[629] The steady state concentration of (NO) is determined by its rate of formation and its rate of decomposition. Consequently, the half-life is not a constant value and is inversely proportional to the concentration of (NO), so the half-life becomes much longer as nitric oxide becomes more dilute.[630] It is an omnipresent intracellular messenger modulating blood flow, thrombosis, and neural activity. It is also an important element in host defense not directly but after it combines with the superoxide anion to form peroxynitrite. Peroxynitrite interacts with

---

[625] Calabrese, V. et al., (October 2007) "Nitric oxide in the central nervous system: neuroprotection versus neurotoxicity"; *Nature Reviews neuroscience;* 8:766-755

[626] SoRelle, R., "Nobel Prize awarded to scientists for nitric oxide discoveries," *Circ;* 98: 2365-2366

[627] Moncado, S., Erusalimsky, JD, (2001), "Does nitric oxide modulate mitochondrial energy generation and apoptosis?," *Nature;* 3: 214-220

[628] Heslop, RB., Jones, K., (1976), "Inorganic Chemistry" Elsevier, Amsterdam, 1976, pp. 424-432

[629] Lowenstein, CJ., et al, "Nitric oxide: a physiologic messenger" *Ann Intern Med.* 1994 Feb 1;120(3):227-37.

[630] Kelm, M., (1999), "Nitric oxide metabolism and breakdown," *Biochemica et Biophysica Acta;* 1411:273-289

lipids, DNA, and proteins via direct oxidative reactions and via indirect radical mediated mechanisms.[631] These reactions trigger cellular responses ranging from subtle modulations of cell signaling to overwhelming oxidative injury, committing cells to necrosis or apoptosis.[632] Oxidative/nitrosative stress occurs where the steady-state ROS/RNS concentration is transiently or chronically enhanced, disturbing cellular metabolic homeostasis and its regulation and damaging cellular constituents.[633]

Because of the explosion of research into nitric oxide and its intermediates (specifically peroxynitrite) and its role not only in endothelial cells[634] but specifically in the immune system,[635,636] AIDS researchers have had ample opportunity to reassess the question of whether the functional disturbances in the endothelial cells of blood vessels resulting in Kaposi's sarcoma and the imbalance in the immune system giving rise to the "opportunistic infections" of AIDS patients could be the result of an imbalance in nitric oxide–glutathione homeostasis rather than an infectious agent. Certainly, the lack of cytotoxic (NO) gas secondary to the loss of synthesis of type 1 cytokines in T helper cells was decisive in the development of "opportunistic infections." By 1981, clinically, the AIDS problem was clearly defined by a consistent set of parameters: (a.) anergic skin reaction to a DTH stimulus and (b) decrease in the number and capacity for stimulation of T helper cells in the blood serum—both of which indicated an underlying problem with cell mediated immunity, and c.) Increased B-cell activity and specific antibody production—indicative of an intact humoral system.[637,638] Although the AIDS crisis occurred several years

---

[631] Pacher, P, et al., (2007), "Nitric Oxide and perosynitrite in health and disease," *Physiol Rev;* 87:315-424

[632] Pacher, Ibid

[633] Luschak, VI, (2011), "Adaptive response to oxidative stress: bacteria, fungi, plants and animals," *Comparative Biochem & Physiol;* 153(2): 175-190

[634] Ignarro, Op Cit.

[635] Taylor-Robinson, AW., Liew, FY, et al., (1994), "Regulation of the immune response by nitric oxide differentially produced by T helper type 1 and T helper type 2 cells," *Eur J Immunol;* 24: 980-984

[636] Roozendaal, R., et al., (2002), "Interaction between nitric oxide and subsets of human T lymphocytes with differences in glutathione metabolism," *Immunology;* 107: 334-339

[637] Gottlieb, MS, et al., (1981), "Pneumocystis carinii pneumonia and mucosal candidiasis in previously healthy homosexual men-evidence of a new acquired cellular immunodeficiency," *NEJM;* 305: 1425-1431

[638] Masur, H., (1992), "Prevention and treatment of Pneumocystis pneumonia," *NEJM;* 327: 1853-1860

before the work of Mosmann and Coffman[639] demonstrated the identification of functionally distinct T helper cell subsets and cytokine profile response patterns, that the AIDSworld continues to use a test of humoral immunity—the so-called "HIV" antibody test—to assess what is fundamentally a cell-mediated immunity problem speaks volumes to the state of delusional intransigence and the failure to understand the underlying aberrations in metabolic homeostasis in the affected cellular compartments.

The early AIDS patients were unwitting participants in an unregulated medical experiment in which they willingly allowed themselves to be exposed to the long-term inhalation of organic nitrites as well as the repeated exposure to microbial toxins (lipopolysaccharides [LPS]) that separately and/or collectively contributed to the frequent and chronic infections that overwhelmed the ability of the cell-mediated response of the immune system. Because these infectious agents also increase the production of nitric oxide and its metabolites, a feedback inhibition occurred, causing a cytokine profile shift from type 1 to type 2.[640,641] Because of the decrease in the production of inducible nitric oxide synthase in the type 1 immune cells and an increase in the number of type 2 cells that do not produce iNOS, the immune cells were unable to respond appropriately to intracellular parasites with an (NO) gas attack. Rising levels of (NO) gas act as an autofeedback to inhibit the proliferation of Th1 cells and their production of IL-2 and IFN-γ.[642,643] (NO) (and its metabolites) plays a significant role in host defense, acting as a diffusible toxic mediator that can

---

[639] Mossman TR., Coffman RL., (1989), "TH1 and TH2 cells: Different patterns of lymphokine secretion lead to different functional properties," *Ann Rev Immunol;* 7: 145-173

[640] Lucey, DR., (1996), "Type 1 and Type 2 cytokine dysregulation in human infectious, neoplastic and inflammatory diseases.

[641] Kröncke, KD., (1995), "Inducible nitric oxide synthase and its product nitric oxide, a small molecule with complex biological activities," *Biol Chem Hoppe-Seyler;* 376: 327-343

[642] Lincoln, J, et al.,(1997) Nitric Oxide in Health and Disease, Cambridge Univ. Press Cambridge, U.K. p 98

[643] Taylor-Robinson, AW, (1997), "Inhibition of IL-2 production by nitric oxide: a novel self-regulatory mechanism for Th1 cell proliferation," *Immunol Cell Biol;* 75(2): 167-175

attack invading organisms[644,645] and tumors,[646] some of which are too large to be phagocytized.

Certainly, the long-term inhalation of organic nitrites combined with the increased intake of immunosuppressive antibiotics such as trimethoprim/sulfamethoxazole (TMP-SMX) and the repeated exposure to the lipopolysaccharides (LPS)[647] of numerous infectious agents were found to be a consistent part of the recorded histories of the early AIDS patients. When this was combined with AZT, which turned out not to be so much of a reverse transcriptase inhibitor as it is a mitochondrial toxin,[648] the results were another deadly iatrogenic catastrophe. That the consequence of the long-term ingestion and exposure of these known toxic combinations could lead to the AIDS disease spectrum by first the increased formation of elevated levels of (NO) and nitrosamine with resultant cellular damage and finally to the exhaustion of the ability of the type 1 immune cells to upregulate iNOS in response to further challenges seems to have been ignored as an underlying process of immune imbalance by the AIDS paradigm. It certainly explains the constellation of findings in these patients of anergy, failure of immune cell response to mitogenic stimulation, and increased antibody count. While the glutathione issue as a relevant therapeutic option and its relationship to (NO) has also been examined extensively as a perusal of the PubMed website will show, the knowledge of this relationship and the ability to reverse the glutathione deficit unfortunately has not changed the course of clinical intervention.

The Glutathione/Cysteine System

The low-molecular-weight thiol tripeptide glutathione (L-γ-glutamyl-L-cysteinyl-glycine) (GSH), glutathione reductase, and glutaredoxin constitute with the thioredoxin pathway, the two independent arms of the system that

---

[644] Chakravortty, D., Hensel, M., (2003), "Inducible nitric oxide synthase and control of intracellular bacterial pathogens," *Microbes Infect;* 5(7): 621-627

[645] Reiss, CS, Komatsu, T., (1998), "Does nitric oxide play a critical role in viral infection," *J Virol;* 4547-4551

[646] Xu, W., Liu, LZ., (2002), "The role of nitric oxide in cancer," *Cell Res;* 12(5-6): 311-320

[647] MacMicking, J., et al., (1997), "Nitric Oxide and macrophage function," *Ann Rev Immunol;* 15: 323-350

[648] Benbrik, E, et al., (1997), "Cellular and mitochondrial toxicity of zidovudine (AZT), didanosine (ddI) and zalcitabine (ddC) on cultured human muscle cells," *J Neurol Sci;* 149(1): 19-25

assist disulphide bond reduction and redox regulation.[649,650] The GSH tripeptide has many biological roles including protection against reactive oxygen and nitrogen species. It is the most abundant nonprotein thiol in the thiol system, being found in the millimolar range (3 to 10 mM) in most cells and has a low redox potential of -240mV[651]. As the carrier of an active thiol group in the form of a cysteine residue, it acts as an antioxidant either by directly interacting with reactive oxygen/nitrogen species and electrophiles or by operating as a cofactor for various enzymes.[652,653] The reduced and oxidized forms of glutathione (GSH/GSSH) act in concert with other redox active compounds (e.g., NAD(P)H) to regulate and maintain cellular redox homeostasis.[654] GSH, as a reducing agent, is part of the adaptive response against oxidative injury, and changes in thiol content and metabolism can have effects on signaling pathways. Germane to the AIDS story, the effector phase of cytotoxic T cell responses and IL-2 dependent functions (e.g., upregulation of iNOS) are inhibited even by partial depletion of the intracellular glutathione pool.[655] Studies have shown that HIV positive patients, with or without antiretroviral therapy, experience a mean loss of about 10 g of cysteine per day under the assumption that normal sulfate excretion with a standard Western diet is ~3 g per day.[656]

Diverse functions of eukaryotic cells are optimized and coordinated by the organization of compatible chemistries into distinct compartments defined by the structures of lipid-containing membranes, multiprotein complexes, and oligomeric structures of saccharides and nucleic acids. This structural and chemical organization is partly coordinated through cysteine residues of proteins that undergo reversible oxidation reduction and serve as chemical/structural-transducing elements. The central thiol/disulfide redox couples thioredoxin-1, thioredoxin-2, GSH/GSSH and cysteine/cysteine (Cys/

---

[649] Paget, MSB, Buttner, MJ, (2003), "Thiol Based Regulatory Switches," *Annu Rev Genet;* 37:91-121

[650] Kumar, C., Igbaria, A., et al., (2011), "Glutathione revisited: a vital function in iron metabolism and ancillary role in thiol-redox control," *EMBO J;* 2044-2056

[651] Kumar, Ibid

[652] Duan, D. Chen C., (2007), "S-nitrosylation/denitrosylation and apoptosis of immune cells," *Cell & Mol Immunol;* 4(5):353-358

[653] Moster, MW. et al., (2009), "Protein S-nitrosylation in health and disease," *Trends Mol Med;* 14(9):391-404

[654] Jones, D.P., et al., (2011), "Dietary sulfur amino acids effects on fasting plasma cysteine/cystine redox potential in humans"; *Nutrition;* 27(2): 199-203

[655] Dröge, W., et al, (1994), "Functions of glutathione and glutathione disulfide in immunology an immunopathology," *FASB J;* 8:1131-1138

[656] Breitkreutz, R., Holm S., (2000), "Massive loss of sulfur in HIV infection," *AIDS Res Hum Retroviruses;* 16(3): 203-209

CySS), are not in equilibrium with each other and are maintained at distinct nonequilibrium potentials in mitochondria, nuclei, the secretory pathway and the extracellular space.[657] Thus, controlled changes in GSH/GSSG redox potential are associated with the functional state of the cells, varying with differentiation, dedifferentiation, proliferation, or apoptosis and necrosis. The thioredoxin system plays a key role in cellular homeostasis under both oxidative stress and type 2 counterregulatory conditions as it can reduce needed transcriptions factors as the prerequisite for enhanced DNA-binding and -activating activity. It is highly expressed in many cancers.[658]

Cysteine only accounts for ~2 percent of the amino acid content of cells (protein bound, peptide bound, free), making it the least-used amino acid in biology.[659] Even though it seems to have limited use, it is one of the most conserved amino acids in proteins. This is likely because of unique properties that allow cysteine to fulfill crucial functions in cells. Often, the target cysteine is located between an acidic and basic amino acid that supports the general acid/base chemistry of S-nitrosylation/denitrosylation reactions.[660] Sulfur is a large, polarizable, and electron-rich atom and is thus very reactive and able to adopt multiple oxidation states.[661] Cysteine residues are used in enzyme-active sites and play structural roles in iron-sulfur (Fe-S) assembly, heme, as well as zinc finger motifs.[662,663] Cysteine SH can react with neighboring SH groups to form a disulfide bridge; and SH activity also influences whether or not it can adopt other oxidation states, i.e., be reactive enough to sense changes in redox through interactions with H_2O_2. Because mitochondrial GSH is not synthesized in mitochondria, it must rely on synthesis in the cytoplasm and transport into the organelle.[664,665] Transport of GSH is determined by the GSH/GSSH redox

---

[657] Go, YM., Jones, DP, (2008), "Redox compartmentalization in eukaryotic cells," *Biochim Biophys Acta;* 1789(11): 1273-1290

[658] Karlenisu, TC, Tonissen, KF, (2010), "Thioredoxin and cancer: a role for thioredoxin in all states of tumor oxygenation," *Cancers;* 2: 209-232

[659] Huang, B., et al., (2009), "Shear flow increases S-nitrosylation of proteins in endothelial cells," *Cardiovasc Res;* 83(3): 536-546

[660] Stamler, JS, et al., (2001), "Nitrosylation: the prototypic redox-based signaling mechanism," *Cell;* 106: 675-683

[661] Grek, CL, et al., (2013), "Causes and consequences of cysteine s-glutathionylation"

[662] Chepelev, NL, et al., (2011), "Regulation of iron pathways in response to hypoxia," *Free Radic Biol Med;* 50(6): 645-666

[663] Lill, R., (2009), "Review Article function and biogenesis of iron-sulphur proteins," *Nature;* 460: 831-838

[664] Griffith OW, Meister A.(1985), "Origin and turnover of mitochondrial glutathione" *PNAS USA;* 82: 4668–4672

[665] Kurosawa K, Hayashi N, et al., (1990) "Transport of glutathione across the mitochondrial membranes" *Biochem Biophys Res Commun;*167:367–372

state and stimulated by mitochondrial substrates, e.g., malate or pyruvate, and inhibited by excessive glutamate or disruption of the protonmotive force with proton ionophores.[666]

The calculated midpoint potential for GSH to glutathione disulfide (GSSG) ratio in the cytosol is

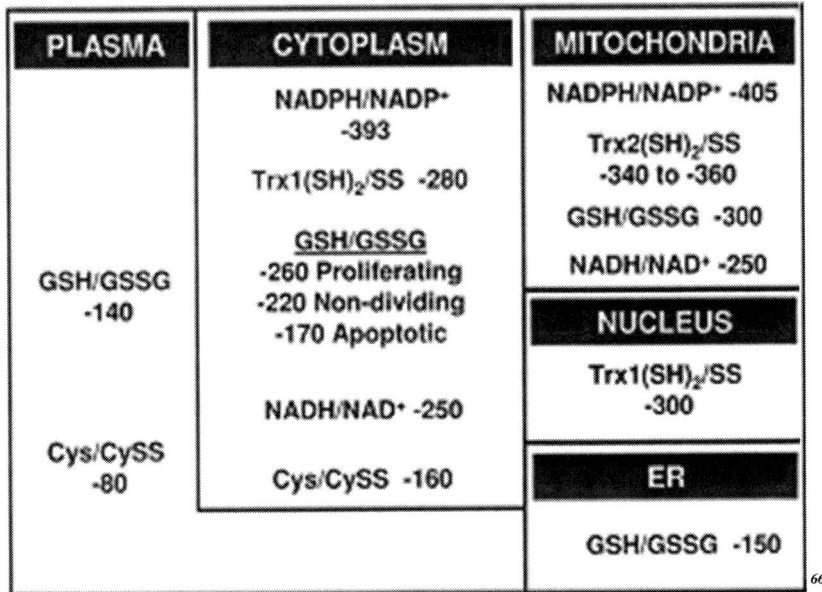

Figure 1

−240mV.[668] Because redox potentials are further influenced by pH, the alkalinity of the matrix lowers the potential even further (figure 1).[669] The interaction of the cysteine/glutathione system with ROS and RNS is required for redox signaling.

In addition to these functions, GSH plays organelle-specific roles in the mitochondria including apoptosis. Because mitochondria produce the lion's share of cellular ROS (~90 percent), glutathione acts as a pivotal molecule in cellular homeostasis. GSH may either directly bind some ROS species or serve as a source of reductive power for certain antioxidant systems. The inner mitochondrial membrane is rich in cardiolipin, a lipid, whereas it is virtually

---

[666] Go, YM., Op cit.
[667] Kemp, M. Op cit. chart requires author's permission for use
[668] Go, YM., Op cit
[669] Kemp, M, et al., (2008), "Nonequilibrium thermodynamics of thiol/disulfide redox systems: a perspective on redox systems biology," *Free Radic Biol Med;* 44:921-937

absent from other membranes and only the outer mitochondrial membrane contains minor amounts of this phospholipid. When mGSH levels are compromised, cardiolipin is one of the important targets of oxidative damage. Because of its unique chemical structure among phospholipids, cardiolipin supports both stability and fluidity to the mitochondrial membrane and plays an important role in energy metabolism, mainly by providing stability for the individual enzymes and enzyme complexes involved in energy production. In addition, cytochrome c is normally bound to the inner mitochondrial membrane by its association with cardiolipin. By protecting cardiolipin from oxidative damage, GSH prevents changes in the physicochemical properties of the mitochondrial inner membrane that lead to membrane destabilization and the dissociation of cytochrome c. ROS may also induce an increase in permeability of the internal mitochondrial membrane for calcium. Enhanced ROS and calcium levels, acting together, may trigger the cell death signals, leading to apoptosis or necrosis.[670]

There are any number of conditions that are known to change intracellular GSH content: presence of heavy metals,[671] heat shock,[672] high glucose concentrations,[673] exposure to reactive oxygen and nitrogen species including H_2O_2,[674] nitric oxide and its congeners,[675] and compounds that can generate ROS.

---

[670] Lushchak, VI., (2011), "Glutathione homeostasis and functions: potential targets for medical interventions," *J Amino Acids;* 2012: 1-26

[671] Woods, JS., Ellis, ME, (1995), "Up-regulation of glutathione synthesis in rat kidney by methyl mercury. Relationship to mercury induced oxidative stress," *Biochem Pharmacol;* 50: 1719-1724

[672] Kondo, T., et al, (1993), "γ-Glutamylcysteine synthetase and active transport of glutathione S-conjugate are responsive to heat shock in K562 erythroid cells"; *J Biol Chem:* 268: 20366-72

[673] Urata, Y. et al., (1996), "Long exposure to high glucose concentration impairs the responsive expression of gamma glutamylcysteine synthetase by interleukin-1 beta and tumor necrosis factor-alpha in mouse endothelial cells," *J Bio Chem:* 271: 15146-52

[674] Rahman, I., et al, (1996), "Transcriptional regulation of γ-glutamylcysteine synthetase-heavy subunit by oxidants in human aveolar epithelial cells," *Biochem Biophys Res Commun:* 229L832-837

[675] Moellering, D., et al., (1999), "The induction of GSH synthesis by nanomolar concentrations of NO in endothelial cells: a role for gamma-glutamylcysteine synthase and gamma-glutamyl transpeptides," *FEBS lett:* 448: 292-306

The Slow Death of the AIDS/Cancer Paradigm and the Apocrypha of the Eukaryotic Cell

By 1989, it was well established that there was a systemic glutathione deficiency in even symptom-free HIV positive individuals.[676,677] They were found to have subnormal glutathione levels in plasma,[678] lung epithelial lining fluid,[679] individual CD4+T cells,[680] and peripheral blood mononuclear cells.[681] A 1997 study by Herzenberg, et al., found that glutathione deficiency is associated with impaired survival in HIV disease[682] and argued that unnecessary or excessive use of drugs known to deplete GSH levels should be avoided by HIV-infected individuals. Even though it was discovered that one of the mainstay "antiretroviral" drugs in the AIDS armamentarium, azidothymidine, decreased both ATP production and GSH in vitro, MOLT 4 human lymphoid cells[683] and other studies indicate that AZT's toxic interactions result from the generation of ROS that react with and deplete intracellular glutathione levels, it continues to be used in the HAART treatment protocol. [684,685,686] There has been no effort in treatment protocols for replacement therapy. Protease inhibitors were likewise discovered to decrease ATP production and GSH levels in pancreatic

---

[676] Buhl, R., et al. "Systemic glutathione deficiency in symptom free HIV seropositive individuals," *Lancet.* 1989 Dec 2;2(8675):1294-8.

[677] Eck, HP, et al, (1989), "Low concentrations of acid soluble thiol (cysteine) in the blood plasma of HIV-1 infected patients," *Biol Chem Hope Seyler;* 370(2):101-8

[678] Helbling, B., et al., (1996) "Decreased release of glutathione into the systemic circulation of patients with HIV infection," *Eur J Clin Invest;* 26:38-44

[679] Buhl, R., et al., (1989) "Systemic glutathione deficiency in symptom-free HIV-seropositive individuals"; *Lancet;* 2(865):1294-8

[680] Staal, F.J., et al., (1992) "Glutathione deficiency and human immunodeficiency virus infection," *Lancet;* 339(8798):909-12

[681] de Quay, et al., (1992) "Glutathione depletion in HIV-infected patients: role of cysteine deficiency and effect of oral N-acetylcysteine," *AIDS;* 6(8):815-9

[682] Herzenberg, LA., et al., (1997), "Glutathione deficiency is associated with impaired survival in HIV disease," *Proc Natl Acad Sci USA;* 94: 1967-1972

[683] Yamaguchi, T., et al., (2002), "Azidothymidine causes functional and structural destruction of mitochondria, glutathione deficiency and dHIV-1 promoter sensitization," *Eur J Biochem;* 269(11) 2782-8

[684] de la Asuncion, JG., et al., (1998), "AZT treatment induces molecular and ultrastructural oxidative damage to muscle mitochondria. Prevention by antioxidant vitamins," *J Clin Invest;* 102(1): 4-9

[685] Gogu, SR., et al., (1991), "Protection of zidovudine induced toxicity against murine erythroid progenitor cells by vitamin E," *Exp Hematol;* 19: 649-652

[686] Prakash, O, et al., (1997), "The human immunodeficiency virus type 1 Tat protein potentiates zidovudine induced cellular toxicity in transgenic mice," *Arch Biochem Biophys;* 343(2): 173-180

beta cells,[687] as well as primary astrocytes.[688] The key role of glutathione in the reduction of reactive oxygen and nitrogen species and the finding that this key antioxidant was consistently deficient in HIV positive and AIDS patients was a clue to not only the expressed immune imbalance but the underlying energy deficit as well.

The question that has not been asked and answered by the AIDS research literature is how the depletion of the thiol pool could lead to the chain of events that presented both as dedifferentiation of vascular endothelial cells (Kaposi's sarcoma) and a depletion of a subset of CD4+T cells, allowing for the rise of opportunistic infections (PCP)? Any theory of disease causation would have to have a logical explanation for these seemingly incongruous phenomena that the HIV/AIDS theory has not been able to provide.

The Discovery of NO Versatility in Mammalian Cells Was Hailed as a Phenomenon

The discovery of the various roles of nitric oxide was received with considerable excitement once it was realized and demonstrated that this molecule had such a versatility of functions and wide-ranging effects on numerous subsystems. Not only is it an autocrine and paracrine signaling molecule and acts as a cytotoxic gas in immune cells, it is now understood that nitric oxide plays a central role in the dynamic energy flows of the organism. At every level of the cell, whether it is the water in the coherent domains, the persistent generation of reactive oxygen/nitrogen species—which generate the energy of electronic excitation, the role of the mitochondria in the production of ATP, or the transfer of energy production to glycolysis in the cytoplasm—it is the disruption of these flows that are primary to the material manifestations of the consequent regulation of genes and proteins. It is the disruption of the energy flows that determine whether or not a tissue remains healthy or becomes diseased. As expressed by Bauer's theory of the living state discussed in the introduction, it is the underlying energy available as defined as a stable nonequilibrium state that sustains the work a living system performs against sliding toward equilibrium. According to Bauer, a living system extracts matter and energy from its environment, expending its resources to obtain them,

---

[687] Chandra, Surabhi, et a., (2008), "HIV-1 protease inhibitors suppress insulin secretion in pancreatic β cells: role of oxidative stress and endoplasmic reticulum stress and protection by thymoquinone (TQ)," *FASEB J;* 22: 1131.2

[688] Arend, C. et al., (2013), "The antiretroviral protease inhibitor ritonavir accelerates glutathione export from cultured primary astroyctes," *Neurochem Res;* 38(4): 732-741

and transforms this energy/matter into higher-quality energy of excitation of its own structures. It is by the creation of these energy flows that the material system is organized, taking it far from thermodynamic equilibrium by raising its energy level, producing gradients and cyclic flow patterns of materials (and energy).[689] This is done by constant electron transfer. NO plays a significant role in the energy cycle of the cell by participating in the cycling of ROS/RNS and the regulation of oxygen consumption in the mitochondria. By competing with oxygen, NO is able to inhibit the heme/copper enzyme cytochrome c oxidase in both an oxygen-competitive and an oxygen-independent manner.[690] Thus, the function of NO has to be considered contextually not only in its role as gatekeeper for the rate of oxidative phosphorylation and energy production as ATP in the mitochondria but for its cytotoxic role in the adaptive immune system.

NO is an intermediate between molecular oxygen (O_2) and nitrogen (N_2). All three have low solubility and readily diffuse through membranes as easily as through cytoplasm.[691] Molecular oxygen has two unpaired electrons in separate orbitals, which inhibit its reactivity with most biomolecules; however, these unpaired electrons make it possible for molecular oxygen to strongly bind to metals such as the iron in hemoglobin and in cytochrome c oxidase. Molecular oxygen has a rapid reaction time with unpaired electrons on other free radicals and can initiate a chain reaction of cascading free radicals. This can be beneficial in creating the energy of electronic excitation that helps maintain cellular structural integrity.[692] However, if not able to be adequately reduced, it may contribute to structural damage by way of oxidative stress.

In contradistinction, nitrogen gas (N_2) is one of the most inert molecules. Because NO is a hybrid between molecular nitrogen and oxygen (has only one unpaired electron), NO is generally less reactive than molecular oxygen but is also able to strongly bind to the iron in heme groups.

This characteristic is the key to its biological activity in activating guanylate cyclase and slowing mitochondrial respiration by binding to cytochrome-c oxidase.[693] Like molecular oxygen, NO may react with free radicals, but as

---

[689] Ho, MW, "The Rainbow and the Worm, the Physics of Oranisms" World Scientific, New Jersey 2008 p 40

[690] Cooper, CE., Giulivi, C., (2006), "Nitric oxide regulation of mitochondrial oxygen consumption II: molecular mechanism and tissue physiology," *Am J Physiol Cell Physiol;* 292: C1993-C2003

[691] Pacher, P. et al., (2007), "Nitric oxice and peroxynitrite in health and disease," *Physiol Rev;* 87: 315-424

[692] Voeikov, V., (2001), "Reactive oxygen species, water, photons, and life," *Rivsta di biol/Bio Forum;* 193-214

[693] Pacher, Ibid

oxygen is a free radical chain initiator, NO is chain terminating. NO can convert thiol radicals (R-SH) into nitrosothiols (RSNO) by acting as a chain terminating agent: RS• + •NO → RS-NO.[694] The chain-terminating reactions explain some of the antioxidant properties attributed to NO. NO does not directly repair radical damage as traditional antioxidants (ascorbate, glutathione, tocopherol) but forms transient intermediate products that can often be repaired by antioxidants to regenerate the original compound.[695] Depending on cellular conditions, e.g., availability of reducing agents, nitrosative stress can be oxidative or antioxidative. This distinction will become central to the understanding of type 2 cellular dis-symbiosis as opposed to type 1. In type 1 cellular dis-symbiosis, an overload of acute oxidative/nitrosative stressors overwhelms the counterregulation of the thiol pool and other antioxidant systems. Depending on the disposition of the patient, acute type 1 dis-symbiosis may be short lived—a week or so—before there is a return to a more balanced homeostatic state.

However, type 2 cellular dis-symbiosis is a more chronic situation in which increased nitrosylation of thiol proteins can lead to a decrease in mitochondrial OXPHOS energy production with a concomitant rise in glycolytic energy production, a decrease in the reducing capabilities for RONS, a decreased transfer of hydrogen ions from the glycerol-3-phosphate, and malate aspartate shuttles to the mitochondria with a consequent surplus of hydrogen ions diffusing from mitochondria to the cytoplasm, creating an "antioxidant" stress and a different set of (mostly reductive) signals, which can augur cellular degeneration, dedifferentiation, and repeated mitotic events. Clinically, this can present with a variety of chronic and degenerative diseases including AIDS and cancer.

More on Nitric Oxide

Nitric oxide is generated in many mammalian tissues and is an important mediator of both physiological and pathological responses.[696] It is derived from the oxidation of one of the terminal quinidine nitrogens of L-arginine.[697,698] It

---

[694] Pacher, Op cit.
[695] Pacher, Op cit.
[696] Carafoli, E., "Intracellular Calcium Homeostasis," *Ann Rev Biochem;* 56:395-433 July 1987
[697] Moncada S., et al., (1991), "Nitric oxide: physiology, pathophysiology and pharmacology," *Pharmacol Rev;* 45: 109-113
[698] Nathan, C., Xie. QW., (1994), "Nitric oxide synthases: roles, tolls, and controls," *Cell;* 78: 915-919

is synthesized by a family of three isoforms of the enzyme nitric oxide synthase (NOS).[699] This family of enzymes converts arginine and molecular oxygen to citrulline and NO in the presence of NADPH and tetrahydrobiopterin (BH_4), FAD, FMN, calmodulin, heme, and O_2.[700] In mammals, NO has a number of physiological functions, both beneficial and detrimental. The beneficial properties of NO have been noted in the regulation of vascular relaxation, platelet aggregation, neurotransmission, cellular respiration, and modulation of immune responses. Detrimental effects of NO include severe vasodilation and myocardial depression during bacterial sepsis,[701] cytotoxic tissue damage associated with autoimmune and chronic allergic inflammation,[702] pathological production of misfolded proteins, and abnormal mitochondrial dynamics including mitochondrial fission and fusion events.[703]

NO, as a signaling molecule, communicates information in a variety of ways. The production of cGMP by guanylate cyclase is the major signal transduction mechanism of NO. Soluble guanylate cyclase contains the same heme protoporphyrin IX as hemoglobin with iron in the ferrous form that binds NO[704] with great affinity. Deoxyhemoglobin binds NO with a ten-thousand-fold greater affinity than molecular oxygen.[705] NO can also diffuse from where it is synthesized into surrounding cells where it will activate soluble guanylate cyclase to produce cGMP, which can then activate cGMP-dependent kinases in the target tissue that modulates intracellular calcium levels.[706] Unlike other signaling molecules that may be recognized by receptors by their shape, NO, with only two atoms, transfers information not by shape but by local concentration. The longer NO is present, the greater the amount of cGMP formed. This system depends on NO being constantly removed, or else, guanylate cyclase will remain fully activated.[707]

---

[699] Rizzuto, R., et al., "Mitochondrial Ca2+ homeostasis in intact cells," *J Cell Biol.* 1994 Sep;126(5):1183-94.

[700] Marletta, MA., (1993), "Nitric oxide synthase structure and mechanism," *J Bio Chem;* 268: 12231-12234

[701] Darwich, SS., (2012), "Inducible Nitric oxide synthase contributes to immune dysfunction following trauma," *Shock;* 38(5): 499-507

[702] Bogdan C., (2001), "Nitric oxide and the immune response," *Nat Immunol;* 2:907-916

[703] Nakamura, T., Lipton, SA, (2011), "S-mitrosylation of critical protein thiols mediates protein misfolding and mitochondrial dysfunction in neurodegenerative diseases," *Antiox Redox Signal;* 14(8): 1479-1491

[704] Pacher, op cit.

[705] Sharma, VS., et al., (1987), "Reaction of nitric oxide with heme proteins and model compounds of hemoglobin," *Biochem;* 26:3837-3843

[706] Pacher, op cit.

[707] Pacher, op cit.

NO is a small hydrophobic molecule that crosses cell membranes without channels or receptors as readily as molecular oxygen and carbon dioxide. The diffusion coefficient of NO in water at 37 degrees is slightly faster than oxygen and carbon dioxide,[708] which allows for the rapid transmission of information over short distances. The average molecular velocity of a molecule with the mass of NO is ~400 m/s at room temperature. The trajectory of NO in solution is repeatedly changed, making ~10 billion collisions each second, but the signaling generally takes place in the confines of subcellular compartments.

NO is generated by at least three (and, with the recognition of mtNOS, possibly 4) isoforms of NO synthases (NOS): nNOS (also known as type I), first identified as being expressed in neuronal cells of the central and peripheral nervous systems and now known to be expressed also in other types of cells, e.g., skeletal muscle and some epithelial cells; eNOS (also known as type 3), first identified in vascular endothelial cells; and iNOS (also known as type 2), which, unlike nNOS, eNOS, and mtNOS, is usually not constitutively expressed but can be induced in a wide range of cell types. Unlike eNOS and nNOS, it is Ca^{2+} independent but is tightly bound to calmodulin. It is absent from resting cells but is expressed in response to proinflammatory cytokines (e.g. IFN-γ, TNF-α and IL-1β and IL-2) and/or microbial stimuli (LPS). Again, unlike nNOS and eNOS, the activity of iNOS is independent of the extracellular calcium concentration in the physiological range.[709] A mitochondrial NOS isoform (mtNOS) has been described similarly to nNOS and eNOS as constitutively expressed as a preformed protein of the mitochondrial inner membrane that generates NO in a Ca^{2+} dependent reaction, binding to calmodulin.[710] NO is pleiotropic and mediates multiple different functions by acting on most cells via interaction with various molecular targets from superoxide anion to protein macromolecules, which can be activated or inhibited through the oxidation of thiols, hemes, Fe-S clusters, and other nonheme prosthetic groups of macromolecules.[711,712,713]

---

[708] Wise, DL. et al., (1968), "Diffusion coefficients of neon, drypton, xenon, carbon monoxide and nitric oxide in water at 10-60° C," *Chem Eng Sci;* 23: 1211-1216

[709] Moncada, S. et al., Nitric Oxide and the cell, proliferation, differentiation, and death 1998 Portland Press Ltd., London p 1

[710] Ghafourifar, P., Cadenas, E. (2005) "Mitochondrial nitric oxide synthase." *Trends Pharmacol Sci* 26:190-195

[711] Nathan, C., (1992), "Nitric oxide as a secretory product of mammalian cells," *FASEB J;* 6: 3051-3064

[712] Kolb, H, Kolb-Bachofen, V., (1992), "Nitric oxide: a pathological factor in autoimmunity," *Immunol Today;* 13: 157-160

[713] Nathan, Xie, Op cit.

Inducible NOS has been generally described as the immunological NOS, and macrophages are the prototypes iNOS-expressing cells.[714] Within the immune system, iNOS is also expressed in monocytes/macrophages from the blood, bone marrow, lung, peritoneum, liver (Kupffer cells), kidney (mesangial cells) and central nervous system (microglia), as well as neutrophils and T lymphocytes.[715] Two subsets of the CD4+ Th cells, Th1 and Th2, have been classified based on the differential pattern of cytokine secretion and the production of iNOS.[716] Th2 cells that secrete IL-4 tend to suppress the inflammatory state of macrophages but are thought to be active in the production of antibodies by B lymphocytes. Th1 cells that secrete IL-1β and IL-2 stimulate macrophages to release inflammatory mediators.[717] Type 2 NOS can be induced in Th1 cells to produce large amounts of NO but not Th2 cells.[718] NO exerts a self-regulatory effect on Th1 cells by inhibiting the production of IL-2 and IFN-γ in these cells in a balanced feedback loop. IL-2 is an essential growth factor for T cells, particularly Th1 cells and CD8+ cells. It should be noted that NO exerts its antiproliferative effect only at relatively high concentrations. Thus, NO operates as an important autoregulatory molecule, preventing the overexpression of Th1 and CD8+ T cells and the excessive overproduction of NO. Th2 cells can proliferate in the presence of IL-4, the production of which is not affected by NO. NO produced in Th1 cells also contributes directly toward microbicidal and tumoricidal effects and tissue destruction attributed to the NO produced by activated macrophages.[719]

NO can be converted to NO_2, NO_2^-, NO_3^-, and other reactive nitrogen intermediates (RNI), among which are S-nitrosothiols (S-NO), peroxynitrite (OONO⁻), and nitrosyl-metal complexes, which are directly implicated in the NOS-mediated post-translational regulation of proteins S-nitrosylation of cysteines, nitration of tyrosines, and nitrosylation of these respective prosthetic

---

[714] Stuehr, DJ., et al., (1991), "Purification and characterization of the cytokine induced macrophage nitric oxide synthase: An FAD and FMN containing flavoprotein," *Proc Natl Acad Sci USA;* 88:7773-7777

[715] Lincoln, J. et al, (1997) "Nitric Oxide in health and Disease" Cambridge University Press p 85

[716] Roitt, I (1994), Essential Immunology, 8th ed. London: Blackwell Scientific Publications

[717] Barnes, PJ, & Liew, FY, (1995), "Nitric oxide and asthmatic inflammation," *Immunology Today;* 16: 128-30

[718] Ibid

[719] Taylor-Robinson, AW., et al., (1994), "Regulation of the immune response by nitric oxide differentially produced by T helper type 1 and T helper type 2 cells," *Eur J Immunol;* 24: 980-984

groups.[720] The products of some of these reactions are then able to react further at nucleophilic centers, of which thiols are a major group. Thus, the main target sites for NO within the cell are metal- and thiol-containing proteins and low-molecular-weight thiols.[721] This, of course, provides a wide range of targets, many of which are biologically active and are involved in a diverse array of metabolic pathways. The seemingly random nature of the interactions that NO can undergo does not appear conducive to its producing a predictable response either as a physiological messenger or as a cytotoxic agent. However, there are two factors that are likely to have a major influence on the final outcome. First, the reactions that can occur are likely to be dependent on the concentration of NO present. Thus, the high levels of NO produced by iNOS will trigger a set of reactions that will not occur during low level of NO synthesis by eNOS and nNOS. Second, the internal environment of the cell can substantially alter the nature of the reactions that can occur. Together with the level of NO, this probably determines whether the overall effect is toxic or not.

It is not known whether there is any selectivity with regard to the thiol groups with which NO interacts. However, under conditions of oxidative/nitrosative stress, the available intracellular thiol pool is depressed. It may be that in these circumstances, additional thiol proteins may become susceptible to NO. The high levels of NO produced by iNOS have been shown to cause nitrosylation of the glycolytic enzyme, glyceraldehyde-3-phosphate dehydrogenase (GDAPH).[722] Following nitrosylation, GDAPH can undergo ADP-ribosylation. This is an irreversible process resulting in inhibition of enzyme activity. It has been suggested that NO may mediate some of its cytotoxic effects by this mechanism since it would reduce the capacity of the target cell for energy production.[723]

Under stable homeostatic conditions, NO can react with O_2 to produce nitrite, and it is by this pathway that NO is excreted.[724] NO also reacts with superoxides to form peroxynitrite (OONO⁻), which subsequently produces hydroxyl radicals.[725] It has been proposed that a major factor in determining whether or not NO is cytotoxic is the intracellular concentration

---

[720] Hess, DT., (2005), "Protein S-nitrosylation: Purview and parameters," *Nat Rev Mol Cell Biol;* 6:150-166

[721] Stamler, JS., "Redox signaling: nitrolysation and related target interactions of nitric oxide" *Cell'* 78:931-6, 1994

[722] catalyzes the 6th step of glycolysis, also involved in transcription and apoptosis

[723] Brüne, et al., "Nitric Oxide, a signal for ADP-ribosylation of proteins"; 1994 *Life Sciences;* 54:61-70

[724] Änggård, E. 1994, "Nitric Oxide: mediator, murderer, and medicine" *Lancet;* 343:1199-1206

[725] Beckman, JS, et al, 1994 "Oxidative chemistry of peroxynitrite: *Methods in Enzymology* 233:229-40

of superoxides.[726] Superoxide levels within cells are normally low. However, activated macrophages and neutrophils can produce NO and superoxides at similar rates.[727] Increased levels of both of these reactive species will also deplete the thiol pool. A combination of these events would provide an environment where NO would be more likely to form peroxynitrite and hydroxyl radicals, and these are more toxic than NO itself.[728,729] The hydroxyl radical is a powerful mutagen, and peroxynitrite causes extensive protein tyrosine nitration. The nitration of tyrosine residues to 3-nitro-tyrosine represents an oxidative post-translational modification that disrupts nitric oxide signaling and skews metabolism toward pro-oxidant processes.[730]

Cells possess protective mechanisms in the face of oxidative stress and for internal homeostasis that includes superoxide dismutase (SOD, the superoxide scavenger) and catalase (peroxide scavenger), two enzymes that help to maintain redox homeostasis. However, ROS have a much bigger role to play in cell metabolism. They participate in most if not all cellular reactions upon external stimuli. The particular reaction of a given cell depends not only on the interaction of the specific molecular signal with the specialized receptor but also on the "context"—previous history of a cell, its current state—and also on the background level and composition of ROS. The latter preconditions depend both upon the manner in which ROS are generated by a cell itself or on their incoming flow and on the rate of their elimination.[731] Thus, clinically, someone who has reduced their glutathione levels to greater than 30 percent as was found in AIDS and pre-AIDS patients could never be considered to be "previously healthy." If there is a continuation of intake of toxic stressors, in the form of poppers and other street drugs or trimethoprim/sulfamethoxazole or antiretrovirals, the clinical consequence will be continued energy reduction and immune suppression—no virus need apply.

It will be considered in the next chapter on the discussion about mitochondrial energy production that these enzymes (SOD, catalase) also have a much bigger role to play in cellular energy production. The turnover numbers

---

[726] Lipton, SA., et al, 1993, "A redox based mechanism for the neuroprotective and neurodestructive effects of nitric oxide and related nitroso compounds" *Nature;*
[727] Beckman, Op Cit
[728] Dinerman, JL, et al, "Molecular mechanisms of nitric oxide regulation: potential relevance to cardiovascular disease" 1993 *Circulation Research;* 73:217-22
[729] Lincoln, J, et al, "Nitric Oxide in health and disease" 1997 Cambridge Univ. Press, Cambridge, UK 23-25
[730] Radi, R., (2013), "Protein tyrosine nitration: biochemical mechanisms and structural basis of functional effects," *Acc Chem Res;* 46(2): 550-559
[731] Voeikov, V., (2001), "Reactive Oxygen Species, water, photons, and life," *Revista di biologia/Biology Forum;* 94: 193-214

for SOD and catalase exceed 10^6 cycles/sec.[732] The question becomes might such an excessive rate of radical production have a function other than cellular structural damage? As it happens, "ROS are major participants of continuous flows of highly non-linear processes in which electron excited species emerge. These processes play a significant role in energy and informational flows in all living systems. . . . Energy released in such reactions is used as an activation energy for the specific biochemical processes, for the continuous 'pumping' of the non-equilibrium state of inter and intracellular structural components."[733] Interestingly, certain cytokines can also induce or inhibit SOD[734]/catalase;[735] therefore, it has been speculated that the cells that generate high levels of NO via type 2 (iNOS) may have a natural defense in place against the toxic effects of NO. However, targets for NO-mediated toxicity (invading microorganisms or tumor cells) could be less resistant.[736]

High levels of NO produced by activation of macrophages have been shown to attack a number of enzymes that contain Fe-S groups. Enzymes in the mitochondrial electron transport chain (NADH:ubiquinone oxidoreductase and NADH:succinate oxidoreductase) are both inhibited by NO.[737] In addition, the activity of cis-aconitase[738]—which has an active Fe-S cluster, a cytoplasmic enzyme forming part of the tricarboxylic acid cycle—is reduced by NO. In this case, inhibition appears to occur via peroxynitrite rather than NO itself.[739] NO acts as a double-edged sword as NO-induced changes may alternatively improve cellular energy dynamics or cause energy depletion within the target cell.

---

[732] Fee, JA, Bull, C, (1986), "Steady state kinetic studies of superoxide dismutases. Saturative behavior of the copper and zinc containing protein," *J Biol Chem;* 261:13000-13005

[733] Voeikov, V., (2001), op cit.

[734] Kemp, K., (2010), "Inflammatory cytokine induced regulation of superoxide dismutase 3 expression in human mesenchymal stem cells," *Stem Cell Rev;* 6(4): 548-559

[735] Chen, H., Li, X, Epstein, PN., (2005), "MnSOD and catalase transgenes demonstrate that protection of islets from oxidative stress does not alter cytokine toxicity," *Diabetes;* 54(5): 1437-46

[736] Stamler, Op Cit

[737] Stuehr, DJ., 1989 "Nitric Oxide: a macrophage product responsible for cytostasis and respiratory inhibition in tumor target cells: *J Exp Med;* 169:1543-55

[738] another Fe-S protein, In the tricarboxylic acid cycle, catalyses the isomeration of citrate to isocitrate

[739] Hibbs, JB., et al. 1988 "Nitric oxide: a cytotoxic activated macrophage effector molecule" *Biochemical and Biophysical Research Communications,* 157:87-94

Ribonucleotidase activity is also reduced by NO resulting in cytostasis in tumor cells.[740] Both DNA damage and NO itself activate poly ADP ribose synthetase (PARS).[741] Rapid activation of this enzyme depletes the intracellular concentration of its substrate, nicotinamide adenine dinucleotide (NAD), thus slowing the rate of glycolysis, electron transport, and, subsequently, ATP formation, a process that can result in cell dysfunction and death.[742] Finally, under conditions where fewer thiol groups are available for interaction (e.g., oxidative stress as in the long-term use of poppers and exposure to various and repeated infectious agents), nucleophilic centers on DNA become potential targets for NO.

Because immune cells produce cytotoxic NO gas, the question of crucial interest to AIDS research was that if NO synthesis is inhibited in mammalian immune cells, would this lead directly to a measurable reduction of the immune defense against microbial agents? The question central to infectious disease medicine, in fact, was raised and tested in any number of experiments.[743]

Several research groups have blocked the synthesis of iNOS in mice by either blocking the gene responsible for the expression of the inducible NOS enzyme or by using iNOS inhibitors. These experiments have demonstrated that without sufficient production of NO, the immune cells lose their ability to restrain or kill microbial agents and that these mice were very susceptible to viral, bacterial, and parasitic infections.[744,745,746]

It is a principle of complex organisms that they must have available energy at will, whenever and wherever required, and in a perfectly coordinated way. Much of the energy supplied is by electron transfer, which is accomplished by redox reactions. Since the energy that is available is in the form of electrons,

---

[740] Lepoivre, M, et al., 1990 "Alterations of ribonucleotide reductase activity following induction of the nitrite generating pathway in adnocarcinoma cells: *J of Biological Chem;* 265:(14)143-9

[741] Zang, J, et al., 1994 "Nitric oxide activation of poly(ADP-ribose) synthetase in neurotoxicity" *Science;* 263:687-9

[742] Szabó, C., Dawson, VL., (1998), "Role of poly (ADP ribose) senthetase in inflammation and ischaemia reperfusion," *Trends Pharmacol Sci;* 19(7): 287-98

[743] Kremer, Op Cit. 38

[744] Wei, XQ, et al. June 1995, "Altered immune responses in mice lacking inducible nitric oxide synthase"; *Nature;* 375: 408-11

[745] MacMickling, JD, et al., "Altered responses to bacterial infection and endotoxic shock in mice lacking inducible nitric oxide synthase"; *Cell,* Volume 81, Issue 4, 641-650, 19 May 1995

[746] MacLean A., Wei, XQ, et al., (1998), "Mice lacking inducible nitric oxide synthase are more susceptible to herpes simplex virus infection despite enhanced Th1 cell responses," *J Gen Virol;* (Pt 4): 825-30

this implies that there must be an excess of reduced to oxidized molecules. In living cells, this takes place by means of sulfur-containing amino acids, sulfurous peptides of low molecular weight, and other sulfur-containing molecules, collectively known as thiols. Thiols contain sulfur hydrogen bonds that contain an unpaired electron, which allows them to neutralize oxygen and NO radicals. Intracellular glutathione (GSH) and glutathione disulfide (GSSG) levels must be optimally balanced because at low levels, T cells cannot maximally activate the immunologically important transcription factor NF-kappaβ. NF-kappaβ family members control the transcription of cytokines and antimicrobial effectors as well as genes that regulate cellular differentiation, survival, and proliferation, thereby regulating various aspects of innate and adaptive immune responses.[747]

If thiols are consumed (as in AIDS patients) by the continuous formation of oxygen and NO radicals and free radicals can no longer be sufficiently controlled and neutralized, there will be major shifts in the redox status in cellular components, in the cell and in the various involved tissues. The cell, depending on the level of oxidative stress, has options consistent with its evolutionary biological heritage: it can preform its specialized function, change its speciation by differentiation or dedifferentiation, it can enter into the mitotic cycle and proliferate, it can die (by necrosis or apoptosis), or between these extremes of oxidative and nitrosative stress, depending on the cell type and the extracellular environment, it can mount a variety of counterregulatory measures. AIDS patients presented with cells expressing a variety of these options. Under long-term exposure to exogenous nitrites in various forms and subsequent reduced energy supplies, the endothelial cells of the blood vessels had an option to dedifferentiate and enter into a mitotic cycle consistent with the Warburg effect. The immune cells had the evolutionary biological option to counterregulate with the overexpression of a type 2 response over a type 1 response with a consequent decrease in the ability of these cells to produce iNOS to meet the intracellular pathogen challenge. The expressed medical conditions, Kaposi's sarcoma and opportunistic infections, can therefore be explained not by invoking viruses but by understanding the nature of energy metabolism, the complementary nature of the relationship between NO/O_2 and cysteine, and the subsequent predictable responses cells will mount in an attempt at self-preservation under these external challenges. It is the interaction of the glutathione/thiol system with NO and its congeners including the superoxide anion that informs the fluidity of the cellular environment in an

---

[747] Hayden, MS, West AP, Ghosh, S., "NF-kappaB and the immune response"; *Oncogene.* 2006 Oct 30;25(51):6758-80.

interrelated and highly complex manner with all the energetic, metabolic, and informational processes of not only the cell but the entire organism.

After more than 30 years, AIDSworld has refused to make the connection between the long-term inhalation of organic nitrites combined with medicines (including antibiotics and antiretrovirals) that increase the formation of NO and nitrosamine that could lead to superelevated amounts of NO and its metabolites. They have discounted the exposure to microbial toxins from chronic infections as a contributing factor in increasing levels of NO and nitrosamine. They have not examined the role of the imbalance of cytokine synthesis and its role in contributing to even more production of NO gas, and finally, they have not examined whether the binding of overproduced NO and nitrosamine or sulfonamide decay products could form nitrosothiols and result in the long-term exhaustion of the thiol pool[748] leading to the cellular changes that have mistakenly been called AIDS. But more than anything, they have contributed to the problem by intervening with drugs that exacerbate the initial metabolic condition.

---

[748] Kremer, H, op cit. p 32

CHAPTER 7

Biological Evolution of the Endosymbiotic Event

If what has been called HIV disease is, in fact, a functional mitochondrial illness, then it is fundamentally a systemic illness that originates from the disruption of the energy metabolism of the mitochondria and the complex consequences of that disruption. The primary cause for beginning the chain reaction is thiol exhaustion → cytokine switch → NO inhibition → type 2 cell dissymbiosis → HIV/AIDS cancer, wasting syndrome, myopathy, encephalopathy, polyneuropathy, enteropathy, etc., in AIDS risk groups.[749] Even AIDSworld research has recognized, without being able to contextualize, that glutathione deficiency in "AIDS" risk groups is associated with impaired survival[750] and that it is not any "HIV" that determines T immune cell response patterns to either Th1 or Th2 but rather the glutathione levels in the antigen-presenting cells.[751] Given just that basic understanding, it reached the level of malevolent intent to treat these proton-deficient patients first with the mitochondrial toxic drug AZT and then to compound and magnify the problem by suggesting and using long-term therapy with the double folate inhibitor trimethoprim/sulfamethoxazole. Not only is folate metabolism important in proliferating cells for producing one-carbon atoms for nucleic acid synthesis, it also has the crucial function of generating reducing power.[752] Depletion of either the cytosolic or

---

[749] Kremer, H., (2008), "The Silent Revolution in Cancer and AIDS medicine," Xlibris
[750] Herzenberg, LA., et al., (1997) "Glutathione deficiency is associated with impaired survival in HIV disease," *PNAS USA*, 94: 1967-1972
[751] Peterson, JD., (1998) "Glutathione levels in antigen-presenting cells modulate Th1 versus Th2 response patterns," *PNAS USA*, 95: 3071-3076
[752] Fan, J, et al., (2014), "Quantitative flux analysis reveals folate dependent NADPH production," *Nature;* 510: 298-302, doi: 10.1038/nature13236.

the mitochondrial methylenetetrahydrofolate dehydrogenase enzyme leads to a decrease in cellular $NADPH/NADP^+$ and reduced/oxidized glutathione ratios (GSH/GSSH) and an exacerbation of the above chain of events.

To gain a deeper understanding of the various manifestations of the thiol deficiency syndrome, it is crucial to examine the multiple functions of the mitochondria in cellular metabolism not only at the molecular level but at the bioenergetic level of microwave frequencies and biophoton communication networks. Biomolecules in the organism are predominantly present in the excited state. As a result, the energetics of living systems are based on energy differentials produced by redox reactions.[753] Because of these energy differentials, living tissues have dielectric properties[754] that are also causal in terms of electromagnetic field propagation.[755] It is the propagation of this field that allows complex molecular groupings to work as interacting networks of nested cycles.[756] For example, it has been demonstrated that proteins recognized their targets not on the basis of the "lock and key" model but on the basis of resonant energy transfer through oscillations of an electromagnetic field.[757,758] In this resonant recognition model (RRM) in which the charge is electromagnetic and the discharge is chemical, it has been demonstrated that certain periodicities within the distribution of energies of delocalized electrons along a protein molecule are critical for protein target interaction.[759]

Mitochondria also have a strong static electric field, form a proton space charge layer, and water ordering in the contiguous cytosol. These established patterns are the necessary conditions for the generation of coherent electrodynamic fields by the attached cytoskeletal architecture. This electromagnetic field establishes both order and stability to the cell structure as well as orderly motion during the cell division cycle. The order and cytoskeletal

---

[753] "Integrative Biophysics-Biophotonics," (2003) Ed. Popp, F.A., & Beloussov, L., Kluwer Academic Publishers, Boston, pp. 66-68

[754] Gabriel, C., et al., (1996), "The dielectric properties of biological tissues: I. Literature survey," *Phys Med Biol;* 41: 2231-2249

[755] Hyland, GJ., (2003) "Bio-electromagnetism" In: Integrative Biophysics, Biophotons, Ed. Popp, FA., Beloussov, L., Kluwer Academic Publishers, Boston, Mass. pp117-148

[756] "Coherent Electromagnetic Fields and Bio-Communication," in Electromagnetic Bio-Information, Ed. Popp, FA., Warnke, U., Konig, H, and Peschka, W., (1989) Urban & Schwarznberg pp. 1-17

[757] Ćosic, I. et al., (1989), "Prediction of hot spots in IL-2 cased on information spectrum characteristics of growth regaling factors," *Biochemie;* 72: 333-342

[758] Ćosic, I., (1994), "Macromolecular bioactivity: Is it resonant interaction between macromolecules? Theory and application," *IEEE Trans on biomed Eng;* 41(12): 1101-1114

[759] Ćosic, I, Ibid

stability has become known as tensegrity.[760] It is this tensegrity that allows for integrated signal transmissions through a complex network of cellular constituents, which control cell behavior. In comparison to bond and cohesive forces, these electrodynamic forces are of a long-range and coherent nature. Thus, mitochondrial dysfunction leads to an increase in entropy by disturbances of the electromagnetic field, diminishing its power and coherence as well as its frequency spectrum.[761] This may result in a change in numerous integrated metabolic networks,[762] for example, altered electrodynamic interaction forces between cancer and healthy cells. Schamhart and van Wijk[763] observed a kind of photon-induced photon absorption in normal cell cultures of high cell density, but the effect disappeared completely in tumor cell cultures. This inability of tumor cells to reabsorb emitted energy coherently underscores the connection between organization and communication as tumor cells have a diminished capacity for intercommunication and socially cohesive behavior.

Because the focus of the dominant paradigm has been to elevate the function of the central nucleus, until recently, the fundamental role played by mitochondria in the dynamic functionality and stable nonequilibrium/redox homeostasis processes of the eukaryotic cell has been undervalued. The maintenance of electrochemical potentials and ionic concentration gradients across cellular boundaries in large part comes from the energy generation of the mitochondria, not only because of the energy produced by ATP but the energy derived from the constant churning of ROS and one-electron oxygen reduction in the coherent domains of surrounding water—a virtual circuitry of coupled oscillating frequencies. Mitochondrial oscillations are dependent on the frequency and amplitude patterns of electron-excited states generation and their relaxation—the processes with ROS participation taking place in an aqueous environment.[764] The energy released in these reactions is used not only for the continuous driving of the nonequilibrium state of inter- and

---

[760] Ingber, DE, (2003), "Tensegrity I. Cell Structure and hierarchical systems biology," *J Cell Sci;* 116(Pt 7): 1157-1173

[761] Pokorny, J., (2012), "Mitochondrial metabolism—neglected link of cancer transformation and treatment," *Prague Med Report;* 113(2): 81-94

[762] Jeong, H., et al., (2000), "The large-scale organization of metabolic networks," *Nature;* 407: 651-654

[763] Schamhart, DHJ., van Wijk, R., (1987), "Photonemission and the degree of differentiation, in: *Photon Emission from Biological Systems,* B Jezowska-Trzebiatowska, B. Kochel, J. Slawinski, (eds.), World Scientific, Singapore, 137-152

[764] Voeikov, V., (2001), "Reactive oxygen species, water, photons, and life," *Rivista biologia/bio forum;* 94: 193-214

intracellular structural components but also for activation energy for specific biochemical processes.[765]

Although most textbooks are still teaching that the dominant role of the mitochondria is the efficiency of its ATP energy production from glucose oxidation by way of pyruvate[766] and the resultant so-called high-energy phosphate bonds, the mitochondrial story is much more complex. This organelle participates in a number of other vital functions only partially or indirectly related to energy production via hydrolysis of the phosphate bond: heat production, detoxification, cellular redox state, mitochondrial membrane potential, cell proliferation, apoptosis/necrosis, steroid synthesis (e.g., adrenal cortex, gonads) that is determined by cholesterol import into the mitochondria, heme synthesis, and production of ROS as second messengers.[767] Mitochondria not only synthesize heme but also assemble iron sulfur (Fe-S) proteins and participate in cellular iron regulation.[768]

A high prevalence of elevated serum and red cell ferritin has been reported in asymptomatic AIDS patients (and cancer patients[769]) and those treated with AZT.[770] AIDSworld has been unable to account for this finding as the elusive virus has not been shown to be implicated in this pathology. There is, of course, the possibility of impaired heme synthesis in mitochondrial pathology and the consequent need to store elevated iron, which can be cytotoxic. This iron is able to act as a catalyst in the formation of ROS.[771] Thus, elevated ferritin levels in AIDS patients can be identified as another marker for mitochondrial metabolic disruption. Finally, the production of urea in the liver as a method of removing toxic ammonia is known as the ornithine-urea cycle and partially occurs in the mitochondria. This cycle becomes crucial to understanding the muscle-wasting cachexia that has come to characterize not only AIDS but other systemic illnesses including cancer, sepsis, surgical trauma, ulcerative colitis, chronic fatigue syndrome, and overtrained athletes. The coincidence of these symptoms in diseases of different etiology suggests a causal relationship.

---

[765] Voeikov, Ibid

[766] ~30-32 ATP vs 2 via the glycolytic pathway

[767] Zorov, DB, et al., (1997), "Mitochondria revisited. Alternative functions of mitochondria," *BioSci Reports;* 17(6): 507-520

[768] Lill, R., et al., (2012), "The role of mitochondria in cellular iron-sulfur protein biogenesis and iron metabolism," *Biochim Biophys Acta;* 1823(9): 1491-1508

[769] Alkhateeb, AA., Connor, JR., (2013), "The significance of ferritin in cancer: antioxidation, inflammation and tumorigenesis," *Biochim Biophys Acta;* 1836(2): 245-154

[770] Riera, A., et al., (1994), "Prevalence of high serum and red cell ferritin levels in HIV-infected patients," *Haematologica;* 79(2): 165-167

[771] Dixon, SJ, Stockwell, BR., (2014), "The role of iron and reactive oxygen species in cell death," *Nat Chem Bio;* 10:9-17

It is the cysteine level (which is significantly diminished in both AIDS and cancer patients[772]) itself that is the physiological regulator of nitrogen balance and body cell mass.[773] It is the catabolism of cysteine to sulfate and protons that determines the rate of carbamoyl-phosphate synthesis, the rate-limiting step of urea biosynthesis. The pathology of cachexia differs substantially from starvation in which the body attempts to save protein. With protracted hunger, unlike cachexia, the degradation of protein is reduced as well as the need for nitrogen export via the ornithine-urea cycle not by cysteine but by the ketone bodies of acidosis.[774,775] In cachexia, patients lose both adipose tissue and skeletal muscle mass.

Human cells carry none[776] (red blood cells) to over one hundred thousand mitochondria in mature oocytes.[777] On average, most eukaryotic cells harbor between one thousand and two thousand of these organelles. However, mitochondria, consistent with their bacterial ancestral origin, are not stationary organelles. They frequently change their shape and position within the cell, and they grow and divide by a process of fission. They have the ability to fuse with other mitochondria. They can then separate and go elsewhere as the need for increased localized energy arises. These regulated changes in mitochondrial morphology are associated with cell survival or cell death.[778] As it is currently understood, the morphology of mitochondria is a key element in mitochondrial-nuclear communication. Except during the glycolytic phase of the cell cycle, mitochondria not only produce ~86 percent of ATP, they consume up to ~90 percent of the oxygen used for both the production of ATP and ROS/RNS. The combination of the energy transduction potential of ATP and the energy of electromagnetic excitation produced by RONS from the electron transport chain contributes to the range of frequencies that allow for

---

[772] Hack, V., et al., (1997), "Cystine levels, cystine flux, and protein catabolism in cancer cachexia, HIV/SIV infection, and senescence," *FASEB J;* 11(1): 84-92

[773] Droge, W., Holm, E., (1997), "Role of cysteine and glutathione in HIV infection and other diseases associated with muscle wasting and immunological dysfunction," *FASEB J;* 11: 1077-1089

[774] Aoki, T., et al., (1972), "Hormonal regulation of glutamine metabolism in fasting man," *Adv Enzyme Regul;* 10:145-151

[775] Smith, RS., et al., (1974), "Nitrogen and amino acid metabolism in adults with protein-calorie malnutrition," *Metabolism;* 23: 603-618

[776] Zhang, ZW, et al., (2011), "Red blood cell extrudes nucleus and mitochondria against oxidative stress, *IUBMB Life;* 63(7): 560-665

[777] Shoubridge, EA., Wai, T. (2007), "Mitochondrial DNA and the mammalian oocyte," *Curr Top Dev Biol;* 77: 87-111

[778] Gomes, LC., et al., (2011), "Mitochondrial elongation during autophagy," *Nature Cell Biol;* 13: 589-596

the maintenance of normal cellular structural/functional organization and associated frequencies and biorhythms.

The mitochondria has an inner and outer membrane. The inner membrane contains the respiratory complexes involved in OXPHOS and ATP production. This membrane also contains a large number of gated channel-forming proteins including some forty-nine different metabolite transporter proteins.[779] During normal mitochondrial respiration, the electrons gained from the oxidation of respiratory substrates are transferred along a chain of carriers that are located in the inner mitochondrial membrane. The energy derived for ATP synthesis is from electrons donated from NADH and $FADH_2$ (products of Krebs cycle) to complexes I and II of the electron transport chain (ETC).

At complexes I, III, and IV, the free energy released by the fall in redox potential of the passing electrons is used to translocate protons from the mitochondrial matrix into the intermembrane space. This process, known as the proton-motive force, generates a proton electrochemical potential gradient across the inner mitochondrial membrane. There are two components of the PMF: the membrane potential, which occurs from the net movement of positive charge across the inner mitochondrial membrane, and the pH gradient. The membrane potential contributes the most energy of ~150–180 mV that is stored in the gradient.[780] According to this Mitchell hypothesis, the stored energy in $\Delta\Psi m$ is then used to synthesize ATP. As protons flow back into the matrix through a proton channel in complex V, ADP and Pi are bound, forming ATP (oxidative phosphorylation). Matrix ATP is then exchanged for cytosolic ADP. The process is as follows: the respiratory complexes I (NADH-ubiquinone reductase), complex II (succinate-ubiquinone reductase), complex III (ubiquinol-cytochrome c reductase), and complex IV (cytochrome c oxidase) are embedded in the inner mitochondrial membrane. The four complexes are linked by ubiquinone (Q) and cytochrome c, which can diffuse through the membrane. Q acts as transport molecule for electrons from complexes I and II to complex III while it is cytochrome c that transports electrons from III to IV. This transportation of electrons is thought to provide energy to the hydrogen pumps in complexes I, II, and IV. The hydrogen ions are channeled through canals in the inner membrane. The hydrogen ion gradients, powered by the electrons, activate the coupling of ADP and P_i to form ATP. Oxygen acts as an electron dump at the end of the chain of complex IV and is immediately reduced to water.

---

[779] Ryan, MT, Hoogenraad, NJ, (2007), "Mitochondrial-nuclear communications," *Annu Rev Biochem;* 76: 701-722

[780] Moncada, S. Erusalimsky, JD., (2002), "Does nitric oxide modulate mitochondrial energy generation and apoptosis?

MITOCHONDRIAL SUBCOMPARTMENTS

Outer Membrane
Protein imports
Metabolite influx & efflux
Fission, Fusion & distribution
Apoptosis factors (e.g., Bcl-2, Bax)
Signaling molecules
Intermembrane Space
Electron transfer (cytochrome c)
Cristae remodeling
Redox enzymes
Protein imports
Apoptosis factors (e.g., cyto c, etc.)
Inner Membrane
Oxidative phosphorylation
Metabolite transport
Protein imports
Protein assembly
Protein degradation
Matrix
TCA cycle enzymes
Fatty acid oxidation
mtDNA replication
mtDNA transcription/translation
Fe-S biogenesis
Protein folding & degradation
Urea cycle enzymes (liver & small intestine)
Gluconeogenic enzyme system (liver & kidney)

chart 1

The mitochondrial membrane, which is highly polarized, has an integral role to play in cellular homeostasis. The disruption of the $\Delta\Psi_m$ has been specifically attributed to the balance shift in ROS generation versus ROS scavenging.[781]

Mitochondria have their own DNA; however, more than 98 percent of the total protein complement of the organelle is encoded by the nuclear genome. Thus, mitochondrial biogenesis requires a coordination of expression of two genomes.[782] The regulation of biogenesis and cell death is influenced by external stressors such as nutrients, hormones, temperature, exercise, hypoxia, electromagnetic fields, toxins, and aging.[783]

Early in programmed cell death, the mitochondrial membrane depolarizes and the permeability increases, which may be due in part to the opening of the permeability transition pore (PT). The mitochondrial PT has been described as a Ca^{2+} dependent pore, which is a contact site between the inner and outer mitochondrial membranes. It is the method by which the genetically reduced mitochondria is able to import/export necessary solutes across the inner membrane.[784] The permeability transition pore (PT) is said to be a nonselective voltage-dependent anion channel (VDAC) that modifies the permeability of the inner mitochondrial membrane. It is a dynamic multiprotein complex probably located at the contact site between the inner and outer mitochondrial membranes.[785] Although the structure has yet to be completely defined, it is thought to contain cytosol (hexokinase), the outer membrane (VDAC), the inner membrane (the adenine nucleotide translocator [ANT]), and the matrix cyclophilin D.[786] The PT pore complex is regulated by thiol-reactive agents, calcium, cyclophilin D ligands, apoptosis-related endoproteases (caspases), and the Bcl-2—family of proteins.[787,788] The PT pore participates in the regulation

---

[781] Aon, MA., et al., (2008), "Mitochondrial oscillations in physiology and pathophysiology," *Adv Exp Med Biol.;* 641: 98-117

[782] Ryan, MT., Hoogenraad, NJ, (2007), "Mitochondrial-nuclear communications," *Annu Rev Biochem;* 76: 701-722

[783] Ibid, Ryan

[784] Halestrap, AP, et al., (2002), "The permeability transition pore complex: another view," *Biochimie;* 84: 153-166

[785] Beutner, G., et al., (1998), "Complexes between porin, hexokinase, mitochondrial creatine kinase and adenylate translocator display properties of the permeability transition pore. Implication for regulation of permeability transition by the kinases," *Biochim Biophys Acta;* 1368(1): 7-18

[786] Susin, SA., et al., (1998), "Mitochondria as regulators of apoptosis: doubt no more," *Biochim Biophy Acta;* 1366: 151-165

[787] Marzo, I., et al.,(1998) "The Permeability Transition Pore Complex: A Target for Apoptosis Regulation by Caspases and Bcl-2–related Proteins," *JEM;* 187(8): 1261-1271

[788] Tsujimoto,Y, Shimizu, S., (2000), "VDAC regulation by the Bcl-2 family of proteins," *Cell Death Diffeent;* 7(12): 1174-1181

of matrix Ca^{2+}, pH, $\Delta\Psi_m$, and volume with several levels of conductance. At its high level of conductance, it can provoke irreversible $\Delta\Psi_m$ dissipation.[789] ADP and ATP are the physiological ligands of the adenine nucleotide translocator (ANT) and function as endogenous inhibitors of PT. Therefore, the depletion of these molecules facilitates PT as does a reduction of the $\Delta\Psi m$ and matrix alkalinization. It follows that the uncoupling or inhibition of the respiratory chain leading to a decrease in $\Delta\Psi m$ or inhibition of ATPase (which causes matrix alkalinization) may favor PT.

While the OXPHOS system can be fueled by several different nutrients, it mainly uses carbohydrates and fats. Glucose is reduced to pyruvate enzymatically by a metabolic chain. This path from glucose to pyruvate is called glycolysis. Glycolysis is an anaerobic breakdown of glucose to lactic acid and pyruvate. This process arose early in evolution in the anaerobic atmosphere of early Earth to produce a net of 2 ATP. It is still the primary system of energy generation used by the eukaryotic cell during the cell division cycle and during times of hypoxic or pseudohypoxic stress.[790] Pyruvate then flows into the citric acid cycle of the mitochondria and is oxidized to form six molecules of carbon dioxide. In this process, the coenzyme NAD+ and FAD are reduced after which their hydrogen ions are delivered to the respiratory chain. NAD+ contains the vitamin niacin from tryptophan and FAD, riboflavin. Thiamin and pantothenic acid are also coenzymes in the cycle. There are at least five nested metabolic pathways during the oxidative process of gaining 29–30 ATP from a molecule of glucose:

1. Glycolysis in the cytoplasm
2. The malate aspartate and glycerol phosphate shuttles for transport of electrons across the inner membrane
3. The citric acid cycle in the mitochondria
4. The respiratory chain and
5. The OXPHOS system

NADH+H⁺ is formed by a special enzyme reaction, and NAD has to be made from another metabolic path of glucose beforehand. The formation of NADH+H⁺ does not take place in the inner membrane of the mitochondria, but special shuttle molecules act as transports to the mitochondria, taking on hydrogen in reduced form from NADH+H⁺. The transport molecules are converted and then returned to the cytoplasm to begin the cycle again. The

---

[789] Susin, SA., Op cit.
[790] Brand, K, (1997), "Aerobic glycolysis by proliferating cells: protection against oxidative stress at the expense of energy yield," *J Bioener Biomembr;* 29(4): 355-364

production of ATP and the maintenance of the respiratory chain are able to continue by the continuous supply of hydrogen ions from NADH+H$^+$ and FADH$_2$.

This pared-down version of OXPHOS system simply demonstrates the highly regulated import/export system between the mitochondria and the cytoplasm and to underscore its functional similarities to what manufacturing has come to call the "just in time" system. If the transport or production pathways in the cell are interrupted at any point in the chain of integrated cycles, the entire cell may be affected. This just-in-time system is the hallmark of the cooperative trend of the chimeric nucleus and the mitochondrial symbiont. This system also makes the targeting of isolated reactions as is currently conceived by the drug/kill paradigm both illogical and dangerous without consideration of a systems analysis of consequent networked metabolic events.

To understand the multiple functions of the mitochondria and its impact not only on the genesis of what has been called AIDS but a variety of other disease states, it is useful to consider the massive gene transfer from the ancestral prokaryote that preceded the formation of the eukaryotic cell that led to the development of the chimeric nucleus.[791] Eukaryote nuclei contain genes of both eubacterial and archaebacterial origin, and these genes have different functions within the eukaryotic cell.[792] Support for the fusion event that occurred ~2 billion years ago[793] derives from the fact that extant eukaryotic nuclear genomes contain genes that manifest sister-group phylogenetic relationships with both eubacterial and archaebacterial genes.[794] This ancient marriage unravels (dis-symbiosis) under biologically stressful conditions and manifests clinically as various disease states. To understand the context in which this happens and why this happens, it is useful to review the evolutionary theory of endosymbiosis and the dynamic advantages that drove this fusion event.

The Endosymbiotic Theory

The endosymbiotic theory was advanced by biologist Lynn Margulis in the 1960s and officially in her 1970 book *Origin of Eukaryotic Cells* and in a later

---

[791] Rivera, MC., et al., (1998), "Genomic evidence for two functionally distinct gene classes," *PNAS USA;* 95: 6239-6244

[792] Cotton, JA., McInerney, JO., (2010), "Eukaryotic genes of archaebacterial origin are more important than the more numerous eubacterial genes, irrespective of function," *PNAS;* 107(40): 17252-17255

[793] Brocks, JJ, et al., (1999), "Archean molecular fossils and the early rise of eukaryotes," *Science;* 285: 1033-1036

[794] Esser, C, et al., (2004), "A genome phylogeny for mitochondria among α-proteobacteria and a predominantly eubacterial ancestry of yeast nuclear genes," *Mol Bio Evolu;* 21(9): 1643-1660

1981 publication, *Symbiosis in Cell Evolution*. Margulis revisited an idea that had been early proposed in 1883 by Andreas Schimper and again in 1905 by a young Russian biologist Constantin Mereschkowsky,[795] arguing that mitochondria (and chloroplasts) evolved from free-living bacteria via symbiosis within a eukaryotic host cell. Although now accepted in some form as a well-supported theory, when she made her observations, most biologists had never heard of endosymbiosis; and both she and the theory were ridiculed by mainstream biologists for a number of years. The discovery in the 1960s of DNA within these organelles and the recognition that they contain a translation system distinct from that of the cytosol were two of the observations that Margulis used in support of the endosymbiont hypothesis of organelle origins.

Additional Observations in Support of the Endosymbiotic Theory

By the use of remote controlled vehicles in the exploration of ocean depths and the discovery of new types of deep-water organisms by 1977, Woese and associates[796] were able to begin to do research on various newly discovered organisms that were previously unknown prokaryotes. Initially, these organisms were classified as a new form of bacteria. However, when comprehensive sequence comparisons of 16S ribosomal nucleic acid (rRNA) of many diverse prokaryotes and the corresponding small subunit rRNA of eukaryotes were completed, it was surmised that living systems represent one of three aboriginal lines of descent: Archaea, single-celled organisms lacking nuclei containing methanogenic bacteria; bacteria, which also lack nuclei, comprising all typical bacteria; and eukarya, organisms with nuclei (single-cell protists, single- and multicelled algae, single- and multicelled fungi, plants, animals, and humans).[797] This was a significant breakthrough in the unraveling of the syntrophic evolutionary events that were at the origin of the eukaryotic cell.

Another piece of eukaryotic cell puzzle was resolved when evidence of early prokaryotic use of oxygen was deduced from 2.7 billion-year-old shale

---

[795] "History: the formation of the endosymbiotic hypothesis," 18 Feb. 215 https://endosymbiotichypothesis.wordpress.com/history-the-formation-of-the-endosymbiotic-hypothesis/

[796] Woese, CR, Fox, GE., (1977), "Phylogenetic structure of the prokaryotic domain: The primary kingdoms," *Proc Nat Acad Sci, USA;* 74(11): 5088-5090

[797] Fox, FE., Stackebrand, RB, et al., (1980), "The phyolgeny of prokaryotes," *Science;* 209: 457-463

that contained Archaean molecular fossils. These fossils indicated the presence of abundant 2α-methyl hopanes (which are not detected in archaea[798]) characteristic of cyanobacteria, indicating that these organisms evolved to use oxygen for energy production well before the atmosphere became oxidizing.[799] This discovery gave credence to the idea that early eubacterium were capable of both aerobic and anaerobic biochemistry.[800]

Eukaryotes are characterized by size—about one-thousand-fold bigger by volume than a typical bacterium or archaeon, and function under different principles: free diffusion has less of a role in eukaryotic cells but has an overarching role in prokaryote metabolism.[801] The compartmentalization of eukaryotic cells is supported by an elaborate endomembrane system and by the actin-tubulin-based cytoskeleton.[802] The hallmark of the eukaryotic cell is the presence of mitochondria, which have a central role in energy transformation, cell signaling, and cell death.[803]

The concept of endosymbiosis was a revolutionary realization that led to a very different and dynamic understanding of cell metabolism away from the genetic determinism model—that is, all eukarya, including the cells found in humans, owe their existence to a single evolutionary thermodynamic event: the unique act of fusion, namely, the critical event of the colonization of a voluminous type of archaea as host/stem cell by a single-cellular α-proteobacterial organism. This formation of an intracellular symbiosis from members of two different species of bacteria that used two different types of energy systems and the integration of the two inherently incompatible alien genome cultures into a common nucleus are thought to have been a singular syntrophic event that occurred ~ 2.1 billion years ago.[804]

The archaebacteria are thought to have been methane-producing bacteria. In most instances, the compounds that serve as substrates for methanogenic

---

[798] Larry L Barton (2005). Structural and Functional Relationships in Prokaryotes. Springer.

[799] Brocks, J, et al., (1999), "Archean molecular fossils and the early rise of eukaryotes," *Science;* 285: 1033-1036

[800] Martin W, Müller M. (1998), "The hydrogen hypothesis for the first eukaryote"; *Nature* 392: 37–41

[801] Guigas, G., et al, (2007), "The degree of macromolecular crowding in the cytoplasm and nucleoplasm of mammalian cells is conserved," *FEBS Lett;* 581: 5094-5098

[802] Dacks, JB, et al., (2009), "Evolution of specificity in the eukaryotic endomembrane system," *Int J Biochem Cell Biol;* 41: 330-340

[803] Koonin, EV., (2010), "The origin and early evolution of eukaryotes in light of phylogenomics," *GenomeBiology;* 11:209

[804] Kremer, H, http://ummafrapp.de/skandal/heinrich/kremer_the_concept_of_cellsymbiosis_therapy.pdf

bacteria, including H_2, formate, acetate, methanol, and methylamines, are produced as end products of various eubacterial and eukaryotic fermentations and anaerobic oxidations of both complex and simple organic compounds.[805]

The Hydrogen Hypothesis or Hydrogen Transfer as the Metabolic Driver of the Endosymbiotic Event

An alternative hypothesis from the idea that the host cell for the endosymbiotic event was not a eukaryote but specifically an archaeon has recently been advanced.[806] It has been observed in every eukaryotic amitochondrial lineage that has been carefully investigated there are evolutionary remnants of mitochondria (mitochondrion-related organelles or MROs).[807] Two types of MROs have been identified: hydrogenosomes and mitosomes. Hydrogenosomes are double-membrane-bounded, pyruvate-metabolizing organelles that produce ATP anaerobically. The inner membrane of the hydrogenosome neither forms cristae nor contains detectable cytochromes or cardiolipin as found in mitochondria.[808] They are also different from mitochondria as most do not contain their own DNA or the citric acid cycle.[809] Instead, they contain enzymes typically found in anaerobic bacteria and are capable of producing molecular hydrogen. In amitochondriate eukaryotes that harbor hydrogenosomes, cytosolic pyruvate is imported into the organelle, where pyruvate ferredoxin oxidoreductase (PFO) converts it to CO_2 and acetyl-CoA and reduces ferredoxin. Ferredoxin is reoxidized by hydrogenase-producing H_2. Per mol of glucose, pyruvate metabolism in hydrogenosomes yields two additional mol ATP and two mol each of H_2, CO_2 and acetate as waste products.[810] Phylogenetic analysis of

---

[805] Wolf, RS., Higgins, IJ, (1979), "Microbial biochemistry of methane—a study in contrasts," *Int Rev Biochem;* 21:267-350

[806] Koonin, Op cit

[807] Gray, MW., (2012), "Mitochondrial Evolution," *Cold Spring Harbor Perspect Biol;* 4: a011403

[808] Honigberg, BM, Volkmann, D. et al, (1984), "A freeze-fracture electron microscope study of Trichomonas vaginalis Donné and Tritrichomonas foetus (Riedmüller)," *J Protozool;* 31(1): 116-131

[809] Clemens, DL, Johnson, PJ, (2000), "Failure to detect DNA in hydrogenosomes of *Trichomonas vaginalis* by nick translation and immunomicroscopy," *Mol Biochem Parasitol;* 106: 307-313

[810] W Martin, M Muller, 1998, "The hydrogen hypothesis for the first eukaryote"; *Nature* 392: 37-41

several hydrogenosmal heat-shock proteins has established that mitochondria and hydrogenosomes have a common eubacterial ancestor.[811]

Several typical mitochondrial proteins have also been identified in mitosomes, which are more highly reduced than the hydrogenosomes. As a result of the discovery of these proteins, mitosomes have been identified as evolutionary derivatives of conventional mitochondria.[812] These organelles are able to generate H_2 by an ATP-producing, hydrogenase-mediated pathway. They have a very limited metabolic capacity but contain the Fe-S cluster formation, suggesting that the Fe-S cluster formation (which is redundant in the electron transport chain molecules of the mitochondria) and its ability to transfer electrons may have been the raison d'etre of the mitochondria rather than the OXPHOS system.[813] This may be because whenever O_2 acts with Fe-containing proteins, ROS, such as the superoxide anions, peroxide anions, and hydroxyl radicals can be generated,[814] increasing the available energy output.

The "hydrogen hypothesis" proposed in 1998 by Martin and Muller observed that there was a *"symbiotic association of an anaerobic, strictly hydrogen-dependent, strictly autotrophic archaebacterium [the host] with an eubacterium [the symbiont] that was able to respire, but generated molecular hydrogen as a waste product of anaerobic heterotrophic metabolism. The host's dependence upon molecular hydrogen produced by the symbiont is put forward as the selective principle that forged the common ancestor of eukaryotic cells."*[815]

Over time, the hydrogen- and gene-donating proteobacteria transformed into the mitochondria, and an improved energy yield resulted as now the host's energy-rich pyruvate could be transferred into the bacterial symbiont for further oxidation. In essence, endosymbiosis was not simply a physical event but a syntrophic event in which the hydrogen product of the symbiont served as an essential nutrient for its Archaea partner. However, to be able to increase the energy yield, the hydrogen from the hydrogenosomes could no longer diffuse through the membrane into the cytoplasm but would now concentrate in the intermembrane space as an energy source for the increased production of ATP as pyruvate was transferred into the endosymbiont. For this

---

[811] Bui, ETN, et al., (1996), "A common evolutionary origin for mitochondria and hydrogenosomes," *Proc Natl Acad Sci USA;* 93: 9651-9656

[812] Hjort, K, et al, (2010), "Diversity and reductive evolution of mitochondria among microbial eukaryotes," *Philos Trans R Soc Lond B Biol Sci;* 365: 713-727

[813] Tovar, J., et al., (2003), "Mitochondrial remnant organelles of *Giardia* function in iron sulphur protein maturation," *Nature;* 426: 172-176

[814] Brand, K., (1997), "Aerobic glycolysis by proliferating cells: protection against oxidative stress at the expense of energy yield," *J Bioenergetics and Biomembr;* 29(4): 355-364

[815] W Martin, M Muller, Op cit.

to occur, the membrane potential of the symbionts had to be structured in such a way that the diffusion of hydrogen ions (protons) was inhibited. As a result, the mitochondrial oscillator, dependent on reactive oxygen species, became a frequency- and/or amplitude-modulated signaling mechanism that could now connect bioenergetics to ROS-activated signal transduction pathways, including those responsible for regulating gene transcription.[816]

The flow of hydrogen, which was the impetus to the combination," and was initially directed out of the symbiont to the Archaea as an additional fuel source, was now reversed to remain within the symbiont, which allowed for an improved energy yield by using the now electron transport chain with oxygen as the final electron receiver. A feature of the hydrogen hypothesis is its explanation of the simultaneous origin of both aerobic and anaerobic energy metabolism in eukaryotes, the assumption being that both pathways were contained in and contributed to the hybrid cell by the α-Proteobacterial partner, which is thought to have been a facultative anaerobe.[817] It is posited that the two pathways would have been differentially expressed in the free-living bacterial symbiont when it encountered the appropriate environmental conditions.

The question of competitive advantage of this symbiotic event seems to be resolved by the hydrogen hypothesis. The conventional hypothesis is that it was the production of increased amounts of ATP. The hydrogen hypothesis challenges this premise by suggesting that it carries several tenuous assumptions:

1. That the host was unable to synthesize sufficient amounts of ATP by itself
2. That the symbiont synthesized ATP in amounts exceeding its needs and
3. That the symbiont could export ATP to its environment so that the host could realize the benefit[818]

The hydrogen hypothesis suggests that in the case of hydrogenosomal metabolism, it was the waste products, CO_2, H_2 and acetate, that were of benefit to the host. Many archaebacteria are strictly dependent upon H_2 for their ATP production.[819] Furthermore, for many methanogens, H_2O and CO_2 are the sole

---

[816] Aon, MA., et al., (2006), "Fundamental organization of cardiac mitochondria as a network of coupled oscillators," *Biophys J;* 91: 4317-4327
[817] Martin, WF., (2010), "The origin of the mitochondria," *Nature.com;* http://www.nature.com/scitable/topicpage/the-origin-of-mitochondria-14232356
[818] Martin & Muller, Op cit
[819] Schönheit, P, Schäfer, T., (1995), "Metabolism of hyperthermophiles," *World J Microbiol Biotechnol;* 11:26-57

source of both energy and carbon[820] whereas others can utilize alternate carbon sources such as methylamine, formic acid, and acetate (all of which are waste products of eubacterial metabolism); and a few can grow on acetate alone.[821] For methanogens, all three waste products of the symbiont's anaerobic metabolism are fuel for life. This energetic addition (by the hydrogen- and gene-donating proteobacteria) was then used to merge some of the genome of the eubacteria with the genome of the Archaea to form a nucleus with its own membrane.[822] The packaging of genes from both bacteria into a membrane-bound nucleus supported the functional division of transcription within the nucleus and translation outside the nucleus onto special structures called ribosomes.[823]

The Human Genome Retains Relics of Its Prokaryotic Ancestry: Syntrophy or Metabolic Symbiosis at the Origin of Eukaryotes

When an end product of one partner's metabolism (e.g., hydrogen) serves as an essential nutrient for the other partner, syntrophy or metabolic symbiosis occurs.[824] The syntrophy hypothesis also proposes that symbiosis was mediated by interspecies' hydrogen transfer but considers that the organisms involved were δ-proteobacteria—ancestral sulfate-reducing myxobacteria and methanogenic Archea.[825] Both the hydrogen hypothesis and the syntrophy hypothesis explain the mosaic character of eukaryotes—the archeal-like genetic machinery and a eubacterial-like metabolism as well as eukaryotic characteristics resulting from the symbiotic event.[826] The minutiae of these differences will be left to the evolutionary biologists; however, analysis of complete genomes indicates that a massive prokaryotic gene transfer (or transfers) preceded the formation of the eukaryotic cell.[827] The genes that have been inherited from both prokaryotic ancestors remain distinguishable. Despite being fewer in number, human genes of archaebacterial origin are more widely expressed across tissues, are more

---

[820] Thauer, RK, et al., (1993), Methanogenesis: Ecology, Physiology, Biochemistry and Genetics (ed. Ferry, J.G.) 209-252; Chapman & Hall, New York
[821] Thauer, Ibid
[822] Gray, MW, et al., (1999), "Mitochondrial evolution," *Science;* 283: 1476-1481
[823] Gray, Ibid
[824] Gray, MW., (1999), "Evolution of organellar genomes," *Curr Opin Genetics Devel;* 9: 678-687
[825] Lopez-Garcia, P. Moreira, D., (1999), "Metabolic symbiosis at the origin of eukaryotes,"
[826] Lopez-Garcia, Ibid
[827] Rivera, MC., et al., (1998), "Genomic evidence for two functionally distinct gene classes," *Proc Natl Acad Sci USA;* 95: 6239-6244

likely to be lethal, and encode for shorter and more central proteins in the protein-protein interaction network than eubacterium-like genes and tend to be involved in informational processes.[828] This informational archaebacterial lineage of genes are more likely to be involved in transcription, translation, and replication (i.e., informational processes that begin to occur in the late S phase of mitosis and are more likely to respond to reductive signaling[829]) and include GTPases, vacuolar ATPase homologs, and most tRNA synthetases.[830]

Eubacterial genes are preferentially involved in the operational processes of higher order cellular metabolism.[831] These genes are more likely to code for amino acid synthesis, biosynthesis of cofactors, cell envelope, energy metabolism, intermediary metabolism, fatty acid and phospholipid biosynthesis, nucleotide biosynthesis and regulatory functions [832] (and are more likely to be responsive to oxidative signaling). Consistent with the endosymbiotic theory and their evolutionary heritage, proteins continue to segregate themselves into functional units. It was found that proteins tend to interact with those encoded by genes of the same ancestry.

Eubacterial proteins are more likely than archaebacterial to be targeted to the mitochondria, and mitochondrion-targeted proteins tend to interact with each other.[833] It was demonstrated that proteins also tend to interact with those within the same functional category (i.e., informational interact with informational and operational with operational).[834] After billions of years, the eukaryotic cell is still essentially two independent cells that continue the cooperative trend under a specific limited range of metabolic conditions. However, this cooperative trend, which is redox sensitive, operates near the border of entropy. The trend is a metabolic electrodynamic state that can exhibit several possible outcomes, which are input dependent. The metabolic trend of the chimeric nucleus and its mitochondrial partner have three options:

---

[828] Alvarez-Ponce, D., McInerney J.O., (2011), "The human genome retains relics of its prokaryotic ancestry: human genes of archaebacterial and eubacterial origin exhibit remarkable differences," *Genome, Biol & Evol;* doi:10.1093/gbe/evr073

[829] Brand, K., (1997), "Aerobic glycolysis by proliferating cells: protection against oxidative stress at the expense of energy yield," *J Bioener & Biomembranes;* 29(4): 355-364

[830] Rivera, Op Cit

[831] Cotton, JA., McInerney, JO, (2010), "Eukaryotic genes of archaebacterial origin are more important than the more numerous eubacterial genes, irrespective of function," *Proc Natl Acad Sci USA;* 107: 17252-17255

[832] Rivera, Op cit

[833] Alverez-Ponce Op cit.

[834] Rual, JF., et al., (2005), "Towards a proteome-scale map of the human protein-protein interaction network" *Nature;* 437: 1173-1178

it can continue at various readjusted homeostatic levels, it can collapse, or it can reverse.

Of particular relevance to the nature of the symbiotic relationship is the noted switch in the energy system from OXPHOS to aerobic glycolysis used by normal cells in the late S phase of cell division and by proliferating tumor cells. Several studies by Brand,[835,836] using rat thymocytes and proliferating human promyelocytic HL-60 cells as models have outlined the mechanism by which normal proliferating cells and proliferating transformed cells preferentially use aerobic glycolysis. This strategic transition in energy production is evolutionarily conserved in the chimeric genome. This research demonstrated that the oxidation of the cysteine residues in the activating transcription factor Sp1 (and others) caused a low-binding efficiency to the cognate DNA element, indicating that nuclear extracts from resting cells were responsive to oxidative signals and consequently decreased the transcription of glycolytic enzymes. However, proliferating cells were responsive to reductive signals, which led to enhanced binding of Sp1 to the GC boxes, thereby increasing gene expression of glycolytic enzymes during the proliferation phase (S phase) of the cell cycle. The Brand studies indicate that cellular redox changes can regulate gene expression by reversible oxidative inactivation of Sp-1 binding.

Confirmation of this process comes from an evaluation of the thioredoxin system. Thioredoxin is a small redox-regulating protein that is crucial to stabilizing cellular redox homeostasis and cell survival under stress.[837] Thioredoxin can directly reduce transcription factors and other antioxidant systems that are upregulated in response to oxidative stress. The main target genes are involved in anaerobic metabolism, angiogenesis, and haematopoiesis. All these target genes ensure that either the cell is restored to normal oxygen homeostasis (e.g., after cell division) by surviving with reduced energy production or that the cells die because of a persistent energy deficit.[838]

An important part of the control strategy is also the role played by pyruvate. The rate of pyruvate formation during aerobic glycolysis increases. This is part of the evolutionarily conserved process by which the required reductive signals are provided during aerobic glycolysis. It has been well documented

---

[835] Brand, K., (1997), "Aerobic glycolysis by proliferating cells: protection against oxidative stress at the expense of energy yield. *J Bioenerg Biomembr;* 29(4): 355-364

[836] Brand, K., Hermfisse, U., (1997), "Aerobic glycolysis by proliferating cells: a protective strategy against reactive oxygen species," *FASEB J;* 11(5): 388-395

[837] Lar;emois. TC. Tpmossem. KF, (2010), "Thioredoxin and cancer: a role for thioredoxin in all states of tumor oxygenation," *Cancers;* 2" 209-232

[838] Roch, S., (2007), "Gene regulation under low oxygen: holding your breath for transcription," *Trends Biochem Sci;* 32: 389-397

that pyruvate is an effective scavenger or ROS.[839,840] Thus, the transition to aerobic glycolysis by proliferating cells results in two cooperative functions: (1) the generation of antioxidative pyruvate (and the thioredoxin system) and (2) the prevention of excessive ROS production by diminishing oxidative glucose metabolism.[841] It is thought that by this method of cell division, using mostly aerobic glycolysis as an energy source, the central genome is protected from the deleterious consequences of oxidative stress. In essence, the transition from the OXPHOS system to aerobic glycolysis is evolutionarily conserved in the archeabacterial genes that are still more responsive to reductive signals (aerobic glycolysis) and the eubacterial genes that are still more responsive to oxidative signals consistent with their original ancestral metabolic pathways. Thus, the redox status of the cell acts as a type of railroad switch sensor for the cell's energy status and therefore[842] determines which genes will be maximally functional (the information or operational genes) depending on whether the cell is resting or dividing.[843]

Early in the AIDS crisis, it was established that these patients had both acute and long-term exposures to a variety of known biological stressors that resulted in a massive loss of sulfur. The issue then as now should not have been to do the called-for human experimentation but to raise questions about the metabolic consequences that arise from a deficiency in the thiol pool. It, in fact, has been the key to solving what did not have to be a thirty-year war on the unsuspecting public. Why? Because it is this proton deficiency that is the missing factor that prohibits the required change in the redox status from acting as the decisive sensor for initiating the protective switch between the mitochondria and the host cell in the early phases of cell division. In addition to pyruvate acting as an antioxidant, hydrogen ions—which are generated by the glycerol phosphate and malate aspartate shuttles and are usually transferred into the mitochondria to fuel the OXPHOS system—are now directionally reversed and remain in the cytosol, enhancing the reductive environment. Under most stable metabolic conditions, if sufficient reducing equivalents are available to transfer to the ETC, the cell will maintain its ability to leave the proliferative

---

[839] Andrae, U. et al., (1985), "Pyruvate and related alpha ketoacids protect mammalian cells in culture against hydrogen peroxide induced cytotoxicity," *Toxicol Lett;* 28: 93-98

[840] O'Donnell—Tormey, J. et al., (1987), "SSecretion of pyruvate—an antioxidant defense of mammalian cells," *J Exp Med;* 165: 500-514

[841] Brand, Hermfisse, Op cit.

[842] Brandes, N, et al., (2008), "Thiol-based redox switches in eukaryotic proteins," *Anioxid Redox Signal;* 11(5): 997-1014

[843] Bauer, CE., et al., (1999), "Mechanisms for redox control of gene expression," *Annu Rev Microbiol;* 53: 495-523

cycle and return to the resting phase. However, stress conditions, involving thiol depletion, which can either be acute or chronic, can alter cellular homeostasis and the chimeric trend of the eukaryotic nucleus by the reversal of the flow of protons. If acute, this will result in collapse of the mitochondrial membrane potential and either necrosis or apoptosis. If chronic, as in AIDS and cancer, the cooperative trend of the chimeric nucleus unravels. It allows the cell to survive but at a lower energy (electromagnetic) level. The mitochondrial symbiont is the driving force in the maintenance of the cell's electromagnetic fields and thus the cooperative trend of the chimeric nucleus.

Stress and the Immune Response

Another factor to consider in metabolic disturbances of AIDS patients was the role that psychological stress played in the development of their altered immune/energy status both before and certainly after the diagnosis. The psychological stress was bolstered by the climate of fear created by both the gross incompetence and outright fraud that was generated around this issue. Recent studies examining the relationship among stress, immunity, and infection have shown that the nervous, endocrine, and immune systems communicate tridirectionally via shared messenger molecules whether neurotransmitters, cytokines, or hormones[844] and that neuroendocrine hormones also influence the regulation of immune function, in particular, Th1/Th2 balance and diurnal variation.[845] It is now understood that the neuroendocrine/immune system operates in a holistic and seamless manner. T cells express over twenty neuroendocrine receptors and at least as many cytokine receptors, underscoring the level of complexity of intracellular cross-talk. T cell responsiveness under different conditions is therefore likely to originate in this receptor cross-communication involving both cytokine and neuroendocrine receptors. Therefore, reductionist experiments, as have been carried out by AIDS researchers, examining the role of individual factors in T-cell subset differences may be less important than examination of the overall cytokine and hormonal milieu *in vivo* at the time of T-cell activation.[846]

Although there has been a great deal of focus on the role of the immune cell network as a defense against foreign proteins, it has a much broader function.

---

[844] Petrovsky, N,(2001) "Towards a unified model of neuroendocrine—immune interaction," *Immun Cell Biol;* 79: 350-357
[845] Petrovsky, Ibid
[846] Petrovsky, Op cit.

The immune cell network is comprised of particularly redox-sensitive cells, whose diverse functions are to ensure a balance in energy flows. If this can no longer be maintained on a cellular or intracellular level by too many immune and nonimmune cells becoming necrotic or apoptotic, then the immune cells switch, consistent with the evolutionary rules of intracellular self-defense of bioenergetic balance (based on redox equilibrium), to an extracellular safeguard that is done largely by increasing antibody production as an emergency measure.[847] The active strategy of immune cells is determined by the health and level of function of the cell symbiotic relationship. "The immune cell network is thus an early warning system for the organism as a whole. The immune cells are feelers and executors, sensors and effectors, that continuously measure and modulate the redox milieu as control variables for the continual perfusion of energy and substance flows."[848] In fact, the extracellular safeguard of increased antibody production was suggested as early as 1982 when it was noted that patients with AIDS might have an immune disregulation rather than an immune deficiency. In a study by Mildvan, et al.,[849] the B-cell compartment of AIDS patients appeared to be relatively intact compared with T-cell function. It is of interest that these researchers considered that the immune defect of AIDS patients might be contained in a subpopulation of helper cells involved mainly in cellular responses. This observation was made four years before the Mosmann and Coffman studies of T-cell subset heterogeneity[850,851] (see chapter on the heterogeneity of the immune system).

If the cell's energy loss is acute as the result of increased oxides, the cell has the option of dying by necrosis. Necrosis is a passive process of unregulated cell demise typified by gross damage and spillage of intracellular contents. If the energy loss is slower and there is still enough energy to dismantle the nucleus and remaining cell contents by programmed cell death when the cell membrane is still intact, then the more controlled apoptosis will occur. Apoptosis then is a controlled process that avoids inflammation and damage to the surrounding

---

[847] Kremer, H., (2008), "The Silent Revolution in Cancer and AIDS medicine," Xlibris pp. 164-165

[848] Kremer, Ibid

[849] Midvan, et al., (1982), "Opportunistic infections and immune deficiency in homosexual men," *Ann Intern Med;* 96(6 Pt 1): 700-704

[850] Mossman, TR, Coffman RI, (1987), "Two types of mouse T helper cell clones: implications for immune regulation," *Immunol Today;* 8: 223-226

[851] Mossman, TR, Coffman RI, (1989), "TH1 and TH2 cells: different patterns of lymphokine secretion lead to different functional properties," *Ann Rev Immunol;* 7: 145-173

tissue.[852] These are the processes that underlie the clinical presentations in acute infections, inflammatory processes, and autoimmune illnesses and have been classified as type 1 overregulation. Type 1 overregulation is dominated by the expression of a type 1 cytokine profile (IL-2, IL-12, IFN-γ, TNF-β).[853] It occurs after an acute load of oxidative stressors and a rapid breakdown of the counterregulation of the thiol pool and other antioxidant systems.

If the stressors are chronic and lead to the activation of the hypothalamic pituitary adrenal (HPA) axis with an increased sustained glucocorticoid output as well as nitrosylation of the thiol proteins and a decreased production of oxidative signals, another series of evolutionary programmed counterregulatory measures occurs, leading ultimately to decreased OXPHOS ATP production and a reversal of the "hybrid impulse" of the central genome and the relationship to the mitochondria. As was the process in the ancient hydrogenosomes, hydrogen begins to diffuse from the mitochondria to the cytoplasm, decreasing the OXPHOS production of ATP and increasing the reductive signals that provoke repetitive mitotic events. This has been termed type 2 counterregulation and offers a plausible mechanism for, depending on the cell type, degeneration or dedifferentiation and proliferation. The cytokine signals are IL-4, IL-10, and TGF-β along with glucocorticoids, which together impart a selective bias toward a Th2 response. This is the pattern consistently encountered in AIDS patients.[854,855,856]

The regulators of these processes are the redox-sensitive mitochondria symbionts. An intensive communication takes place between the immune cell network and the neuroendocrine system as both systems synthesize and respond to the same signaling molecules: neurotransmitters, cytokines, and hormones.[857,858] Accordingly, the immune cells process all stress factors found in the blood or lymph pathways, in extracellular liquids, or those mediated by cell-to-cell contact or transmitted through neural pathways. Whether the disruption is caused by psychic

---

[852] Steller, H., (1995), "Mechanisms and genes of cellular suicide," *Science;* 267: 1445-1449

[853] Lucey, DR. et al., (1996), "Type 1 and Type 2 cytokine dysregulation in human infections, neoplastic, and inflammatory diseases," *Clin Microbiol Rev;* 532-562

[854] Barcellini, WGP, et al., (1994), "Th1 and Th2 cytokine production by peripheral blood mononuclear cells from HIV infected patients," *AIDS;* 8: 757-762

[855] Meyaard, LSA, et al, (1994), "Changes in cytokine secretion patterns of CD4+T cell clones in human immunodeficiency virus infections," *Blood;* 84: 4262-4268

[856] Navikas, VJ, et al., (1994), "Increased levels of interferon-gamma (IFN-gamma), IL-4 and transforming growth factor (TGF-β) mRNA expressing blood mononuclear cells in human HIV infection," *Clin Exp Immunol:* 6:59-63

[857] Petrovsky, Op cit.

[858] Shi, Y., et al., (2002), "Stressed to death: Implication of lymphocyte apoptosis for psychoneuroimmunology," *Brain, Behavior, Immunity;* 17: S18-S26

trauma, pain, protein deficiency, microbial antigens or alloantigens, or antioxidant impairment as a result of malnutrition, nitrites or nitrosamines, bacterial toxins, serious burns or injuries, operations or organ transplants, pharmacological toxins, microwave radiation, drug abuse, doping agents, contaminated coagulating proteins or multitransfusions, antibiotics or vaccines, or congenital or acquired factors, the T helper cells and other cell systems will always react, readjust, and/or adapt by following the same evolutionary biological principles.[859]

Type 1 Cell Dis-symbiosis: Hypercatabolic Response to Acute Stressors

Under an acute stress load, the mitochondria has a system of evolutionary biological response patterns. An overwhelming acute stress load (NO and its congeners, the superoxide radical and hydrogen peroxide) can lead to a rapid breakdown of the counterregulation of the thiol pool and other antioxidant systems. The acuteness and rapidity of this response will lead to the opening of the mitochondrial transition pore, which has been demonstrated to induce a depolarization of the transmembrane potential ($\Delta\Psi m$). Depolarization of the $\Delta\Psi m$ can then lead to the release of apoptogenic factors including the protein-splitting caspase enzymes as well as decrease of the efficiency of oxidative phosphorylation. In normal physiology, and remembering that most of the genetic material of the symbiont has been transferred to the central genome, the PT is important for the transport of metabolites, which help to generate the $\Delta\Psi m$ as well as structural molecules, which have to be regulated and tightly controlled. If these functions are not correctly regulated, mitochondria could suffer irreversible damage.

The idea that PT can be a trigger for both apoptosis and necrosis is compatible with the finding that many drugs induce necrosis at high doses and apoptosis at lower doses. When PT is induced in a massive and rapid manner, which can quickly alter calcium fluctuations and other metabolic events, necrosis occurs before apoptogenic proteases can act. However induction of PT in a more controlled and protracted fashion allows proteases to be activated before ATP depletion causes cell death. Once the PT channel is affected, there follows release of calcium ions[860] followed by Ca^{2+} reuptake (Ca^{2+} cycling)[861] and

---

[859] Kremer, Op cit

[860] Giorgi, C., et al., (2012), "Mitochondrial Ca(2+) and apoptosis," *Cell Calcium;* 52(1): 36-43 doi: 10.1016/j.ceca.2012.02.008. Epub 2012 Apr 3.

[861] Richter, C., (1998), "Nitric Oxide and its congeners in mitochondria: implications for apoptosis," *Environ Health Perspectives;* 105(5): 1125-1130

the release of mitochondrial proteins. Because proton extrusion is generally a function of the respiratory chain, Ca2+ fluxes across the mitochondria divert protons away from the ATP synthase and thus uncouple respiration from ATP production.[862] Nuclear DNA and cell structures are then degraded by a cascade of protein-splitting enzymes. Pro-apoptotic factors and cytochrome c are released from the mitochondria. This is the consistent pattern that is evolutionarily conserved of the decompensated dis-regulation of cell symbiosis. This pattern is also is dependent on a type 1 cytokine profile.[863]

Type 2 Cell Dis-symbiosis: Counterregulation Under Chronic Stress Loads

However, in chronically stressed cells, including cancer cells, it is not a depolarization but hyperpolarization (more negative than normal) of the mitochondrial membrane potential that has been linked to malignant transformation:[864] $\Delta\Psi m$ in cancer cells $=\sim220mV$ as compared to $\sim140mV$ in normal cells.[865] Thermodynamically, the optimal $\Delta\Psi m$ for optimal ATP production is between 130–140mV.[866] A 10 percent value alteration in the $\Delta\Psi m$, above or below optimum results in an ~90 percent decrease in ATP synthesis and an ~90 percent increase in ROS.[867] When this occurs, it stalls respiration via the OXPHOS chain, shifting energy production to the cytoplasm via aerobic glycolysis. Thus, the hyperpolarization in cancer cells is suboptimal for efficient mitochondrial ATP production and mitochondria can no longer induce apoptosis. Experimentally, when cancer cells are switched out of aerobic glycolysis and into aerobic respiration, their $\Delta\Psi m$ returns to that of normal cells.[868,869]

---

[862] Demaures, N, et al., (2008), "Regulation of plasma membrane calcium fluxes by mitochondria," *Biochimica Biophysica Acta;* 1787(11): 1383-1394

[863] Lucey, et al., Op cit.

[864] Hockenbery, DM, (2010), "Targeting mitochondria for cancer therapy," *Enviorn Mol Mutagen;* 51(5): 476-489

[865] Forrest, MD., (2015), "Why cancer cells have a more hyperpolarised mitochondrial membrane potential and emergent prospects for therapy," *bioRxiv;*

[866] Bagkos, G., et al., (2014), "ATP synthesis revisited: new avenues for the management of mitochondrial diseases," *Curr Pharm Design;* 20(28): 4570-4579

[867] Bagkos, Ibid

[868] Fantin, VR, et al. (2006), "Attenuation of LDH-A expression uncovers a link between glycolysis, mitochondrial physiology, and tumor maintenance," *Cancer Cell;* 9(6): 425-435

[869] Bonnet, S., et al., (2007), "A mitochondria K+ channel axis is suppressed in cancer and its normalization promote apoptosis and inhibits cancer growth," *Cancer Cell;* 11(1): 37-51

Hyperpolarization of the ΔΨm has been associated with a decrease in Ca2+ cycling. The decrease in Ca2+ cycling is associated a reduced release of this ion from intracellular storage sites and Ca2+ accumulation into the mitochondrial matrix and with a decrease in the malate-aspartate shuttle of protons into the mitochondrial matrix. In apoptosis/necrosis, the mitochondrial release of cytochrome c is a crucial event in the cell-death pathway. The family of Bcl-2 proteins, located on the outer mitochondrial membrane, can prevent this release and are able to maintain some level of mitochondrial homeostasis. This family of proteins has been recently shown to regulate the integrity of the mitochondrial outer membrane via regulation of the outer membrane protein VDAC. The family of caspase enzymes becomes demobilized by the nitrosylation of a cysteine residue, thereby reducing the cells' entry into the apoptotic process.[870,871] If the outer membrane loses permeability after VDAC closure, metabolic anions such as ADP and malate will no longer be available to the mitochondria. This would slow ATP synthesis, the citric acid cycle, and the NAD+/NADH shuttles, leading to falling ATP and NAD+ levels, decreasing the cells OXPHOS energetic capacity, as well as a drop in CO_2 levels, which could affect the cell's pH balance.

Much of the early work on the hyperpolarization of cancer cell membranes was done by Dr. Lan Bo Chen at the Dana-Farber Institute in Boston using mitochondrial-specific rhodamine-based dyes. He demonstrated that the majority of cancer cells have hyperpolarized mitochondria compared with noncancer cells. He wrote: "The results of a six year systematic study overwhelmingly indicates that all normal epithelial cells tested have low mitochondrial potential, hence, low rhodamine 123 uptake and retention. In contrast, screenings of 200 cell lines/types derived from tumors of kidney, ovary, pancreas, lung, adrenal cortex, skin, breast, prostate, cervix, vulva, colon, liver, testes, esophagus, trachea, and tongue show that a great majority of adenocarcinoma, transitional cell carcinoma, squamous cell carcinoma, and melanoma have high rhodamine 123 uptake and retention."[872]

---

[870] Kim, YM, et al., (2000), "Nitric oxide prevents tumor necrosis factor α-induced rat hepatoyte apoptosis by the interruption of mitochondrial apoptotic signaling through S-nitrosylation of caspase-8," *Hepatology*; 32: 770-778

[871] Parrish, AB, et al., (2016), "Cellular mechanisms controlling caspase activation and function," *CSH Perspectives*; pp. 1-24

[872] Chen, LB., (1988), "Mitochondrial Membrane potential in living cells," *Ann Rev Cell Biol;* 4: 155-181

PROTEIN	CELLULAR FUNCTION	FUNCTIONAL EFFECT
Capase 3	↑ apoptosis	↓ enzymatic activity
Capase 8	apop. activation Cap. 3	↓ enzymatic activity
Bcl-2	inhibition of Cyto. C	Inhibits Bcl-2 degradation
c-FLIP	caspase 8 inhibitor	Inhibits c-Flip degradation
TRX	redox reg. and apoptosis	↓apoptosis, ↑ ROS
ASK1	Apoptosis	Inhibits ASK1 activity and binding to MKK-3 and 6
Src	proto-oncogene	↑ auto-phosphorylation
P21^{Ras}	GTPase	↑cellular GTPase activity
PTEN	phosphatase	↑ stability & activity of HIF-1α
HIF-1α	angiogenesis	↑stability and transcriptional activity
MMP-9	Proteolysis of ECM	↑ migration & invasion of cells
Dynamin-2	GTPase	↑ PGK activation & survival
Albumin	SNO reservoir	↑ cytoprotective & anti-bacterial effect
GRK2	negative regulator of-β-AR	↑ activity of β-AR signaling
NOS	multiple effects	Inhibition of NOS activity and NO production
Glucokinase	glucose metabolism	↑ in GK activity
JNK 1	apoptosis	↓ activation of cJun, apop.
Ap-1	transcription factor	↓ binding of c-Fos and c-Jun
NF-κβ p65	transcription factor	↓ iNOS negative transcription
Estrogen receptor	transcriptional regulator	↓ transcriptional activity

Chart 2
S-Nitrosylation of Protein Targets:[873] Type 2 Cell Dis-symbiosis

---

[873] Nitric Oxide and Cancer, Prognosis, Prevention and Therapy, (2010) ED. Benjamin Bonavida, Humana Press, Springer New York, pp. 91-92

Dichloroacetate: Reversal of the Metabolic-Electrical Remodeling and Apoptosis Resistance in Cancer Cells

A question that researchers have been addressing is what would happen to cancer cells if this hyperpolarization (as well as the S-nitrosylation of various thiol proteins) could be reversed and there could be a normalization of the mitochondrial membrane potential? Cancer progression and its resistance to therapy has been associated with the suppression of apoptosis and a suppression of mitochondrial activity. The PT channels close. As a result, there is a decrease of entry of pyruvate that results in a decreased flux of electrons in the ETC and therefore decrease in mitochondrial ROS production. Simultaneously, with the reduced entry of pyruvate (leading to a decline in glucose oxidation), glycolysis increases. The by-products of glycolysis (e.g., lactate and acidosis) contribute to the breakdown of the extracellular matrix, allow for the increase in cell mobility, and increase metastatic potential. All these elements are known to be upregulated in cancer and contribute to apoptosis resistance. Increased hexokinase 2 and Bcl-2 levels may also contribute to the apoptosis's suppressive capacity by the hyperpolarization of the mitochondrial membrane. Hexokinase directly interacts and promotes an "open" configuration of the VDAC in the outer mitochondrial membrane. Bcl-2 helps to inhibit cytochrome c release and inhibits K+ channel Kv1.5.[874]

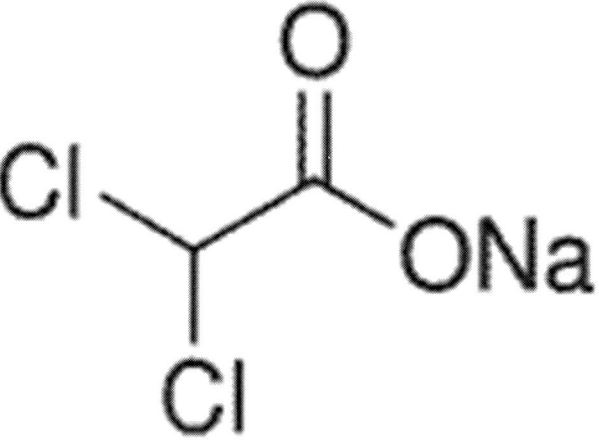

Sodium dichloroacetate

---

[874] Potassium channel, voltage dependent, Kv1.5 downloaded 2.27.2015 http://www.ebi.ac.uk/interpro/entry/IPR004052

The Slow Death of the AIDS/Cancer Paradigm and the Apocrypha of the Eukaryotic Cell

Salts of dichloroacetate (DCA) have been shown to depolarize mitochondria, returning the $\Delta\Psi m$ toward levels of noncancer cells without affecting the mitochondria of non-cancerous cells. DCA inhibits mitochondrial pyruvate dehydrogenase kinase (PDK), which normally inactivates the enzyme pyruvate dehydrogenase (PDH), which catalyzes the conversion of pyruvate to acetyl-CoA, thus allowing the shift in metabolism from cytoplasm-based glycolysis to mitochondria-based glucose oxidation. This allows for a decrease of the $\Delta\Psi m$, an increase in the production of mitochondrial ROS (H_2O_2), and activation of the PT channels in cancer cells but not normal cells. The flux of electrons down the ETC is associated with the production of ROS and with the efflux of H+, which contribute to a negative $\Delta\Psi m$. DCA has been shown to induce apoptosis, decrease proliferation, and tumor growth without apparent toxicity.

What this demonstrates is that glucose oxidation was increased by DCA and clearly shows that cancer mitochondria undergo a metabolic electrical remodeling that is an adaptive response and therefore may not be irreversibly damaged as has been previously thought. This further raises the possibility that in cancer there is an active and dynamic suppression of mitochondrial function in order to suppress apoptosis. The refueling of mitochondria by driving pyruvate inside this organelle, reverses this suppression, reactivates the apoptotic pathway (increased ROS, decreased $\Delta\Psi m$, open PT), and unlocks the cancer cells from a state of apoptosis resistance. Inhibiting glycolysis (especially in the proximal stages) will not reactivate mitochondria. It will be toxic to several noncancerous tissues that depend on glycolysis for energy production. The issue is to improve the glycolysis to glucose oxidation coupling, not inhibit glycolysis.

The switch in energy production from oxidative phosphorylation to glycolysis has been termed the Warburg effect and has been confounding researchers steeped in the dogmas of material scientism, genetic determinism, and Darwinism. Medical molecular biology has failed in explanation of disease development and progression as a consequence of genetic disruption because it has not been able to rationally construe the consequences of the intersection of deep phylogenetics with the geochemistry of early Earth. The central genomes of eukaryotes developed billions of years ago as a fusion event involving an archaebacterium and an eubacterium. The eubacterium became the mitochondria that transferred most of its genetic capability to the central genome. As a result of this event, current eukaryotic genomes are chimeras of genes inherited from both endosymbiotic partners: the archaebacterium and the eubacterium. It is not the interactions of these two organisms and their genomes per se but the energetic links that created the initial drive toward fusion that can give insight into most of the chronic disease manifestations plaguing modern civilization. The crucial issue has always been how do these two genomes communicate and how is cell metabolism altered when those communication channels began to falter? Under conditions of both acute and long-term stress, it is the evolutionary biological energetic/metabolic delinking of the trend of the initial fusion event that can lead to the reversal of the "hybrid impulse." It is this evolutionary biological programmed response that seeks a homeostatic niche for survival by switching energy production from the more efficient OXPHOS to the less efficient and more ancient aerobic glycolysis consistent with the information functions (translation, transcription, and replication) of the ancestry of the archaebacterial genome. The acute loss of energy fluctuations or the energy switch from OXPHOS to glycolysis and the consequent change in cellular metabolism then are what manifest as certain disease states, including AIDS and cancer. Both AIDS, which includes in the syndrome two types of cancers and cancer without the AIDS diagnosis, are electrochemical metabolic processes and can only be identified and resolved in the context of the synthrophic evolutionary origin of the eukaryotic cell.

Life is a process of harnessing energy, from the sun or from the energy released by one-electron oxygen reduction. These processes can start chain reactions of free radicals, which allowed open systems in water to self-organize, thus producing order out of chaos and giving rise to dramatic decreases in entropy. From the beginning, life occurred on Earth because it was able to harness these energy sources. Because the radicals created are highly reactive, a method was needed to balance what could be a deleterious process by the counterbalance of reduction. Living systems have used sulfur to quell the radical fires. Both of these elements, oxygen and sulfur, belong in the same column of the periodic table and can exchange electrons. The driving force, mainly the interspecies hydrogen transfer[875] that created the evolutionary process of cell symbiosis, was a nonlinear, complex, and quasi-deterministic thermodynamic energy-fluctuating event. The methanogen consumed the hydrogen and carbon dioxide liberated from the eubacteria, and the eubacteria benefited by being able to speed up its metabolic rate because it now had a ready hydrogen sink.[876] The mitochondrial endosymbionts and the chimeric nucleus allowed for the evolution of ever increasing complexity, including humans who have the possibility of being both self-aware and in alignment with the natural flow of the universe. However, current environmental/political trends that have increased in intensity since the beginning of the Industrial Revolution

---

[875] Lopez-Garcia, P, Moreira, D., (1999), "Metabolic symbiosis at the origin of eukaryotes," *Trends Biochem Sci;* 24(3): 88-93
[876] Lopez-Garcia, Ibid.

The Slow Death of the AIDS/Cancer Paradigm and the Apocrypha of the Eukaryotic Cell

challenge the symbiont and the chimeric nucleus with an ever-increasing array of environmental, electromagnetic, pharmacological, and psychological toxins. The question is, to what degree will the current economic/war paradigm push the boundaries of the limits of endosymbiotic homeostasis?

According the National Cancer Institute, cancer will affect one in two men and one in three women in the United States, and the number of new cases is projected to double by 2050. Until midtwentieth century, physicians were treating patients primarily for acute complaints (type 1 overregulation). Chronic diseases have now become the leading causes of death and disability in the United states.[877] Seven of the top ten causes of death in 2010 were chronic diseases including hypertension, CAD, stroke, diabetes, cancer, COPD, and kidney failure. This disease spectrum reflects a clear pattern of the type 2 dis-symbiosis of the hybrid impulse of the eukaryotic cell. With an insight into the evolutionary biology of the eukaryotic cell, AIDS and cancer and many of the chronic diseases that are plaguing society are not the great conundrums of modern civilization but simply overcompensated type 2 counterregulation of the cell network—predictable (and often reversible) from an evolutionary biological point of view.

---

[877] http://www.cdc.gov/chronicdisease/overview/index.htm?s_cid=ostltsdyk_govd_203 20 May 2014

CHAPTER 8

The Versatility of the Mitochondrial Endosymbiont Is Consistent with Its Evolutionary Heritage

Free radicals provide activation energy for biological processes as well as biochemical and physiological rhythmic modes

By 1956 Denham Harman advanced the free radical theory of aging before most other scientists understood the role of free radicals in biological processes.[878] At the cellular level, all the biological stressors, including those of chemical and physical (abiotic) or of infectious (biotic) or of an emotional (psychological) nature, can cause an increase in endogenous free radical production and can overwhelm the various antioxidant defenses, causing both cellular and extracellular matrix damage.[879] This hypothesis has been widely accepted, and free radicals are now commonly thought of as pathogenic agents. However, as is generally true in complex nonlinear biological systems, ROS are neither all bad nor all good but must be considered contextually as they play a much more starring role in the vital functions of normal physiology.[880] What role ROS play will depends on the previous history of the cell, its current state (reductive capacity), and also background level and composition of ROS. As

---

[878] Harman, D., (1956), "Aging: a theory based on free radical and radiation chemistry," *J Gerontol;* 11(3): 298-300

[879] van Wijk, R.,(1992) "Biophoton emission, stress and disease," *Experientia;* 48: 1029-1030

[880] Dröge, W., (2002), "Free radicals in the physiological control of cell function," *Physiol Rev;* 82: 47-95

discussed in the chapter on nitric oxide, the composition of ROS depends both upon the mode of ROS generation by the cell itself and their incoming flow from both internal and exogenous sources and on the rate of elimination.[881] In the early AIDS patients, as construed from their long histories of toxin exposures, not only was the influx of ROS/RNS increased over time by previously named conditions, but the rate of elimination was significantly reduced as a result of specific known antioxidant deficiencies.

Therefore, the various functions of free radicals must be considered contextually beyond their destructive capabilities. Free radicals help to maintain redox homeostasis, mediate physiological responses, initiate signaling cascades,[882] and are indispensable participants of fluxes in which a valuable form of energy—high-density energy of electromagnetic excitation (EEE, as the result of rapid fluctuations of oxygen reduction from its excited to ground state)—is constantly generated in the biologic system. Energy released by these reactions can then be used as an activation energy for specific biochemical processes and for the continuous "pumping" of the nonequilibrium state of inter- and intracellular structural components. This ROS energy pumping, which is oscillatory, not only drives the activation of biochemical processes but also develops structural patterns that determine biochemical and physiological rhythmic modes.[883]

ROS liberate enough energy to generate electronically excited states of carbonyls, excited pigments, and singlet molecular oxygen.[884,885] These reactions are unique in their energy output as they are accompanied by the release of energy quanta equivalent to electronic excitation. The ROS, produced in great abundance, may also act as oscillatory sparks of low-power/high-density energy impulses that are quickly produced and then eliminated by certain enzymes (SOD and catalase at a rate exceeding 10^6 cycles/sec) running in aqueous systems. Energy that is generated in reaction to ROS elimination is not dissipated as heat but may be stored and used both as energy of activation of particular biochemical reactions and as regulatory signals.[886] According to some estimates, 10 percent and as much as 20 percent of oxygen consumed by

---

[881] Voeikov, V., (2001), Op cit.
[882] Dröge, W., Ibid
[883] Voeikov, V., (2001), Op Cit.
[884] van Wijk, Op cit.
[885] Pospisil, P, et al., (2014), "Role of reactive oxygen species in ultra-weak photon emission in biological systems," *J Photochem Photobiol;* 139: 11-23
[886] Voeikov, VL., (2006), "Reactive oxygen species (ROS): pathogens or sources of vital energy? Part 2. bioenergetic and bioinformational functions of ROS," *J Alt Complem Med;* 12(3): 265-270

an animal at rest is routed to the univalent pathway of reduction along which ROS are generated.[887]

All aerobic animals, including humans, gain most of our energy from the oxidation of different substrates. Nervous tissue and brain have an especially high oxygen utilization. The human brain, which is approximately 2 percent of body weight, uses more than 20 percent of oxygen consumed. But there is an unanswered question. Biochemistry textbooks claim that most oxygen utilization takes place in the mitochondria where the energy potential of oxygen is transferred into the production of ATP. But studies have shown that brain cells contain fewer mitochondria than muscle or liver cells.[888] Therefore, there must exist some other pathway for O_2 reduction the brain uses to consume more oxygen than any other tissue. The answer may be found in the energy derived from one-electron oxygen reduction that can occur in the structured water-surrounding-protein complexes.

The Unique Properties of Oxygen

Although there is evidence that the earliest organism developed enzymes able to reduce oxygen,[889] the evolutionary impulse toward greater complexity on Earth was not initiated until there were rising levels of atmospheric oxygen. The oxygen molecule contains a vast reservoir of available energy. It has the identifiably uncommon quantum characteristic of two electrons with parallel spins on its valence orbitals.[890] One of the quantum physical properties of an electron is a spin, which may be either clockwise or counterclockwise in its direction of rotation. The most stable state for two electrons with opposite spins is their pairing. Generally, electrons in a molecule separate into pairs (M $(\uparrow\downarrow)_n$). This is called the ground singlet state. If an electron loses a partner, the molecule becomes unbalanced and turns into a free radical—a particle with an odd number of electrons. However, this is not true for oxygen. Two of its twelve electrons are unpaired and occupy spaces in the highest unfilled orbital of the molecule at opposite ends of the molecule, in essence, creating two free radical centers. Thus, oxygen is a diradical in which the two unpaired electrons

---

[887] Shoaf, AR., Shaikh, AU, et al., (1991), "Extraction and analysis of superoxide free radicals (O_2^-) from whole mammalian liver" J Biolumin Chemilumin; 6: 87-96

[888] David, H, (1977), "Quantitative Ultrastructural Data of Animal and Human Cells," Stuttgart; New York

[889] Mascarelli, AL, (2010), "Methane eating microbes make their own oxygen," *Nature;* doi:10.1038/news.2010.146

[890] Matthews, PCS, (1986), *"Quantum chemistry of atoms and molecules"* Cambridge Univ. Press

have parallel spins in the most stable configuration of the molecule, which is therefore, by definition, in a triplet state, $^3O_2$. Particles in a triplet state are paramagnetic and possess an excess energy over a ground singlet state where all the electrons are paired. Unlike other molecules, however, oxygen in its singlet state is even more excited than a triplet state. Triplet oxygen is a vast energy store, able to release more than 180 kcal/mol of energy upon its reduction to two water molecules after gaining four electrons (together with their carriers, protons).[891] But oxygen cannot be spontaneously reduced, which accounts for the relative stability of the triplet state.[892,893]

There are several ways to activate oxygen. One of them is one-electron oxygen reduction with the subsequent formation of free radicals. An interesting aspect of these free radicals is that they may initiate chain reactions in solutions containing bioorganic molecules. The chain reactions occur because a free radical gains an electron from a molecule and turns into a molecule. The molecule is now a free radical and begins seeking an electron donor. It is in this manner that free radicals may commence the process of chain reactions in solutions containing bioorganic molecules. In vitro, it has been demonstrated that these reactions form more radicals that could have negative effects on cellular constituents.[894] In any case, the production of free radicals becomes a problem in either the acute or chronic persistence in a deficit of available reducing agents. Organisms use multiple mechanisms for a purposeful one-electron reduction of oxygen,[895] and whether these oxygen radicals serve as a source of energy supply or initiate cell damage depends on the context in which they occur. As the energy from these chain reactions may be released as light rather than heat, under certain conditions, oscillations appear. From these conditions, it can be presumed that the oscillatory release of photonic energy may be in principle provided by electron currents in closed circles of free radical transformations.[896]

Water plays a starring role in the generation, transformation, and utilization of energy for the realization of biological functions primarily by the process of

---

[891] Voeikov, V., (2003), "Mitogenetic radiation, biophotons and non-linear oxidative processes in aqueous media" in Integrative Biophysics, Biophotonics (Popp, FA., and Beloussov L, ed.) Kluwer Academic Publishers, Boston
[892] Voeikov, VL, (2006), Op cit.
[893] Khan, Wilson (1995), Op. cit.
[894] Fridovich, I., (1998), "Oxygen toxicity: a radical explanation," *J Exp Biol;* 201: 1203-1209
[895] Voeikov, (2001), Op cit.
[896] Voeikov, (2003), Op cit

one electron oxygen reduction. Its direct involvement in hydrolytic processes in which the formation of proteins, carbohydrates, and lipids are produced, in ATP synthesis, and in energy gain because of ATP hydrolysis is well-known.[897] However, recently, water has been shown to be one of the major sources of high-grade energy—the energy of electromagnetic excitation (EEE) generated when electrons in their excited state drop back to their ground state and in which active oxygen participates. In all reactions of radical recombination and peroxide decomposition, whether they proceed spontaneously or by way of catalysts, electron excited states are generated, i.e., the reaction of spontaneous superoxide dismutation:

$$2O_2^{-}\bullet + 2H^{+} \rightarrow H_2O_2 + {}^1O_2{}^{\bullet}$$

In this reaction, an electron excited singlet oxygen ($^1O_2\,^{\bullet}$) arises, which then converts to triplet oxygen. This causes a release of a quantum of energy of about 1 eV.[898] In the reaction if two molecules of hydrogen peroxide decompose to two molecules of water and a molecule of oxygen, 2 eV are released. The net release of energy of the reduction of one oxygen molecule to two water molecules by consecutive addition of four electrons to it is 8 eV. How does that compare to the energy released by ATP?

Even though the concept of the high-energy phosphate bond was disproved in the mid-1950s,[899] it is still being taught that ATP is the fundamental source of cellular energy. Textbooks continue to claim that upon hydrolysis of the phosphate bond, the ATP molecule releases this high energy stored in the phosphate bond that results from the transport of electrons through the electron transport chain. It is the hydrolysis of this bond that can then be released for work. However, the energy released when a phosphate bond is hydrolyzed yields ~ 6 to 14 kcal/mol[900,901] (equivalent to <0.5 eV or an electromagnetic wave with $\lambda > 2.5$ microns—the middle of the IR spectrum). Interestingly, it has been shown that ATP synthesis from ADP and P_i requires the input of approximately 10 kcal/mol of free energy.[902] Since it takes as much energy to make ATP as

---

[897] Voeikov, VL, (2003), "Fundamental role of water in bioenergetics) pp 89-104 in Biophotonics and Coherent Systems in Biology, Springer

[898] Voeikov, (2001), Op cit.

[899] Podolsky, RJ, Morales, MP, (1956), "The enthalpy change of adenosine triphosphate hydrolysis," *J Biol Chem;* 218:945-959

[900] Podolsky, RJ, Morales, MP, Ibid

[901] Kawaguchi, K, Ishiwata, S., (2001), "Thermal activation of single kinesin molecules with temperature pulse microscopy," *Cell Motility and the Ctoskeleton;* 49: 41-47

[902] Tsong, TY, (1989), "Deciphering the language of cells," *Trends Biochem Sci;* 14(3): 89-92

The Slow Death of the AIDS/Cancer Paradigm
and the Apocrypha of the Eukaryotic Cell

is posited as the energy released by the hydrolysis of ATP, then relying on the molecule as the sole energy source redefines the living state as in equilibrium, i.e., dead. Of course, this is an absurdity, and thus, there is a consideration that there are other methods by which energy is harnessed both from ATP and by the use of ROS and the resultant electronic excited states.

ATP, in addition to not being able to supply sufficient cellular energy needs, is not always at the site where energy is required for work, especially in large proteins with many parts (e.g., myosin). Therefore, one has to consider how energy in the cell is transmitted over distances. Recent research has noted that the cellular architecture, the cytoskeleton, especially microtubules, fulfills the prerequisites for the generation of a quasi-coherent electromagnetic field.[903] The volume fraction of the cell occupied by the microtrabecular network along with the microtubules and intermediate filaments that compose the cytoskeleton has been measured at just under 20 percent.[904] Enzyme clusters self-assemble along these networks.[905] Analysis of high-voltage electron micrographs reveals that within this trabecular lattice, more than half the water lies within 5 nm of some obvious surface.[906] Consequently, the whole biological water is interfacial water, which is almost totally coherent.[907,908]

Interfacial water creating exclusion zones next to molecular surfaces has quasi-polymeric properties and molecular ordering that creates an energy differential available for work. Exclusion zones or EZ water may be used as a source of respiration (one-electron oxygen reduction and the propagation of branched chain reactions)[909]. The structure of the coherent domains of

---

[903] Cifra, M., (2009), "Study of electromagnetic oscillations of yeast cells in kHz and GHz region," Doctoral Thesis, Czech Technical University in Prague

[904] Gershon, BZ., Cohen, D., (1985), "The cytoplasmic matrix: its volume and surface area and the diffusion of molecules through it," *Proc Nat Acad Sci USA*;82(15):5030-5034

[905] Barry, R., Zemer, G. (2011), "Self assembling enzymes and the origins of the cytoskeleton," *Curr Opin Microbiol;* 14(6): 704-711

[906] Clegg, J.S., (1988), "On the internal environment of animal cells," *Microcompartmentation*, CRC Press. Boca Raton

[907] coherence—the property of an ensemble of components of having a well defined value of the phase in tune with a field present in the ensemble—in quantum electrodynamics—which describes the interaction between the electromagnetic field and an ensemble of molecules

[908] Beloussov, LV, Voeikov, VI, Martynyuk, VS, (Editors), *Biophotonics and Coherent Systems in Biology;* Springer 2007, New York, NY

[909] branching chain reactin is a chain reaction which includes a propagation step or steps in which there is an increase in the number of active intermediates; for example $H + O2 \rightarrow OH + O$ is a branching reaction since one of the active intermediates (H) gives rise to two (OH and O).

interfacial water can offer a continuous supply of electrons that work with ATP to supply the stored structural energy of the cell. As such, it might be valuable to reconsider an alternate hypothesis on how ATP might fulfill its energetic function. The concept of the high-energy phosphate bond was disproved as early as the 1950s. There may be no utilizable free energy stored in any of the phosphate bonds of ATP. According to an early model proposed by Riseman and Kirkwood,[910] ATP serves its role for keeping contractile proteins like myosin from collapsing upon themselves and shortening by the method of long-range electrostatic repulsion (transmitted through space). Early in his career, Gilbert Ling proposed a similar salt-linkage hypothesis. According to this hypothesis, the negatively charged β and γ-carboxyl groups of isolated native proteins are largely engaged in salt linkages with fixed cations (e.g., positively charged ϵ-amino groups and guanidyl groups belonging respectively to lysine and arginine residues of intracellular proteins)[911] and are therefore not free to adsorb cations like K^+. In Ling's early model, these β and γ-carboxyl groups can be made available for adsorbing K^+ ions by ATP when ATP occupies key controlling cardinal sights.[912] He later refined this concept by analyzing negative-charge densities and attractions based on the density of an oxygen atom at an oxyacid group and assigning to it a value. He also introduced a positive-charge density that is a measure of the positive-charge density of a fixed cation group. Based on these charge density calculations, he was able to demonstrate that these values had a high predictability for the likelihood of either K^+ or Na^+ being attracted to a protein residue.[913] He identified ATP as the "cardinal adsorbent" that acts, because of a dense negative charge, on the protein-ion-water systems similar to a horseshoe magnet on local nails and iron filings.[914] In fact, it is this binding per se that is the event of primary significance as the electron cloud shifts along through adjacent atoms. In negatively charged proteins, this will allow an extension because negatively charged proteins with

---

[910] Kirkwook, JG., Riseman, J. (1948), "The intrinisic viscosities and diffusion constants of flexible macromolecules in solution," *J Chem Phys;* 16: 565-572

[911] Speakman, JB, Hirst, MC., (1931), "The pH stability region of insoluble proteins," *Nature;*127: 665-666

[912] Ling, G., (2001), Life at the Cell and Below Cell Level, the Hidden History of a Fundamental Revolution in Biology, Pacific Press, NY, p 50

[913] Ling discounts the theory of pumps as unnecessary as solute partitioning can be explained by a combination of association with proteins and reduced solvency of cell water

[914] Ling, Ibid

the negatively charged ATP will induce locally strong repulsive forces that drive the extension.[915]

Imagine a series of iron nails joined head to end with bits of string and lying near randomly placed iron filings. When a strong horseshoe magnet is brought into contact with the head of one nail, a magnetization is propagated. As a result, not only are the tethered nails brought into a more rigid and ordered conformation, but the iron filings also become magnetized and attach themselves singly or in polarized multilayers onto the chain of nails. The magnet together with the nails and iron filings now exists in a higher-energy, lower-entropy state.[916] As an example of this long-range action is the hemoglobin (Hgb) molecule. Hemoglobin's affinity for oxygen is considerably reduced by ATP.[917] The action seems to result only from ATP binding because (a) hemoglobin does not hydrolyze ATP and (b) the ATP-binding site is remote from the four oxygen-binding sites. Therefore, the effect of ATP binding is to induce a type of cooperative phase transition that propagates throughout the hemoglobin molecule.

In the living cell, the protein-ion-water systems are, like the example above, cooperatively linked. The protein (cytoskeleton and attached proteins) can be thought of as the tethered nails, K^+/Na^+ and water molecules are the equivalent of the iron filings, and ATP with a high concentration of negative charge is the equivalent of the horseshoe magnet. As proteins are dynamic systems, they must fluctuate (oscillate) in order to work. Accordingly, ATP then acts as the principal cardinal adsorbent[918] on the cytoskeletal structure, conferring a higher level of structural organization and stored available energy for work in the space-time structure, allowing organelles and motor proteins and protein clusters surrounded by a coherent domain of water molecules to move at will when and where needed in the cell. It is likely that close proximity of the three ATP phosphates confers a high concentration of negative charge on the molecule,[919] creating a focal point of intense charge. Therefore, ATP is one part of the provision of cellular structural energy available for the performance of work, but the other parts are derived from the steady-state level of ROS and

---

[915] Pollack, GH., (2001), "Cells, Gels and the engines of life, a new, unifying approach to cell function," Ebner & Sons, Seattle, WA. p 257888888

[916] Ling Op cit 150

[917] Klinger, RG., Zahn, DP, et al., (1971), "Binding of ATP to human hemoglobin under simulated *in vivo* conditions," *Europ J Biochem;* 18: 171-177

[918] cardinal adsorbent: an adsorbent on a cell protein that critically control the metastable cooperative state of a gang of protein sites

[919] Ling, GN, (2001) Life at the cell and below cell level, the hidden history of a fundamental revolution in biology, Pacific Press, NY

the interaction of singlet oxygen and structured water. These energetic fluxes are part of the nonequilibrium processes that contribute to the creation of the energy of electronic excitation that allows spontaneous organization, fluidity, and oscillatory periodicity, which is characteristic of living cells.[920,921]

The reactive species not only help to drive a multitude of metabolic process but are part of the cells stored structural energy that may address the missing energy needs of the cell, which are not completely answered by ATP and may work cooperatively with ATP to maintain the high-energy, low-entropy state of a normally functioning cell. The key to understanding the thermodynamics of a living system is energy storage under energy flow as first suggested by Gurwitsch in the early part of the twentieth century when he began to examine the phenomenon of mitogenic radiation (photons) on plant cell growth. What he demonstrated in his experiments was that direct activation of oxygen is indispensable for the emergence of such (mitogenic) radiations in the course of biochemical reactions.[922] Thus, activation of oxygen was early in the twentieth century determined to be the necessary factor for the occurrence of cell division, the fundamental process without which no living system can sustain itself.[923]

Mitochondria Play a Versatile Role in Cell Metabolism

Mitochondrial biochemistry is complex and is involved not only in energy production by way of oxygen consumption and oxidative phosphorylation but also in lipid catabolism, heme biosynthesis, calcium homeostasis, apoptosis, and production of ROS, including NO. Mitochondria also play a role in the wasting syndrome experienced by patients in the late stages of thiol deficiency. This is because the first stage of urea synthesis occurs in the liver mitochondria. The wasting syndrome occurs in the latter stages of thiol deficiency when there are elevated levels of the ammonium ion as a result of the degradation of proteins of the peripheral muscles, which are transformed and used as substrates in glycolysis. Several studies have observed that the threshold for

---

[920] Richard, P., (2003), "The rhythm of yeast," *FEMS Microbiol Rev;* 547-557

[921] Popp, FA., (1992), "Some essential questions of biophoton research and probable answers" in Recent Advances in Biophoton Research and its Applications, Ke-hsueh Li and Qiao Gu (eds), Singapore, World Scientific, 1-46

[922] Gurwitsch, AG., Gurwitsch, LD., (1943), "Twenty years of mitogenetic radiation emergence, development and perspectives." *Uspekhi Sovremennoi Biologii;* 16: 305-334

[923] Wieland, H., (1932), "On the mechanism of oxidation," Yale Univ. Press, New Haven

the conversion of amino acids into other forms of chemical energy and the concomitant production of urea are regulated by the plasma cysteine level and hepatic cysteine catabolism.[924,925] The liver detoxifies ammonium by exporting nitrogen as urea via the ornithine cycle. The syndrome is characterized by low cysteine and glutamine levels and elevated levels of glutamate and hepatic urea production with a concomitant negative nitrogen balance. The control of the first stage of nitrogen export via the ornithine cycle occurs in the liver mitochondria by cysteine levels. Under normal metabolic conditions, if cysteine levels in plasma are in range, controlled amounts of urea are produced. However, low cysteine triggers an increasing breakdown of muscle proteins,[926] a characteristic finding in the later stages of the thiol deficiency syndrome. This process cannot simply be reversed, as often advocated, by increased caloric intake but must be addressed at the level of specific sulfur and other nutrient deficiencies.

Much recent research has focused on the dangers of reactive oxygen species to cell structures; but as seen from the above discussion, their steady-state output, largely from the mitochondria, demonstrates how the cell maximizes the use of energy output without dissipation into heat. Mitochondria can be a significant source of cellular ROS, which inherently depends on the metabolic "state" of the mitochondria.[927] According to Peter Mitchell's chemiosmotic theory (for an alternate mechanism, I suggest Gilbert Ling's induction-adsorption hypothesis),[928] the energetically favorable transfer of electrons from NADH to O_2 through the respiratory complexes is coupled to the pumping of protons thorough complexes I, III, IV into the intermembrane space.[929] This creates a temporary form of stored energy termed the protonmotive force (PMF), which is used by complex V to produce ATP from ADP and P_i. Therefore, the

---

[924] Kinscherf, R. et al., (1996), "Low plasma glutamine in combination with high glutamate levels indicate risk for loss of body cell mass (BCM) in healthy individuals: the effect of N-acetyl cysteine on BCM, *J Mol Med;* 74: 393-400

[925] Hortin, GL., et al, (1994), "Changes in plasma amino acid concentrations in response to HIV-1 infection," *Clin Chem;* 40: 785-789

[926] Kremer, H, (2008), The Silent Revolution in Cancer and AIDS Medicine, XLibris, pp. 320-321

[927] Brown, GC., Borutaite, V., (2012), "There is no evidence that mitochondria are the main source of reactive oxygen species in mammalian cells." *Mitochondrion;* 112:1-4

[928] For a rebuttal of this theory, I suggest Gilbert Ling, (1981), "Oxidative phosphorylation and mitochondrial physiology: a critical review of the chemiosmotic theory, and reinterpretation by the association induction hypothesis," *Physiol Chem & Physics;* 13: 29-96

[929] Saier, MH., (1997) "Peter Mitchell and his chemiosmotic theories" *ASM News;* 63(1): 13-21

production of ATP from nutrient oxidation in mitochondria depends on a multitude of redox reactions and the production of ROS.

ROS produced in mitochondria and one-electron oxygen reduction in structured water combine to form the energy of electronic excitation.

Although ATP cannot supply the total energy needs of the cell, the role of ROS produced in the mitochondria must be considered as another potential energy source under normal physiological conditions. Because of the ubiquitous presence of enzymes belonging to the NADPH-oxidase family (combined with other means of direct oxygen reduction—see below), even under resting conditions, up to 20 percent of all oxygen consumed is directly reduced and goes to ROS production.[930] It can increase up to 70 percent when metabolism is enhanced.[931]

Oxygen can only accept one electron at a time during its reduction to water, and electrons from complexes I and III can "spin off" prematurely, univalently reducing O_2 to produce proximal ROS superoxide anion radical (O_2^-).[932] Superoxide anion radical is then quickly dismutated (recombined) to H_2O_2, which is considered to be the major ROS signaling molecule because of its longer half-life and capacity to diffuse through membranes. There are other mitochondrial sources for these molecules, but complexes I and III are the most well characterized.[933]

From the dynamic point of view, normal ROS metabolism in an organism represents an intense flux of oxygen reduction to water—$4O_2 + 2H_2 \rightarrow 2H_2O + 3O_2$—and occurs not only enzymatically in the mitochondria but nonenzymatically in the interfacial EZ water.[934] The reaction consists of several

---

[930] Souza, HP, Liu, X., et al., (2002), "Quantitation of superoxide generation and substrate utilization by vascular NAD(P)H oxidase'" *Am J Physiol Heart Circ Physiol;* 282:H466-H474

[931] Trimarchi, JR., Liu, L., (2000), "Oxidative phosphorylation dependent and independent oxygen consumption by individual preimplantation mouse embryos," *Biol Reprod;* 62: 1866-1874

[932] Mailloux, RJ, Harper, M.E., (2011), "Uncoupling proteins and the control of mitochondrial reactive oxygen species production," *Free Rad Bio Med;* 51: 11061115

[933] Mailloux, R.J., et al., (2013), "Unearthing the secrets of mitochondrial ROS and glutathione in bioenergetics," *Trends Biochem Sci;* 38: 592-632

[934] Voeikov, VL, (2006), "Reactive Oxygen species—pathogen or sources of vital energy: Part 1. ROS in normal and pathological physiology of living systems," *J Alt Comp Med; 12(2):* 111-118

steps requiring a fourfold excess of oxygen to reduce one-oxygen molecule to two water molecules. Otherwise, the intermediate ROS accumulate and may initiate uncontrolled chain reactions with bioorganic molecules.[935] First, an adequate supply of oxygen and active hydrogen are the necessary conditions to keep ROS and other free radical particles at a low stationary level. Second, all these reactions imply recombination of unpaired electrons.[936] These reactions are accompanied by the release of energy quanta equivalent to electronic excitation. This means that the molecule is fluorescent. Fluorescence thus becomes an indicator of qualities that may have a major biological importance, indicating that the molecule can accept energy without dissipating it.[937]

The energy of electronic excitation (EEE) is equivalent to energy of photons belonging to the visible and ultraviolet (UV) range of the electromagnetic spectrum. Energy production in the reaction of dismutation of two superoxide radicals is ~22 kcal/mol,[938] equal to the energy gap between triplet and excited singlet states of oxygen and equivalent to the near IR photon of $\lambda \sim 1269$ nm.[939] When two singlet oxygen particles transit to triplet state simultaneously, EEE may be "pooled," and a doubled quantum of energy (equivalent to 44 kcal/mol or $\lambda \sim 635$ nm red light) is released.[940] This may happen when a double dismutation takes place. Because of the high turnover numbers of dismutase and catalase, quanta of high-density energy should be generated with some megahertz frequencies. This provides favorable conditions for energy pooling to even higher quanta and saves it from immediate dissipation into heat. Thus, oxygen activation is a prerequisite condition for the emergence of these fields.

Until recently, the role of EEE—a high-density valuable form of energy—has not been considered in biochemistry except for vision and photosynthesis. However, evidence has long supported a key role of EEE and related photon emissions in the regulation of vital process. In the early part of the last century, the Gurwitsch experiments demonstrated that cell division was being triggered by mitogenic processes.[941] He suggested that amplification of the initial signal is

---

[935] Voeikov, VL, (2006), "Reactive Oxygen Species (ROS): Pathogens or sources of vital energy? Part 2. Bioenergetic and bioinformational function of ROS," *J Alt and Comp Med;* 12(3): 265-279

[936] Voeikov, Ibid

[937] Szent-Györgyi, (1956), "Bioenergetics," *Science;* 124(3227): 873-875

[938] 1 eV = 23.06035 kcal mol^{-1}

[939] Voeikov, Op cit

[940] Cadenas, E., Sies, H, (1984), "Low level chemiluminescence as an indicator of singlet molecular oxygen in biological systems," *Meth Enzymol;* 105:221-231

[941] Gurwitsch, AG., Gurwitsh, LD, (1943), "Twenty years of mitogenetic radiation: emergence, development and perspectives," *translation from Russian in 21st Century*, Fall 1999; 41-53

caused by secondary emission: a cell happened to catch a photon then becomes a secondary emitter of mitogenic radiation. He found that the cell itself may not enter into mitosis but may serve to "multiply" photons by a branching chain reaction mechanism, which has been proven experimentally.[942] New data demonstrates that very weak emissions in the range from the UV to the near IR range of the electromagnetic spectrum affect activity of enzymes,[943] activity, and morphology of cells and tissues;[944] regulate locomotion and mutual orientation of cells;[945] and determine the rate of development of embryos and their morphologic features.[946]

Although the concept of structured water has sparked much controversy, it was the scientific basis for the invention of a breakthrough technology with which most physicians are familiar—magnetic resonance imaging (MRI)—for which Raymond Damadian holds the patent. Water molecules are moving and changing positions constantly. However, if one takes a snapshot at any given instant, most of the molecules are attached more strongly to their neighboring water molecules and indirectly to their ultimate protein-anchoring sites. The attachment to neighboring water molecules restrains and slows both their translational and rotational movements. The MRI works by assessing the rotational correlation time of hydrogen atoms or protons of water molecules and their relaxation times. Damadian showed that the relaxation times of water protons of normal tissues are different among themselves, but the water protons in cancer have longer relaxation times than in normal tissue.[947] In other words, cancer has less water structure (less available energy) as predicted as early as 1957 by Albert Szent-Györgyi.[948] One of the characteristics of cancer cells and their seeming lack of communication and functional coherence with healthy neighboring cells can be measured in their degree of incoherence as it directly relates to the inability of the cancer system to coherently reabsorb emitted photons.[949] Normal cells show decreasing photon emissions with an increasing number of cells, but the photon emission of tumor cells increases in

---

[942] Gurwitsch, AG, Gurwitsch, LD, (1942), "Pecularities of chain reactions and common energy levels in biological systems," *Acta Physicochimica USSR;* 16: 288-295

[943] Cilento, G., (1988) "Photobiochemistry without light," *Experientia;* 44: 5720576

[944] Galantsev, VP, et al., (1993) "Lipid peroxidation, low-level chemiluminescence and regulation of secretion in the mammary gland," *Experentia;* 49: 870-875

[945] Albrect-Buehler, G., (1995) "Changes of cell behavior by near infrared signals," *Cell Motil Cytoskeleton;* 32: 299-304

[946] Burlakov, A., et al., (2000), "Distant wave interactions in early embryological development of loach," *Ontognenez* (Moscow); 31(5): 343-349

[947] Ling, Op cit.p 82

[948] Szent-Györgyi, A., (1957), "Bioenergetics," Academic Press, New York

[949] Schamhart, S., van Wijk, R., (1986), "Photon emission and degree of differentiation"

a nonlinear way to higher values, displaying a qualitative as well as a quantitative difference.[950,951]

The Disruption of Oscillatory Frequencies Common in Diseased States

Generally, regulation of biologic functions on the molecular level is regarded as either a binding or chemical modification of the target protein (e.g., hormone → receptor, drug → enzyme, phosphorylation-dephosphorylation of a regulated protein) resulting in a specific change of conformation and, as a consequence, the specific regulated activity.[952] This initial stimulus is believed to initiate a series of downstream events that collectively represent a physiologic response of a cell to the stimulus. However, the "lock and key" model doesn't account for either the speed, oscillatory nature, or long-range characteristics of molecular reactions in the cell. Regulation in physiology often means a change in the parameters of a particular biologic process under the effect of an external influence that is aimed to support vitality of the living system to which this process belongs.[953] A conservative estimate of ten thousand molecular species squared equals potentially 10^8 pairwise interactions. Even if the molecules have very intricate complementary shapes, it would be highly unlikely for the right molecules to find one another in the crowded environment of subcellular compartments in which there will only be a few copies of each type of molecule. It is more likely that the formation of intermolecular response patterns is generated by the universal electromagnetic attractive and repulsive forces as the electromagnetic spectrum is not only huge but has the capability of providing exquisite specificity and selectivity. It is known that molecules with the same intrinsic frequency of vibration not only resonate over long distances and are able to undergo coherent excitations. They can attract one another over long distances with a frequency specificity accuracy within 1 percent.[954,955] One

---

[950] van Wijk, R., et al., (1993), "Light induced photon emission by mammalian cells," *J Phhotochem Photobio;* 4: 87-97

[951] van Wijk, R., et al, (1995a), "Relaxation dynamics of light induced photon emission by mammalian cells and nuclei," *Progress in Biomed Optics, Europto Series;* 2627: 176-185

[952] Voeikov, Op cit

[953] Voeikov, Op cit

[954] Ho, MW., (2008), The Rainbow and the Worm, pp 134-135, World Scientific, New Jersey

[955] McClare, CW, (1972), "A 'molecular energy' muscle model," *J Theor Biol;* 35(3): 569-595

of the more obvious features of all physiologic and biomolecular processes is their nonlinear oscillatory (periodic) and wave-like character.[956] Accordingly, "parameters of an oscillatory process may be regulated by an external oscillatory factor in a resonance like fashion. Essentially, oscillatory behavior is an intrinsic feature of processes with participation of ROS going on in aqueous environment and accompanied with generation of the energy of electronic excitation (EEE)."[957]

This becomes important to the AIDS story because of the consistent histories of the long-term use and exposure to a plethora of metabolic toxins, the use of which was underscored by a consistent finding of decreased cysteine/glutathione as well as other antioxidants. The situation was made iatrogenically worse with the introduction of the highly mitochondrial toxic oxidizing agent, AZT, and the use of the double folate inhibitor, trimethoprim/sulfamethoxazole, both of which acted synergistically to further aggravate an already severe proton deficit. All the biological stressors whether biotic, abiotic or psychological in nature can cause an increase in endogenous free radical production and can overwhelm the various antioxidant defenses.[958] In AIDS patients, the metabolic consequence of these various and prolonged toxic exposures led ultimately to increased nitrosylation[959] of the thiol pool of various antiapoptotic proteins[960] as well as to decreased energy production in the mitochondria (ATP and ROS/RNS) and an increase in aerobic glycolysis. These energy changes had consequences as defined by the three stages of the ongoing thiol deficiency process:

1. The clinically mute phase during which the reserve capacity of cell respiration reaches a critical threshold.
2. The clinically compensated phase when a type 1 to type 2 cytokine dysregulation with a Th1 to Th2 switch, type 1 overregulation of cell dis-symbiosis and/or type 2 counterregulation of cell dis-symbiosis, the point in time of a possible "HIV" test reaction.

---

[956] Voeikov, Op cit
[957] Voeikov, Op cit
[958] van Wijk, R.,(1992) "Biophoton emission, stress and disease," *Experientia;* 48: 1029-1030
[959] Wang, Z., (2012), "Protein s-nitrosylation and cancer," *Cancer Lett;* 320(2): 123-129
[960] Azad, N, et al., (2006), "S-nitrosylation of Bcl-2 inhibits its ubiquitin-proteasomal degradation. A novel antiapoptotic mechanism that suppresses apoptosis," *J Biol Chem;* 281(45): 34124-34134

3. The clinically manifest phase with the development of opportunistic diseases, Kaposi's sarcomas, lymphomas, myopathies, encephalopathies, wasting syndrome.[961]

Reappraisal of the Warburg Effect

Otto Warburg first observed the phenomenon of aerobic glycolysis in tumor cells.[962] From this observation, he postulated that the driver of tumorigenesis (dedifferentiation) is reduced cellular respiration (energy) because of some insult to the mitochondria. Subsequent studies have confirmed the increased rate of glucose degradation to lactate despite the presence of oxygen, which is available to the mitochondria in several types of fast-growing tumor cells. However, the process was not universal in any given cancer colony as it was soon recognized that oxygen consumption may not be quantitatively diminished. Until recently, this was one of the fundamental problems in biochemistry not yet fully understood. As a result of this vacuum, genetic determinists have claimed that cancer starts as a single gene mutation in a somatic cell followed by successive mutations that lead to malignant transformation. This belief is held in spite of the fact that it has been demonstrated that there are often genetic differences among cancer cells as some have acquired mutations that others do not exhibit.[963] This, of course, means that a tumor is not a clone in which cells carry and transmit to their progeny an accumulated set of mutations. In fact, tumors are polyclonal, and their genomic fingerprint has been shown to be very unstable and changing continuously when cultured in vitro.[964] By now, it should be clear that my focus is on the most basic and fundamental problem in cell transformation, not genetic abnormalities but the energetic changes that allow the breaks, deletions, and transcription of alternate reading frames to produce an alternate set of proteins.[965]

---

[961] Kremer, Op., Ci., p 320

[962] Warburg, O, Poesener, K, Negelein E., (1924), "Ueber den Stoffwechsel der Tumoren"; *Biochemische Zeitschrift;* 152: 319-344 Reprinted in english in the book *On metabolism of tumors* by Otto Warburg, Constable, London, 1930

[963] Gerstung, M, et al., (2014), "Subclonal variant calling with multiple samples and prior knowledge," *Bioinformatics;* pp 1-7 doi: 10.1093/bioinformatics/btt750

[964] Shah, SP, et al., (2012), "The clonal and mutational evolution spectrum of primary triple-negative breast cancers," *Nature;* 486:365-399

[965] Ciocca, DR, Calderwook, SK, (2005), "Heat shock proteins in cancer: diagnostic, prognostic, predictive, and treatment implications," *Cell Stress Chaperones;* 10(2): 86-103

The Warburg effect or the method by which the cell transitions from the predominant use of oxidative phosphorylation to glycolysis has also garnered much controversy. It is neither universal nor unique to cancer cells. It is also the process used by normal proliferating cells in the late S phase of cell division in the presence of adequate glucose and oxygen supplies.[966,967] Alteration of partly oxidative to almost completely glycolytic degradation to pyruvate and mainly lactate occurs during the transition from the resting to the proliferative state.[968] During normal cell cycle progression, the rate of glucose conversion to lactate peaks in the late S phase of the cell cycle, which is also characteristic of a variety of tumor cells.[969]

Glycolytic enzymes are some of the most ancient and highly conserved proteins and genes known with a strong conservation of sequences even between higher mammals and bacteria. During the evolutionary process as life developed on Earth, under strictly anaerobic conditions, these enzymes were among the first enzyme pathways to appear. This enzyme system allowed primitive archeabacteria to utilize simple carbohydrates as energy stores and release by coupling the breakdown to higher-energy phosphates. The twelve mammalian glycolytic enzyme genes are genetically unlinked and dispersed around the genome, mainly on different chromosomes.[970]

Recent molecular studies have shown that extant bacterial species (e.g., Archaebacter, termophilic sulfur bacteria) have complex patterns of gene expression under anoxic conditions, including the regulation of bioenergetic

---

[966] Greiner, EF, et al, (1994) "Glucose is essential for proliferation and the glycolytic enzyme induction that provokes a transition to glycolytic energy production," *J Biol Chem;* 269(50): 31484-31490

[967] Barron, JT, Kopp SJ, et al., (1991), "Differential effects of fatty acids on glycolysis and glycogen metabolism in vascular smooth muscle," *Biochim Biophys Acta;* 1093(2-3): 125-135

[968] Brand, KA., Hermfisse U., (1997), "Aerobic glycolysis by proliferating cells: a protective strategy against reactive oxygen species," *FASEB J;* 11(5): 388-395

[969] Baumann, M, Jezussek, D., et al., (1988), "Activities of phosphohexose isomerase and other glycolytic enzymes in normal and tumor tissue of patients with neoplastic diseases: comparison with serum activities and correlation to tumor staging and grading," *Tumour Biol;* 9(6): 281-286

[970] Webster, KA., Murphy, BJ., (1988), "Regulation of tissue specific glycolytic isozyme genes: coordinate regulation by oxygen availability in skeletal muscle cells," *Can J Zool;* 66: 1046-1058

gene expression by elemental sulfur and phosphorus.[971,972,973,974] There is an interesting parallel between sulfur regulation of bioenergetic pathways in the Archaean-era microorganisms and oxygen regulation in eukaryotes. Oxygen replaced sulfur as the terminal electron acceptor of carbohydrate catabolism, but yet after billions of years, it is the oxidation or reduction of the sulfur moieties of certain transcription factors that still determines whether there will be a decreased or an increased expression of glycolytic enzymes.[975] Thus, the fundamental features of biology and genetics, including DNA synthesis, transcription and translation, and their regulation, were established under strictly anaerobic conditions. The archaebacterial genes in the eukaryotic chimeric genome continue to respond to these ancient redox cues. It is for this reason the enzymes in the glycolytic pathway appear to continue to have an absolute requirement for a reducing environment in order to function.[976] These genes that evolved in an anaerobic-reducing environment are still more likely to be involved in the informational process of transcription, translation, and replication.[977] The questions posed by Karl Brand working with rat thymocytes and HL-60 cells was how this energetic transition occurs.[978]

---

[971] Fardeau, ML, et al., (1996), "Effect of thiosulphate as electron acceptor on glucose and xylose oxidation by *Thermanaerobacter finnii* and a *Thermoanaerobacter* sp. isolated from oil field water," *Res Microbiol;* 147: 159-165

[972] Kelly, RM, Adams, MW., (1994), "Metabolism in hyperthermophilic microorganisms," *Antonie Van Leeuwenhoek;* 66: 247-270

[973] Segerer, A., et al. (1985), "Two contrary modes of chemolithotrophy in the same archaebacterium" *Nature;* 313: 787-789

[974] Brunner, NA, et al., (1998), "NAD+ dependent glyceraldehyde-s-phosphate dehydrogenase from *Termoproteus tenax*. The first identified archael member of the aldehyde dehydrogenase superfamily is a glycolytic enzyme with unusual regulatory properties," *J Biol Chem;* 273: 6149-6156

[975] Brand, K., (1997), "Aerobic glycolysis by proliferating cells: protection against oxidative stress at the expense of energy yield," *J Bioenerg Biomembr;* 29(4): 355-364

[976] Segerer, A., et al., (1985), "Two contrary modes of chemolithotrophy in the same archaebacterium," *Nature;* 313: 787-789

[977] Alvarez-Ponce, D, McInerney, JO, (2011), "The human genome retains relics of its prokaryotic ancestry: human genes of archaebacterial and eubacterial origin exhibit remarkable differences," *Genome Biol Evol;* 1-24

[978] Brand, K., (1997), "Aerobic glycolysis by proliferating cells: protection against oxidative stress at the expense of energy yield.

Why Tumor Cells and Normal Proliferating Cells Meet Their Increased Energy Demands from the Glycolytic Pathway

Significantly, it was found that there is a nineteen- to twentyfold increase in the rate of glucose degradation to lactate during the transition of rat thymocytes from the resting to the proliferative state. This transition occurs as the result of either (a) an enhanced transcription or (b) a decreased degradation of enzymes and mRNA involved in glycolysis: aldolase A, glyceraldehyde-3-phosphate dehydrogenase, hexokinase type 1 and 2, and pyruvate kinase type M2 with a corresponding increase in the mRNA levels.[979,980] It was observed that the dividing cell required more energy than the resting cell and that this energy demand was met solely by glycolysis. This increased energy demand in dividing cells becomes all the more important to understand as the energy demands in cancer, stage 3 thiol deficiency, and other metabolic conditions (e.g., sepsis, trauma, chronic fatigue syndrome, inflammatory bowel diseases, and after anaerobic exercise) also use the glycolytic pathway for energy production, ultimately requiring the breakdown of skeletal muscle protein to supply the increased glucose demand.

Total ATP yield in proliferating cells revealed that 86 percent is produced by glycolytic glucose breakdown to pyruvate and lactate and only 14 percent by oxidation of pyruvate derived from glucose to carbon dioxide and water in the citric acid cycle and the respiratory chain. In resting thymocytes, these numbers are reversed: 88 percent of ATP arose from oxidative phosphorylation and 12 percent from glycolysis.[981] As seen in figure 1, there is also an increase in ATP yield by a factor of 6 by use of the glycolytic pathway.

	moles ATP	%	moles ATP	%
Glycolysis	41	12	1442	86
Oxidation	302	88	238	14
Total ATP Yield	344	100	1680	100

figure 1

ATP yield during glycolysis and oxidation [982]

---

[979] Brand, Ibid
[980] Brand, K., (1987), "Role of ornithine decarboxylase on glycolytic enzyme induction during thymocyte proliferation," *J of Bio Chem;* 262: 15232-15235
[981] Brand, (1997), Op cit.
[982] Brand, Ibid

To answer the question why this happens, Brand then studied the regulation of cell-cycle-associated gene expression of aldolase A and pyruvate kinase M, representative of glycolytic enzymes. He looked at five binding sites for the activating transcription factor Sp1. Sp1 is a zinc finger transcription factor that binds to GC rich motifs of many promoters. The protein is involved in cell differentiation, cell growth, apoptosis, immune responses, responses to DNA damage, and chromatin remodeling.[983] Sp1 is involved in the mechanism by which the promoter of the aldolase A gene achieves high-level transcription during the S phase of the cell cycle. What was discovered was that the oxidation of the cysteine residues (thiol) in Sp1 causes a low-binding efficiency to the cognate DNA element and that the nuclear extracts from resting cells were responsive to oxidative signals, leading to decreased DNA binding and decreased transcription of glycolytic enzymes. Alternatively, proliferative cells were responsive to reductive signals, leading to enhanced binding to the GC boxes, thus provoking enhanced gene expression of glycolytic enzymes during proliferation.[984] This is consistent with other studies that found that glycolytic enzyme genes are regulated by hypoxia responsive transcription factors, not only Sp-1 but hypoxia inducible factor 1-α (HIF 1-α), AP-1, and possibly metal response elements as well.[985,986,987]

In another study, it was discovered that oxidative signaling in the regulation of gene expression was necessary during the G_0 to G_1 phase transition.[988] In other words, the redox status has been demonstrated to be the controlling switch in the microenvironment that determines whether the cell has the option of primarily using the ancient glycolytic pathway or the mitochondrial endosymbiont oxidative phosphorylation for its energy needs during different phases of the cell cycle. Importantly, the observation was made that as pyruvate

---

[983] Gene ID: 6667, updated 4 May 2014 http://www.ncbi.nlm.nih.gov/gene/6667

[984] Brand (1997) Op cit

[985] Discher, DJ, et al., (1998), "Hypoxia regulates β-enolase and pyruvate kinase-M promotes by modulating Sp1/Sp3 binding to a conserved GC element," *J Biol Chem;* 273: 26087-26093

[986] Hochachka, PW., Lutz, PI., (2001), "Mechanism, origin, and evolution of anoxia tolerance in animals" *Comp Biochem Physiol;* 130B: 435-459

[987] Murphy, BJ, et al., (1999), "Activation of metallithionein gene expression by hypoxia involves metal response elements and metal transcription factor-1; *Cancer Res;* 59:1315-1322

[988] Goldstone, SD., et al, (1996), "Oxidative signaling and gene expression during lymphocyte activation," *Biochimica Biophysica Acta;* 1314: 175-182

acts as an antioxidant.[989,990] Pyruvate acting as an antioxidant combined with the flow reversal of hydrogen ions from the glycolytically generated NADH malate-aspartate and glycerol phosphate shuttles increases the reducing environment. Thus, the process of glycolysis itself reduces the level of ROS produced by the mitochondria, and this energy transfer mechanism is a way for the cell not only to protect the central genome from oxidative attack during mitosis but to signal the upregulation of proteins that support the glycolytic process.

Over the long run, because of a deficit of antioxidants, the disruption of normal energy flows, which are generated largely in the mitochondria by the production of not only ATP but the ROS as well, may lead to evolutionary genetically conserved patterns of cellular responses to a perceived low-oxygen (pseudohypoxia), lower-energy state. If the cell does not acutely die by necrosis or apoptosis (type 1 overregulation), it has the option of reverting to the mechanism of type 2 counterregulation. The counterregulation process results in a series of alternative metabolic processes that result in a decrease in efficient energy output. There is an increase in the nitrosylation of the cysteine moiety of certain proteins and a decrease in the mitochondrial production of ATP and ROS. There is also a decrease in calcium cycling. There follows a consequent hyperpolarization on the mitochondrial membrane potential and the upregulation of both glycolytic and anti-apoptotic proteins (e.g., Bcl-2).[991] The cell nucleus then has the option for the reversal of the "hybrid impulse" away from the cooperation with the endosymbiont mitochondria. This is the default survival mode of the eukaryotic cell. Higher-order functioning involves the cooperation of the proteobacteria operational genes and the archaebacteria information genes working in tandem during the balancing of both the informational and operational systems in the orderly process of cellular homeostasis and cell division. The result of the dis-symbiosis of the hybrid trend is either apoptosis/necrosis or, depending on the length of the insult, reserve capacity of the cell and the cell type, degeneration, or entry into a repetitive mitotic cycle at a lower energy-level with dedifferentiation as the consequence.

---

[989] O'Donnell-Tormey, et al., (1987), "Secretion of pyruvate. An antioxidant defense of mammalian cells," *J Exp Med;* 165(2): 500-514

[990] Andrae, U, et al., (1985), "Pyruvate and related alpha-ketoacids protect mammalian cells in culture against hydrogen peroxide-induced cytotoxicity" *Toxicol Lett;* 28(2-3): 93-98

[991] Hockenbery, DM., (2010), "Targeting mitochondria for cancer therapy," *Environ Mol Mutagen;* 51(5): 476-489

Every eukaryotic cell nucleus has integrated its ancestral genome to create a new hybrid combination.[992] Whether the overregulation or the counterregulation occurs to dismantle the hybrid impulse of the eukaryotic cell when it encounters either acute or long-term biologically stressful situations determines how many chronic diseases will manifest. This has especially proven consistent in the diseases that are called AIDS and cancer.

---

[992] Rivera, MC., et al., (1998), "Genomic evidence for two functionally distinct gene classes," *Proc Natl Acad Sci USA*, 95: 6239-6244

CHAPTER 9

The Binary Strategy of Human Immune Defense— The Essential Absurdity of Counting Total CD4+T cells

In order to complete the bioforensic pathology of deconstructing the AIDS crime and the crimes of the AIDSworld syndicate, it is important to visit the 1986 studies by Mosmann and Coffman and their collaborators who first identified a functional dichotomy in T helper lymphocytes. These researchers reported that cloned murine helper T (Th) lymphocytes could be divided into two different functional subsets on the basis of the immunoregulatory cytokines produced by these clones.[993] While this information was not available at the time of the AIDS theory was advanced, there was knowledge and acknowledgment that AIDS was primarily a problem of cell-mediated immunity. Even though this division of T cell function based on cytokine response patterns has been well defined and has matured over the last thirty years, AIDSworld continues to ignore the information by stubbornly and illogically continuing to use the total CD4+T cell count in patient evaluation.

From early in the AIDS crisis, it was understood that patients exhibited a consistent range of altered immune responses that indicated a problem with cell-mediated immunity. However, these findings could not be explained by the

---

[993] Lucey, DR., et al., (1996), "Type 1 and Type 2 cytokine dysregulation in human infectious, neoplastic, and inflammatory diseases"; *Clin Micro Rev;* 9(4): 532-562

then-extant understanding of immune system complexity or by the imagined HIV vector:[994,995]

1. The blood serum depletion of T helper cells
2. While simultaneously finding increased levels of certain antibodies
3. The lack of immune cell response to mitogenic stimulation and
4. Dermal anergy after provocation with recall antigens in DTH

The lack of immune cell response to mitogenic stimulation and Dermal anergy after provocation with recall antigens in DTH

As early as 1972, Parish observed that there was an inverse relationship between cell-mediated immunity (CMI) and humoral immunity in response to antigenic stimuli.[996] However, the mechanisms of these cross-regulatory properties of Th1 and Th2 cytokines were not fully recognized until 1986 when the research group of Mosmann and Coffman began to elucidate the nature of the heterogeneity of T helper immune cells. They reported that cloned murine helper T (Th) lymphocytes could be divided into two functional subsets on the basis of immunoregulatory lymphokines (cytokines) produced by each group of cells. Th1 clones were characterized by the production of IL 2 and IFN-γ in response to antigen presenting cells (APCs) or concanavalin A (Con A), whereas type 2 helper cells (Th2) clones produced, IL 4.[997] After several years of investigation, the Mosmann and Coffman group concluded that the Th1 cells mainly interacted with the nonspecific macrophages, reciprocally to type 2 cytokines.

The Th2 cells were largely directed to perform helper functions for the antibody-producing B cells (with the exception of a subgroup of B cells, which are activated by Th1 and produce antibodies of a subgroup of immunoglobulin class G). A balance shift to Th1 produced a marked DTH reaction and

---

[994] Gottlieb, MS., et al., (1981), "Pneumocystis carinii pneumonia and mucosal candidiasis in previously healthy homosexual men, evidence of a new acquired cellular immunodeficiency," *NEJM;* 305(24):1425-1431

[995] Masur, H., et al., (1981), "An outbreak of community-acquired Pneumocystis carinii pneumonia: initial manifestation of cellular immune dysfunction," *NEJM;* 305(24): 1431-1438

[996] Parish, CR., (1972), "The relationship between humoral and cell-mediated immunity," *Transplant Rev;* 13: 35-66

[997] Mossman, TR., et al., (1986), "Two types of murine helper T cell clone: I. Definition according to profiles of lymphokine activities and secreted proteins," *J imunol;* 136: 2348-2357

vice versa. A balance shift toward Th2 led to a weak DTH or no response whatsoever.[998,999,1000] This research was beginning to answer the questions of the immune enigma found in the initial cohort of AIDS patients because it discovered a bipolar autofeedback system of self-regulatory cytokines sensitive to redox conditions.

Since 1948, the World Health Organization (WHO) has defined health as "a state of complete physical, mental and social well-being and not merely the absence of disease or infirmity."[1001] This definition is congruent with the concepts advanced by some of the best medical minds of the last century: of internal and external milieus developed by Claude Bernard;[1002] of homeostasis advanced by Walter Cannon;[1003] and of the general adaptation syndrome suggested in 1950 by Hans Selye.[1004] Ignoring not only the accepted definition of health but the foundational precepts of allopathic clinical medicine, the first 1981 CDC MMWR report on five young homosexuals who presented to three separate hospitals in Los Angeles with a variety of illnesses indicating that they were severely immunosuppressed and had been so for at least several months prior to admission yet were described as being, "previously healthy." The patients were between the ages of twenty-nine and thirty-six, all were diagnosed with P. carinii pneumonia, and laboratory confirmed previous or current cytomegalovirus (CMV). Two had elevated liver enzymes, all had oral candidiasis, and all had reported being ill for several months prior to admission. "The patients did not know each other and had no known common contacts or knowledge of sexual partners who had had similar illnesses. Two of the 5 reported having frequent homosexual contacts with various partners. ALL 5 REPORTED USING INHALANT DRUGS AND 1 REPORTED PARENTAL DRUG ABUSE. Three patients had profoundly depressed in vitro proliferative responses to mitogens and antigens. Lymphocyte studies were not performed

---

[998] Mossman, Ibid

[999] Mossman, TR, Coffman RI., (1989), "Th1 and Th2 cells: different patterns of lymphokine secretion lead to different functional properties" *Ann Rev Immunol;* 7: 145-173

[1000] Mossman, TR., Coffman, RI., (1989), "Heterogeneity of cytokine secretion patterns and functions of helper T cells," *Adv Immunol;* 46: 111-147244

[1001] http://www.who.int/about/definition/en/print.html

[1002] Gross, CG., (1998), "Claud Bernard and the constancy of the internal environment," *The Neuroscientist;* 380-385

[1003] Cannon, W., (1963), *The wisdom of the body;* W.W. Norton & Co., Rev. and Enl. Ed edition

[1004] Selye, H, (1950), "Stress and the general adaptation syndrome," *BMJ;* 1384-1392

on the other 2 patients" (emphasis added).[1005] The report continued, "All the above suggest the possibility of a cellular immune dysfunction related to a common exposure that predisposes individuals to opportunistic infections such as pneumocystis and candidiasis."[1006]

First, the fact that they had "no common contacts or knowledge of sexual partners who had similar illnesses" should have immediately suggested an environmental exposure rather than an infectious process. Second, that they all had a common history of homosexuality and prior histories of a compendium of a variety of common infectious diseases and the universal use of volatile nitrites was further evidence that should honestly have been construed as a new environmental risk. The common history of consistent environmental exposure to agents historically known to be immunosuppressive was the red flag that was ultimately ignored in the search for an infectious agent. Had the social histories of this subset of the urban gay population in the 1970s been actively explored as the unique initiator, it would have uncovered several lifestyle factors that brought about an abrupt change in group behavior that had profoundly negative effects: (1) the increased use of nitrites as sexual doping agents, (2) the random but persistent use of immune-suppressing antibiotics, (3) the increase in the use of immune-suppressing narcotics, (4) a high rate of sexual promiscuity, and (5) the consequence of recurrent bowel, liver, and venereal infections—bacterial, parasitic, and viral.[1007]

Six months after that first report, the NEJM[1008] identified eleven cases of Pneumocystis carinii (PCP), which occurred in a cohort of young men between 1979 and 1981. One patient had Kaposi's (KS) sarcoma, seven of the patients were drug abusers, six identified as homosexual, and two were both. Similar to the patients in Los Angeles, these men had depressed lymphocyte counts, but their humoral immunity (antibody) remained intact. By 1982, more clusters were being reported from large urban areas of the United States and Europe. The CDC MMWR[1009] published another paper of nineteen confirmed cases of KS and/or PCP, again claiming that the patients were previously healthy homosexual males. Thus, early in the AIDS era, the syndrome was defined

---

[1005] CDC (June 5, 1981) "Pneumocystis Pneumonia—Los Angeles" *MMWR;* 30(21):1-3
[1006] Ibid
[1007] Levine AS. (1982) "The Epidemic of Acquired Immune Dysfunction in Homosexual Men and Its Sequelae-Opportunistic Infections, Kaposi's Sarcoma, and Other Malignancies:An Update and Interpretation," *Cancer Treatment Reports;* 66:1391
[1008] Masur, H., et al., (Dec. 10, 1981), "An outbreak of community acquired
[1009] CDC (June 18, 1982) "A cluster of Kaposi's Sarcoma and Pneumocystis carinii pneumonia among homosexual male residents of Los Angeles and range counties, California," *MMWR;*31(23):305-7

by these two diseases. This report from the CDC, however, clearly shows that the authors were not thinking through the underlying metabolic process that could address the basic issue: what could cause an outbreak in noncontiguous urban centers of disease clusters in a defined subset of the male homosexual population that indicated the patients had a suppression of cellular immunity yet simultaneously maintained the function of their humoral immune system? Was there a logical explanation separate from the viral quagmire, for the unusual imbalance in the immune system that allowed for the growth of a variety of opportunistic infectious diseases and at the same time the development of an uncommon vascular cancer in a limited cohort of young homosexual men?

In 1981, physicians and immunologists were unaware of the mechanics of the bipolar nature of the immune system or that there were subsets of T helper immune cells. They were not aware that there was one subset that produced NO (and its metabolites as toxic gases) and one that did not. However, considering the then-current immune theory, it was incongruent that the T helper immune cells in AIDS patients could be so drastically reduced yet at the same time the production of certain antibodies could be so consistently elevated to the point of hypergammaglobulinemia.[1010] Any theory of the disease would have to have a congruent and logical explanation of these persistent indicators: anergy, marked decrease in lymphocytes, failure of lymphocyte response to mitogens, yet increased antibodies. The then-current immune theory claimed that in order for the B cells to produce antibodies, they needed to receive an activation signal from the thymus maturing T cells, thus the designation helper. It was not until the 1980s that the mysteries of the T cells began to be unraveled, yet twenty-first-century AIDSworld has continued to resist this knowledge and disastrously continues to employ the technique of flow cytometry to measure total CD4+T cell count, ignoring the vagaries and nondiagnostic capabilities of this measure.

Confining their thinking to a narrow set of options and under the strong influence of the CDC's Epidemic Intelligence Service,[1011] AIDSworld also ignored historical precedents of similar clinical presentations of immune suppression in other types of patients. Physicians, from their cumulative years of clinical experience, for years prior to the AIDS outbreak, had been cataloguing similar symptoms in both general surgery and transplantation

---

[1010] Nagase, H., et al., (2001), "Mechanism of hypergammaglobulinemia by HIV infection: circulating memory B-cell reduction with plasmacytosis," *Clin Immunol;* 100(2): 250-259

[1011] Ellison, B., (1993), "AIDS; Words from the Front," *Spin* http://www.virusmyth.com/aids/hiv/beeis.htm

patients. Finding vascular cancers and opportunistic infections as the result of immune suppression was not a unique historical event.

Yet the early MMWR paper describing the early AIDS patients shows that rather than exploring the environmental angle, they were already emphasizing the possibility of infection by sexual transmission by attempting to find sexual contacts for diseases that have nothing to do with sexual contact per se as it is a great leap of creative imagination to identify a lung infection and a cancer of the blood vessels as sexually transmitted. As they covered their bases, a caveat was introduced by acknowledging that "exposure to some substance [rather than a unique infectious agent] may eventually lead to immunodeficiency among a subset of the homosexual male population that shares a particular life style." The article goes on to quote Marmor, et al., out of England,[1012] who had investigated twenty homosexual men with histologically confirmed Kaposi's sarcoma and compared them to forty controls. The Marmor group discovered that there was a "significant association between Kaposi's sarcoma and use of a number of drugs [amyl nitrite, ethyl chloride, cocaine, phencyclidine, methaqualone, and amphetamine].... Risk-ratio estimates of 12.3 for amyl nitrite [95 percent confidence limits] and 2.0 for sexual activity." Even though as early as 1984 it was evident that HIV does not exist in the cells from the lesions of KS and therefore cannot be the direct cause of KS,[1013] without explanation, it has continued to be listed as one of the CDC's litany of AIDS-defining diseases. It has been demonstrated that in some homosexuals, KS can occur in the complete absence of both CDC defined[1014] immune deficiency and HIV.[1015] Now another "virus," HHV-8, has been tagged as the designated invader.

Because the early cases were all homosexual men (before the addition of hemophiliacs and IV drug users), one can ascertain from reading these early reports that there was a very heavy bias toward thinking that diseases long known and associated with immune suppression and nothing to do with the list of long-known sexually transmitted diseases were miraculously being transmitted through the sexual act of anal intercourse. It was never considered that it was not anal intercourse per se but the frequency and local trauma of anal intercourse (especially from a practice known as fisting) to the rectal and

---

[1012] Marmor, M, et al., (15 May 1982) "Risk factors for Kaposi's sarcoma in homosexual men," *Lancet;* 319(8281):1083-1087
[1013] Shaw MS, et al., (1984),. "Molecular Characterisation of Human T-Cell Leukemia (Lymphotrophic) Virus Type III in the Acquired Immune Deficiency Syndrome," *Science* 226:1165
[1014] Based on total CD4+ T cell counts and not CD4+T cell FUNCTIONS
[1015] Friedman-Kein AE, et al., (1990) "Kaposi's sarcoma in HIV negative homosexual men," *Lancet* 1:168

intestinal mucosa, the rate of exposure to immunosuppressive sperm[1016,1017] and other known STDs, the risk of damage to the intestinal mucosa with the secondary risk of the elevation of enteric pathogens entering the bloodstream, as well as the alteration of normal intestinal pathogens that are an integral part of immune homeostasis.[1018] In this regard, it has been documented[1019,1020,1021] that passive anal intercourse was another environmental risk factor and was the only sexual act that has ever been shown to be directly related to the development of AIDS and KS.

Root-Bernstein,[1022] on completing an extensive literature review on AIDS risk factors, found that every AIDS patient had some subset of immunosuppressive factors at work, including but not limited to "immunological contact with semen components; recreational drugs such as nitrites; addictive drugs such as opiates and cocaine, multiple concurrent infections with viruses, bacteria, amoeba, protozoa and/or fungi; malnutrition due to several causes including malabsorption syndrome associated with 'gay bowel syndrome'; chronic antibiotic use; blood transfusions; the indirect results of drug addiction, anorexia and poverty; and blood factor treatment."

The pieces of the puzzle that had to associate seamlessly in the formulation of any congruent theory of disease causation in these patients were four patterns that physicians were consistently finding that defined the clinical manifestations: anergy (failure to respond to a DTH skin test for multiple antigens; lymphopenia (specifically, depression the the total CD4+T count); the lymphocytes from these patients failed to mount a proliferative response to

---

[1016] Mathur, S., Goust, J.-M., Williamson, H.O., et al. (1981), Cross-reactivity of sperm and T-lymphocyte antigens. Amer. J. Reprod. Immunol., 1, 113-118.

[1017] Mavligit, G.M., Talpaz, M., Hsia, F.T., et al. (1984), Chronic immune stimulation by sperm alloantigens. Support for the hypothesis that spermatazoa induce immune dysregulation in homosexual males. J. Amer. med. Ass., 251, 237-241.

[1018] O'Harra, A.M., Shanahan, F., (2006), "The gut flora as a forgotten organ," *Embro Rep;* 7(7): 688-693

[1019] Marmor M. Epidemic Kaposi's Sarcoma and Sexual Practices Among Male Homosexuals. p 291 in AIDS:The Epidemic of Kaposi's Sarcoma and Opportunistic Infections. (AE Freidman-Kein, LJ Laubenstein, eds) Masson Publishing USA Inc, Chicago 1984.

[1020] Kingsley LA, Detels R, Kaslow R et al. (1987) Risk Factors for seroconversion to human immunodeficiency virus among male homosexuals. *Lancet* 1:345

[1021] Godfried JP, van Griensven G, Tielman R et al (1987). Risk factors and prevalence of HIV antibodies in homosexual men in the Netherlands. *Am J Epidemiol* 125:1048

[1022] Root-Bernstein, R.S., (1990), "Non-HIV immunosuppressive factors in AIDS: a multifactorial, synergistic theory of AIDS Etiology," *Res Immunol;* 141: 815-838

mitogens (PHA) in vitro; but anomalously, even with the thenextant immune theory, had elevated antibodies.

When the AIDS dogma was being formulated, doctors were not aware of the various roles of nitric oxide in the immune system (i.e., redox signaling, immune regulation, energy production, and antipathogen activities) or had the work of Mossman and Coffman[1023] who discovered that CD4+ (helper) T cells differentiate into functional subgroups been completed. However, according to the then-current immune theory, B cells, which mature in the bone marrow, need to receive activation signals from the T helper cells that mature in the thymus. It was simply not only incongruous but inconceivable in the context of that theory that the T helper cells in these patients, which were found to be so drastically reduced, could yet somehow stimulate the B cells to continually produce antibodies and often at an elevated rate. What was producing the activation signals? No one bothered to answer or address this major contradiction.

Also ignored was the fact that the extant immune theory postulated that elevated antibodies to a pathogen indicated that the host had mounted a defense, rejected the invader, and was subsequently protected from future infections. This, of course, is the theoretical basis of the entire vaccine industry. But in AIDSworld, that fact was largely ignored, and continues to remain ignored, as the AIDS protagonists claim that the mysterious 10 plus or minus Kb HIV has powers never before seen in an earthbound infectious agent and well beyond the capabilities possible for its limited genetic inheritance. They have also spent countless hours in human experimentation trying to develop a vaccine that has zero probability of working.[1024,1025] The CDC continues to promote antibody tests for diagnostic purposes, knowing that, in fact, these tests are a measure of the functional congruency of humoral immunity when they have defined AIDS as a problem of cell-mediated immunity. Why physicians have not seen the base of this flimflam is a monument to the concept of cognitive dissonance. It is not only a collective psychosis. It is a hostile and combative and well-funded psychosis.

[1023] Mossman, TR, Coffman RL., (1989), Th1 and Th2 cells: Different patterns of lymphokine secretion lead to different functional propertis," *Ann Rev Immunol;* 7:145-173

[1024] http://www.fiercebiotech.com/story/new-study-confirms-worst-fears-about-mercks-hiv-vaccine/2012-05-21

[1025] Sekaly, RP, (2008), "The failed HIV Merck vaccine study: a step back or a launching point for future vaccine development," *JEM;* 205(1): 7-12

By 1984 Robert Gallo and Luc Montagnier claimed to have "isolated" a new virus that was the causative agent, and the AIDS industry was born based on the assumption that HIV causes AID and that AID is, in fact, the cause of the twenty-nine diseases that comprise the S. They made a further assumption congruent with this theory that all AIDS patients will have evidence of HIV. However, the papers produced by these two laboratories were anything but conclusive for those assertions. In the Montagnier paper,[1026] they reported only a single isolation of "HIV" (reverse transcriptase) from a lymph node of a homosexual male who had lymphadenopathy but who did not have AIDS, and Gallo's "isolate" turned out to be Montagnier's cultures from which he had abstracted the "HIV" characteristic: reverse transcriptase.[1027] Not only that, what Gallo claimed was HTLV-III (later to be renamed HIV) was only found less than half (10/21) of AIDS patients with opportunistic infections and in less than one-third (13/43) with Kaposi's sarcoma.[1028]

Why let these facts get in the way of dogma and a windfall of financial gain to Gallo on the antibody test he patented just a day before the announcement was made that HIV was the "probable" causative agent?

By 1986, the American Academy of Sciences and the Institute of Medicine assembled a rubber stamp committee of medical scientists to address what was considered a growing and soon-to-be worldwide pandemic of AIDS. Like Catholic popes in earlier eras who issued papal bulls and were considered infallible, the committee, chaired by David Baltimore, issued several from-on-high pronouncements. The committee stated that the work of Montagnier and Gallo "led to its [HIV] definitive identification as the cause of AIDS."[1029] Therefore, the committee reached a "consensus" all the while ignoring serious objections raised by scientists who had both more competence and integrity in their respective fields than either Gallo or Montagnier;[1030,1031] and thus, a decree was given to the world that the evidence that HIV causes AIDS is scientifically conclusive! The committee, in another Orwellian thrust, changed from a plurality what clearly is a syndrome of unrelated diseases into to a singularity

---

[1026] Barré-Sinoussi, F., et al.: Isolation of a T-lymphotropic retrovirus from a patient at risk for acquired immune deficiency syndrome (AIDS). Science 1983; 220: 868-871.

[1027] Cohen, J.: H.H.S.-Gallo guilty of misconduct. Science 1993; 259: 168-170

[1028] Connor S. AIDS: Science Stands On Trial. New Scientist 1987; Feb 12:49-54.

[1029] Institute of Medicine: Confronting AIDS. Washington, National Academy Press, 1986.

[1030] Duesberg, P.H.: Retroviruses as carcinogens and pathogens: Expectations and reality. Cancer Res 1987; 47: 1199-1220.

[1031] Booth, W.: A rebel without a cause for AIDS. Science 1988; 239: 1485-1488.

by proposing to rename AIDS, HIV disease.[1032] By this linguistic slight of pen, the world has come to believe that there is a disease HIV/AIDS rather than a syndrome theoretically resulting from HIV causing AID which leads to S. However, after more than thirty years, what has been forgotten in the cloud of dogma is that there is still no viable explanation that can withstand scrutiny. This renaming also hid the fact that AIDS is not a singularity but a disparate collection of twenty-nine diseases. The CDC later claimed that finding a low CD4+T cell count could be added to the disparate collection.

Science is not a democratic process. If it is not fundamentally based on knowable factual information, it can easily fall into fantasy. What this committee failed to understand but with the support of the Epidemic Intelligence Service and the controlled media as their leveraging handmaidens faked was that there is no such thing as a scientific proof; that proofs only exist in mathematics and logic but not in science. Scientific knowledge is tentative and provisional, and nothing is ever final.[1033] A theory of a phenomenon is simply the best explanation among all available alternatives, and it absolutely must have predictive power. Yet it goes without saying that the HIV as the cause of AID as the cause of S is anything but the best alternative.

In immunology, however, two researchers were raising questions about the functioning of the immune system that were being glossed over by the retrovirologists, namely, are B cell help and delayed-type hypersensitivity mediated by different types of CD4+T cells? In other words, are there classes of Th cells analogous to the classes of antibodies made by B cells?[1034]

T Cell Heterogeneity

The body's resistance to disease-causing pathogens has two pathways it can employ. It can use nonspecific (innate immunity) or specific (adaptive immunity), generally in combination. Innate immunity comprises mechanical barriers (e.g., skin and mucous membranes), phagocytosis, fever, inflammation, and acute phase proteins. The acute phase complement proteins opsonize or perforate the invading cell membrane, for example, those of bacteria, resulting in their destruction by phagocytosis.

[1032] Institute of Medicine: Confronting AIDS-Update 1988. Washington, National Academy Press, 1988

[1033] Satoshi, Kanazawa, (Nov. 16, 2008), "Common misconceptions about science I: 'scientific proof'"; *Psychology Today*

[1034] Coffman, RL., (2006), "Origins of the Th1-Th2 model: a personal perspective," *Nat Immunol;* 7(6):539-541

Adaptive immunity has two exquisite qualities: specificity and memory. The two main arms of adaptive immunity include humoral (comprising B cells and effector T cells) and cell-mediated immunity (comprising T cells and macrophages), both with their related cytokines.

In 1986, a new foundation for modern T cell biology was established by Mosmann and Coffman when they individually published two landmark papers that proposed the Th1-Th2 hypothesis.[1035,1036] The theory was based on the observation that distinct subsets of CD4+T helper (Th) cells expressed discrete cytokine profiles after activation that defined their different regulatory and effector functions: Th1 cells induce cell-mediated inflammatory responses and Th2 cells provide B cell help. Importantly, Coffman surmised that the effector cytokines produced by one subset of cells would regulate the development and function of the other.[1037] In other words, the system had built-in counterregulatory controls. The central idea of these findings was that each Th subset has the ability to stimulate one set of coordinated antipathogen effector functions and to promote the development of more cells of the same Th subset while inhibiting both the development of the opposite subset and many of its most important effector functions.

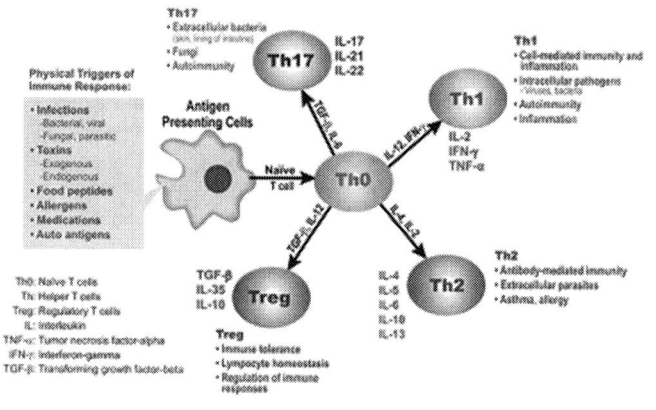

figure 1

[1035] Coffman, R.L, Carty J, (1986) "A T cell activity that enhances polyclonal IgE production and its inhibition by interferon-gamma"; *J Immunol;* 136:949-954

[1036] Mosmann, TR., et al., (1986) "Two types of murine helper T cell clone. I. definition according to profiles of lymphokine activities and secreted proteins," *J Immunol;* 136:2348-2357

[1037] McGeachy, MJ, (2008), "Th17 cell differentiation: the long and winding road," *Immunity;* 28:445-453

[1038] http://www.wellnessalternatives-stl.com/am-i-th1-or-th2-or-th17/ date of download 5.1.2016

Only a few key cytokines were found to be central to both the stimulatory and inhibitory activities of the Th subsets; however, these cytokines are not exclusively produced by Th cells, and many other leucocytes can contribute to a type 1–like or a type 2–like response.[1039] Subsequently, other lineages of CD4+T cells have been identified: Th17, Th9, follicular helper (Tfh), Th22, and T regulatory (reg), etc. But the focus here will be simplified to the role of the dual strategy of the immune system in response to oxidative stress as manifested in AIDS patients. Th1 cells can be stimulated by type 1 cytokines to activate the enzyme iNOS to produce the gas cloud of NO that can diffuse across the bacterial membrane. As previously discussed, iNOS exerts antimicrobial actions through several mechanisms.[1040] The NO (and its congeners) can inhibit bacterial replication by binding directly to double-stranded DNA, causing deamination and breakage, and by disrupting zinc metalloproteins involved in DNA synthesis. NO also impairs bacterial function by disrupting heme-containing bacterial enzymes and oxidizing bacterial lipids. Viral infection is impaired through inhibitory NO actions on replication and activation of proteases involved in virus entry. Type 2 cytokines inhibit the expression of iNOS but simultaneously permit the B cell antibody response.

Th0 clones are described as those that can produce cytokines of both Th1 and Th2 clones. The clones serve as precursors to the other Th clones.[1041] The Th1 subset of CD4+T cells was found to produce mainly Il-2, TNF-α, and IFN-γ, and mediated DTH responses. The Th2 subset was found to help B cells to secrete antibodies by producing a B cell stimulatory factor later named IL-4. Important to the AIDS conundrum was the finding that a shift in balance to Th1 produced a strong DTH reaction while a shift in balance to Th2 led to a weak DTH or no response at all.[1042] IFN-γ blocked Th2 antibody responses, building the initial binary concept of CD4 T helper subtypes (the Th1/Th2 paradigm). The implication being that the subsets regulate each other and that Th1 and Th2 exert distinct and well-defined immune functions. The Th1 cells were active against intracellular bacteria and viruses using inducible NO and its congeners, but they were also involved in tissue damage as the result of fighting chronic infections or promoting autoimmune diseases. Th2 cells, on the other hand, were shown to produce IL-4, IL-5, and IL-13 cytokines and to

---

[1039] Mosmann, TR., Sad. S., (1996), "The expanding universe of T cell subsets: Th1, Th2 and more." *Immunol today;* 17:138–146

[1040] Schonohoff, CM., et al, (2003), "Nitrosylation of cytochrome c during apoptosis," *J Biol Chem;* 278:18265-18270

[1041] Lucey, DR., (1999), "Evolution of the Type 1 (Th1)-Type 2 (Th2) cytokine paradigm," *New vaccines new technology;* 13(1): 1–9

[1042] Mosmann (1986) Op cit

provide help in the IgE production and eosinophilic inflammation that clear extracellular parasites but also cause various forms of allergy.

Type 1 and Type 2 Cytokines and Their Predominant Immune Responses

Type 1 Cytokines Leading to Predominant Cell-Mediated Immunity
IFN-γ
IL-12*
IL-2
TNF-β

Type 2 Cytokines Leading to Predominant Humoral Immunity
IL-4*
IL-10*
IL-5
IL-6
IL-13

*Cytokines that are also cross-regulatory (i.e., IFN-γ and IL-12 inhibit type 2 cytokine responses, and IL-4 and IL-10 inhibit type-1 cytokine response).[1043]

However, it should be noted that there are complexities to this Th1/Th2 dichotomy, e.g., Th1 clones increase production of certain antibody isotypes and therefore do not uniformly mediate cell-mediated immunity. Some cytokines such as IL-12, which is associated with CMI, are not made by T cells whereas many Th1 and Th2 cytokines are made by cells other than CD4+T helper cells. Also, there are many human T cells (Th0) that cannot be slotted in to either Th1 or Th2 as they produce cytokines of both subsets. Further, some T cells produce one but not all the defining Th1-Th2 cytokines, and some cytokines are neither Th1 nor Th2 but rather modulate cellular or humoral responses.[1044] It should also be noted that a relative predominance of type 1 or type 2 cytokine responses may be present without an absolute dichotomy of either cytokine response.

What was important to the AIDS conundrum of how patients with anergy and depressed circulatory CD4+T cells could at the same time have increased antibody production was, however, answered by the findings of the

---

[1043] Lucey (1999), Op cit.
[1044] Lucey, (1999) Op cit.

dual strategy of the immune system and its counterregulatory functions. This information, combined with the knowledge of the counterbalancing roles of the NO/glutathione systems for redox signaling as modulators of pathogen eradication, immune suppression, and tissue restoration and wound healing, answers the AIDS dilemma. This evidence provided a cellular basis for the older observations of differential regulation of delayed-type hypersensitivity and optimum antibody production. To date, the AIDS theorists have acknowledged these findings but have not been able to incorporate these observations into their theory. The knowledge of this dual strategy of the immune system is a central aspect of both understanding the imbalance in the immune system in AIDS and developing appropriate therapeutic interventions, away from the virus/HAART model. It is no longer logical to be continually befuddled by how HIV could manage this immune disbalance, especially since what is being called HIV cannot be expressed in Th1 cells but in the Th0 and Th2 cells.[1045,1046,1047]

History of Immune Suppression in the Twentieth Century: Confused at a Higher Level of Understanding

In the AIDS paradigm, the decrease in circulating CD4+T lymphocytes has been attributed to the progressive destruction caused by HI viruses.[1048] There is still no logical explanation of the mechanism. However, already in the 1970s before the AIDS era, Anthony Fauci's[1049] laboratory had already demonstrated that in persistent hypercortisolism as occurring in long-term stress, an increasing number of CD4+T cells leave the bloodstream and can

---

[1045] Chehimi, J, et al., (1995), "Differential regulation of IL-10 and role of IL-12 during HIV infection of T helper cells," abstr in *Second National Conf on Human Retrovirurses*. Inf Disease Soc. Amer., Alexendria, Va.

[1046] Maggi, E., et al., (1994), "Ability of HIV t promote a Th1 to Th0 shift and to replicate preferentially in Th2 and Th0 cells," *Science;* 265:244-248

[1047] Romagnani, S., et al., (1994), "HIV can induce a Th1 to Th0 shift and preferentially replicate in CD4+T cell clones producing Th2-type clones," *Res Immunol;* 145: 611-618

[1048] Hässig A, Liang WX, Stampfli K. Reappraisal of the depletion of circulating CD4-lymphocytes in HJV-carriers in transition to AIDS. Continuum 1 996;3:1 8-20.

[1049] http://www.niaid.nih.gov/about/directors/Pages/default.aspx

therefore activate B cells in the bone marrow.[1050,1051,1052] When the cortisol levels drop to normal, these lymphocytes then return to the bloodstream. As they have forgotten or simply ignored this research, by 1994, there was still no explanation incorporating these earlier experimental findings for the mechanism of how HIV was making CD4+T cells disappear. A study by Maurizio Carbonari, et al., actually showed by phenotypic analysis that apoptotic lymphocytes were, in fact, not CD4+T cells but mostly CD8+T cells and CD19+ B cells. They surmised that in contrast to what had been previously suggested (that HIV is killing CD4+T cells), the phenomenon of in vitro lymphocyte apoptosis might not be pathogenically related to the depletion of CD4+T cells in acquired immunodeficiency syndrome.[1053] However, the study that showed a decided lack of understanding of the type1/type 2 hypothesis by AIDSworld and should have put the HIV causes AID idea to rest was also published in 1995[1054] when it was found that the marker for HIV expression could only be demonstrated preferentially in Th2 and Th0 cell types and not among the Th1 cells. Contrary to the proposed AIDS hypothesis, the model demonstrated that the "infection" occurs in the cells whose growth actually increases after infection!

There has been silence on why what is being called HIV is found in the progenitor Th0 cells from which Th1 and Th2 evolve and in cells that increase the humoral expression of the immunity but not in the subset that controls cell-mediated immunity. In spite of more than a $300 billion expenditure on AIDS research over the last decades, in an unpublicized scientific declaration of defeat, it was admitted that "the riddle of CD4 cell loss [from the bloodstream] remains unresolved [by the current HIV/AIDS theory]. We are still very confused about the mechanisms that lead to CD4 depletion. . . . But at least we are now

---

[1050] Fauci AS, Dale DC. The effect of in vivo hydrocortisone on subpopulations of human lymphocytes. J Clin Invest 1 974;53:240-246.

[1051] Fauci AS, Dale DC. Ihe effect of hydrocortisone on the kinetics of normal human lymphocytes. Blood 1 975;46:235-243.

[1052] Fauci AS, Pratt KR. Activation of human [3 lymphocytes. 1. Direct plaque-forming cell assay tor the measurement of polydonal activation and antigenic stimulation of human [3 lymphocytes. J Exp Med 1976;1 44:674-684.

[1053] Carbonari M, Cibati M, Cherchi M et al. Detection and characterization of apoptotic peripheral blood Iymphocytes in human immunodeficiency virus infection and cancer chemotherapy by a novel flow immunocyto- metric method. Blood 1 994;83: 1 268-1 277.

[1054] Maggi, E. et al., (1995), "Ability of HIV to promote a Th1 to Th2 shift and to replicate preferentially in Th2 and Th0 cells," *Science*; 265:244-248

confused at a higher level of understanding."[1055] The retrovirus researchers still have no grasp of the mechanism of the biologically programmed Th1 to Th2 functional shift of the T helper cells that drift out of the bloodstream and into the bone marrow and other organs where they carry out their specialized function of supporting B cells in the production of antibodies.

The immune system is both nonlinear and complex, and that complexity indicates that the same type of molecule might have both a beneficial or a deleterious effect. Generally, the nature of the effect will relate to the metabolic condition (redox environment) of the cell/organ when the contact begins and on both how much and how long the cell is exposed to the signal. As an example, NO is able to promote either suppression or activation,[1056] death or survival,[1057,1058] or gene transcription or repression.[1059,1060] It can also act as an oxidative or an antioxidative signal.

It also must be considered that the immune system interacts with the nervous system in an integral way. This integral behavior was brought into focus by Candace Pert,[1061] a molecular biologist who was a key figure in the discovery of the endorphin molecule, the body's natural form of morphine. It was discovered that the cells in both the nervous system and the immune system have opioid receptors. Pert is now widely regarded as the mother of the new field of science known as psychoneuroimmunology, which examines the influence of stress and nervous system functions in relation to immune function, especially in relation to the onset and progression of disease. In biological terms, stressors are not only emotional. They can be defined as psychological, toxic, infectious, traumatic, nutritional, or electromagnetic. Pert has advanced the earlier ideas of Bernard, Cannon, and Selye into modern scientific methodology. It seems that endorphins can produce a beneficial effect of the immune response by

---

[1055] Balter, M., (1997), "How does HIV overcome the body's T cell body guards?," 11th Colloquium of the Cent-Gardes Marnes-la-Coquette, France, 27 to 29 October 1997, *Science,* 287:1399-1400

[1056] Sriskandan, S., et al, (1996), "Bacterial superantigen induced human lymphocyte responses are nitric oxide dependent and mediated by IL-12 and IFN-γ" *J Immunol;* 156:2430-2435

[1057] Schonhoff, Op cit.

[1058] Zech, B., et al., (2003), "Nitric Oxide donors inhibit formation of the Apaf-1/caspase-9 apoptosome and activation of caspases:," *Biochem J;* 371:1055-1064

[1059] Bogdan, C., (2001), "Nitric oxide and the regulation of gene expression," *Trends Cell Biol;* 11:66-75

[1060] Pfeilschifter, J., et al, (2001), "Regulation of gene expression of nitric oxide," *Pflugers Arch;* 442:479-486

[1061] Pert, Candace (1999), "Molecules of Emotion: The science behind mind-body medicine," Simon & Schuster, NY

enhancing the natural killer function of human lymphocytes.[1062] However, it has been well documented that long-term stress and the long-term use of opioids do not enhance but suppress the immune response.[1063,1064]

The immune disbalance found in AIDS patients was by no means a unique event as it is also found in chronic opioid use, malnutrition, organ transplant, and surgical patients.

Opioids, Long Known to Suppress the Immune System

That the immune system was involved in various aspects associated with the chronic use of opioids was suggested as early as 1844[1065] and more recently by others.[1066] The cells of the immune system possess opiate receptors[1067] that when activated induce a variety of functional modifications such as the establishment of profound immune suppression following chronic opiate treatment.[1068,1069] Cloetta, in a study done in 1902, showed that chronic morphine injections resulted in leucopenia (sic) in rabbits, and leucopenia (sic) in morphine addicts was described as early as 1901 by Archard and Loeper. In 1898, Cantacuzene showed that morphine modulated the expression of chemotactic and phagocytic activity both in vitro and in vivo experimental systems. He also showed that morphine-treated guinea pigs had a greater mortality rate than controls after peritoneal injection of cholera bacilli.[1070] More recent studies have shown that

---

[1062] Kay, N, Allen J., Morley, JE., (1984), "Endorphins stimulate normal human peripheral blood lymphocyte natural killer activity," *Life Sci;* 35(1):53-59

[1063] Dhabhar, F.S., (2009), "Enhancing versus suppressive effects of stress on immune function: implications for immunoprotection and immunopathology," *Neuroimmunomodulation;* 16(5):300-317

[1064] Sacerdote, P., (2006), "Opioids and the immune system," *Palliat Med;* 20 suppl 1:a9-15

[1065] Cohen, et al., (1965), "Effect of actinomycin D on morphine tolerance," *Proc So Exp Biol Med;* 119:381-384

[1066] Dafny, N. et al., (1988), "Immune response products alter CNS activity: interferon modulates central opioid functions," *J Neurosci Res;* 19:130-139

[1067] Hazum E., et al., (1979), "Specific non-opiate receptors for endorphin," *Science;* 205:1033-1035

[1068] Jaffe, JH., (1990) "Drug addiction and drug abuse in *The Pharmacological Basis of Therapeutics.* 8th ed., Gilman. AG., Rall, TW., Nies AS., Taylor, P., Eds., Macmillan, NY, 1990 pp. 435-521

[1069] Pellis, NR., Harper, C., Dafny, N.,(1986) "Suppression of the induction of delayed hypersensitivity in rats by repetitive morphine treatments" *Exp Neurol;* 93:92-97

[1070] Freedman, H., Kline, T., Specter. S., (1996) Drugs of abuse, immunity and infection, New York, CRC Press, p 5

morphine induces the expression of the Fas protein, a receptor on the cell surface that triggers the cell's suicide by apoptosis when it binds to its ligand FasL. This induction of Fas expression by opioids appears to prime lymphocytes for elimination by apoptosis.[1071]

Other studies have shown that both psychological and physical stressors impact the intercommunication between the immune and the nervous system. Long-term chronic stress significantly impacts leukocyte cellularity and immune responses and often leads to immunosuppression. It is generally accepted that acute stress could improve the function of the immune system while chronic stress often results in reduction of immune responses.[1072] Just as morphine has been shown to prime lymphocytes for elimination by apoptosis, chronic-stress-induced lymphocyte reduction occurs through endogenous opioid-mediated Fas expression as well.[1073,1074] More recent studies have shown that chronic morphine treatment suppresses cellular immunity and increases T helper cell differentiation into Th2.[1075] IL-2 and IFN-γ (Th1) levels decrease while IL-4 and IL-5 (Th2) level increase. Consonant with this immune shift has been that the DTH response is also reduced.[1076]

Pneumocystis Pneumonia: Consequence of Malnutrition

Malnutrition is either directly or indirectly responsible for 54 percent of the 10.8 million deaths per year in children under five in developing countries.[1077] For centuries, it has been recognized that there is an association between malnutrition and disease. Cicely Williams, a Western pediatrician who worked for seven years in Ghana, first described kwashiorkor in the early part of the

---

[1071] Yin, D., et al.,(1999) "Fas mediated cell death promoted by opoids," *Nature;* 397(218)

[1072] Dhabhar, FS., McEwen, BS., (1997), "Acute stress enhances while chronic stress suppresses cell mediated immunity in vivo: a potential role for leukocyte trafficking," *Brain Behav Immun;* 11:286-306

[1073] Yin, D. et al, (1999), Op cit

[1074] Yin, D., et al, (2000), "Chronic restraint stress promotes lymphocyte apoptosis by modulating CD95 expression," *J Exp Medicine;* 191:1423-1429

[1075] Roy, S., et al, (2004), "Chronic morphine treatment differentiates T helper cells to Th2 effector cells by modulating transcription factors GATA 3 and T-bet," *J Neuroimmunol;* 147(1-2): 78-81

[1076] Bryant, HU, Roudebush, RE., (1990), "Suppressive effects of morphine pellet implants on in vivo parameters of immune function, *J Pharmcol;* 225(2): 410-414

[1077] Blossner, M., de Onis, M., (2005), "Malnutrition: Quantifying the health impact at national an local levels," World health Organization: Geneva, Switzerland

twentieth century as a specific clinical entity.[1078] It was often associated in children with parasitic infestation and acute respiratory and gastrointestinal disease. Scientists began to characterize what later became known as the nutrition/infection synergism.[1079] Recent studies on the influence of infection on metabolism and nutritional status have demonstrated the degree to which preexisting malnutrition may be exacerbated by the anorexia and negative nitrogen balance that frequently accompany infection.[1080] In effect, malnutrition is a common cause of secondary immune deficiency.[1081] It is well-known that it affects T-cell-mediated immune responses. It has recently been demonstrated that the gene expression and intracellular production of cytokines responsible for Th1 cell differentiation are diminished in malnourished children.[1082] Thus, the defect found in AIDS patients, an immune balance shift from Th2 to Th1, is not an uncommon finding in those who suffer from food insufficiency. This, of course, needs to be underscored in reference to what has been called African AIDS and the widespread food insecurity/infection issues that exist in many of the countries on this continent.

One of the classic AIDS-defining diseases is Pneumocystis pneumonia. Pneumocystis carinii (now jiroveci), an atypical fungus, first came to attention as a cause of interstitial pneumonia in severely malnourished and premature infants in orphanages during World War II in Central and Eastern Europe. The WWII cases of "plasma-cell pneumonia" were also later reported in Iranian orphanages. It has been reported that by four years of age, two-thirds of normal children have antibody to P. carinii in titers of 1:16 or greater.[1083]

Subsequent to WWII, it was ascertained that patients with such diseases as treated lymphoma or leukemia, patients on immunosuppressive therapy following organ transplantation, and patients receiving long-term cortical steroids such as severe combined immunodeficiency and agammaglobulinemia or hypergammaglobulinemia typically became likely hosts for this organism as well. Without chemoprophylaxis, rates of PCP are 5 to 25 percent in transplant

---

[1078] Heikens, GT, Manary, M., (2009), "75 years of Kwashiorkor in Africa," *Malawi Med J;* 21(3):96-100

[1079] Scrimshaw, N.S., SanGiovanni, JP., (1997), "Synergism of nutrition, infection, and immunity: an overview," *Am J Clin Nutr;* 66(2):4645-4775

[1080] Kurpad, AV., (2006), "The requirements of protein & amino acid during acute & chronic infections," *Ind J Med Res;* 124:129-148

[1081] Schaible, UE., Kaufmann, SH., (2007), "Malnutrition and infection: Complex mechanisms and global impact," *PLoS Med;* 4, e115

[1082] Gonzalez-Torres, C., et al., (2012), "Effect of malnutrition on the expression of cytokines involved in Th1 cell differentiation," *Nutrients;* 5:579-593

[1083] Pifer, LL, et al, (1978), "Pneumocystis carinii infection: evidence for high prevalence in normal and immunosuppressed children," *Pediatrics;* 61(1): 35-41

patients, 2 to 5 percent in patients with collagen vascular disease, and 1 to 25 percent in patients with cancer.[1084] Thus, while the virus hunters were looking for a virus that would attack the immune system that would lead to AID and cause S, one of which was PCP, they failed to consider the existing medical literature that was not exactly bereft of evidence of the pathophysiology of immune deficiency and its various manifestations, especially in malnourished and immune compromised individuals.

Organ Transplantation

In 1954, at the Brigham Hospital in Boston, Dr. Joseph Murray performed the first successful human kidney transplant in a patient with chronic renal failure. The patient received a kidney from his identical twin brother, which alleviated the problem of transplantation rejection, which had been a major stumbling block to the wide use of this procedure. By the 1960s, Burroughs and Wellcome had developed an imidazole derivative of 6-mercaptopurine (6-MP), which was known to be immunosuppressive in kidney transplantation in dogs. Unlike 6-MP, which had to be given intravenously, azathioprine (brand name Imuran), a nitroso compound, was developed as an oral medication. Surgeons soon found that the combination of prednisone and azathioprine decreased the risk of rejection, but it continued to be a problem that by 1978 the one-year graft survival rate for cadaveric kidneys in the United States was still only ~ 47 percent with a very high mortality rate of 30 percent.[1085] The revolution in transplantation began in 1978 with the introduction of a new immunosuppressive fungal metabolite patented by Sandoz: cyclosporine. With the combination of azathioprine, prednisone, and cyclosporine, the graft survival rate for kidney transplantation increased to more than 70 percent and the mortality rate sank to less than 10 percent with similar numbers for liver transplants and great improvements in heart transplant survival as well.[1086]

Although the combination of these powerful immunosuppressive agents improved both morbidity and mortality in transplant patients, they came with incredible risk: susceptibility to opportunistic infections and cancer[1087] such as Kaposi's sarcoma (KS) and lymphomas. Kaposi's sarcoma is more prevalent

---

[1084] Morris, A., et al., (2004), "Current epidemiology of *Pneumocystis* pneumonia," *Emerg Inf Dis; 10(10)*: 1713-1720
[1085] Klintmalm, G.B., (2004), "The history of organ transplantation in the Baylor Health Care System," *Proc (Bayl Univ Med Cent); 17(1)*:23-34
[1086] Klintmalm, Ibid
[1087] Klintmalm, op cit

in males of Mediterranean, Middle Eastern, and African origin where it can occur in up to 5 percent of the transplant patients from these backgrounds.[1088] A recent study in JAMA[1089] found that organ transplant recipients in the United States have a high risk of developing thirty-two different types of cancer with an overall doubling of cancer risk compared to the general population. This study was not surprising because as early at 1969, the first case of KS in association with immunosuppression in a renal transplant patient was described,[1090] and KS was found to occur in more than 3 percent of all de novo neoplasms in organ transplant recipients, which was 150 to 200 times the expected incidence of this tumor in the general population. Importantly, another study from South Africa of the malignant complications including Kaposi's sarcoma that developed in 5 of 989 renal transplant patients who were prescribed steroids, azathioprine, and/or cyclosporine A and developed disseminated forms of the disease found that four had complete tumor regression at all sites upon withdrawal of the immunosuppressive drugs.[1091] Other reports have confirmed these results.[1092,1093]

These studies have not been widely publicized or understood as they do not easily fit the current acceptance of the notion that metastatic cancer is irreversible. If withdrawing immune-suppressive drugs in transplant patients who are clearly ill even before they receive the transplant can lead to a regression of a tumor that has already widely disseminated, then what can this teach us about HIV positive and AIDS patients who have been labeled "long-term nonprogressors"? Long-term nonprogressors are people who are HIV positive but have at least a ten-year latent period to the onset of AIDS or never develop the syndrome. The common elements in the reports of long-term survivors are that they (1) have avoided taking chemotherapy/antiretroviral drugs such as AZT, ddI, ddC, drT, and 3TC; (2) have stopped all high-risk activities such as drug use and unprotected or high-risk anal sex upon learning of their HIV

[1088] Campistol, JM, Schena, FP.,(2007) "Kaposi's sarcoma in renal transplant recipients—the impact of proliferation signal inhibitors," *Neph Dial Transpl;* 22(Suppl 1):i17-i22

[1089] Engels, EA., et al., (2011), "Spectrum of cancer risk among U.S. solid organ transplant recipients: the transplant cancer match study," *JAMA;* 306(17): 1891-1901

[1090] Penn, I., (1979), "Kaposi's sarcoma in organ transplant recipients: report of 20 cases," *Transplantation;* 27(1):8-11

[1091] Margolis, L, et al., (1994) "Kaposi's sarcoma in renal transplant recipients. Experience at Johannesburg Hospital 1969-1989," *S Afr Med J;* 84(1):16-7

[1092] Moray, G., et al., (2004), "Immunosuppressive therapy and kaposi's sarcoma after kidney transplantation," *Transpl Proc;* 36(1): 168-170

[1093] Zmonarski, SC., (2005), "Regression of Kaposi's sarcoma in renal graft recipients after conversion to Sirolimus treatment," *Transpl Proc;* 37(2): 964-966

status (HIV positive); and (3) have begun taking charge of their lives, including their health.[1094,1095,1096,1097,1098]

According to virologist Peter Duesberg[1099] in his 1996 book Inventing the AIDS Virus, the vast majority of HIV positives are, in fact, long-term survivors. He noted, "Worldwide, they number 17 million, including 1 million HIV positive but healthy Americans and 0.5 million HIV positive but healthy Europeans. . . . Only 6 percent [or 1,025,073] of the 18 million HIV positives [including 17 million without AIDS] have developed AIDS diseases since AIDS statistics have been kept . . . and the actual AIDS risk of an HIV carrier is less than 1 percent per year."[1100] Although it has been almost two decades since the publication of that book, the CDC estimates for people in the United States who "are living with HIV infection" is still ~1.1 million[1101]—the same number estimated at the start of the AIDS era. It is further stated that 15,529 people died with an AIDS diagnosis in 2010; however, "the deaths of persons with an AIDS diagnosis can be due to any cause—that is, the death may or may not be related to AIDS." In essence, at this time, there are no hard numbers for AIDS deaths either in the United States or worldwide.[1102,1103]

The renal transplant patients, like the AIDS patients who had histories of contact with multiple immunosuppressive agents, were exposed to three distinct drugs that act synergistically to suppress the immune system and to create the conditions for the development of cancer: cyclosporine A, a lipophilic

---

[1094] Cao, Yunzhen, et al., (1995), "Virologic and immunologic characterization of long-term survivors of HIV-type 1 infection," *NEJM;* 332: 201-208

[1095] Altman, L, (Jan. 24, 1995), "Long term survivors may hold the clues to puzzle of AIDS," *NYTimes;* Science section

[1096] Pantaleo, G. et al., (1995), "Studies in subjects with long term nonprogressive Human Immunodeficiency Virus infection," *NEJM;* 332:209

[1097] Hogervorst, E., et al., (1995), "Predictors for non and slow progression in HIV type 1 infection: low viral RNA copy numbers in serum and maintenance of high HIV-1 p24 specific antibody levels," *J Inf Dis;* 171:811

[1098] Hoover, D.R., et al., (1995) "Long term survival without clinical AIDS after CD4+ cell counts fall below 200," *AIDS;* 9:145

[1099] Duesberg, PH, (1996), Inventing the AIDS Virus, Regnery Publishing, Washington, D.C.p 425

[1100] World Health Organization, Current Global Situation

[1101] http://www.cdc.gov/hiv/statistics/basics/ataglance.html HIV in the United States: At a Glance, Feb. 26, 2014

[1102] Derbyshire, SW., (1995), "WHO criticised for 'inflating' AIDS figures," AIDS Anal Afr; 5(6): 4-5

[1103] Apr., 18, 2006, "How was the AIDS situation in Africa so greatly overstated?," The Irish Times; http://www.irishtimes.com/news/health/how-was-the-aids-situation-in-africa-so-greatly-overstated-1.1039953 downloaded 31 July 2015

cyclic undecapeptide isolated from a fungus found to inhibit T cell activation by blocking the transcription of cytokines including IL-2 and IL-4;[1104,1105] prednisone, a glucocorticoid that exerts its effects by preferentially inhibiting type 1 cytokines, leading to an eventual shift toward a Th2 profile among CD4+T lymphocytes by interference with cytokine receptor signaling that leads to an increase in T-cell, thymocyte and eosinophil apoptosis, reduced T cell activation, and decreased production of nitric oxide and by down-modulating adhesion molecules on antigen-presenting cells (APCs);[1106] and azathioprine, a nitroso compound, both in vitro and in vivo, metabolized to 6-MP through the reduction by glutathione and other sulfhydryl-containing compounds, ultimately becoming incorporated into replicating DNA, blocking the de novo synthesis of purines,[1107] thereby inhibiting cell proliferation, especially in fast-growing cells such as lymphocytes. Clearly, the immunosuppression in transplant patients was another not-uncommon clinical model from which the AIDS protagonists could have drawn parallels and inspiration, especially from the fact that even cases of disseminated Kaposi's sarcoma was reversible on the withdrawal of immune-suppressing drugs.

Surgical Patients: DTH Skin Test as an Indicator of the Th1/Th2 Imbalance

Although the delayed-type hypersensitivity (DTH) reaction was discovered over one hundred years ago, the exact nature of the reaction has been the subject of contentious debate over the years. The reaction was discovered in 1882 by Robert Koch, but it was not until the 1940s that Landsteiner and Chase proved that the reaction was mediated by the cellular and not the humoral arm of the immune system.[1108] Using this information, in the mid-1970s, hoping to find a way to improve outcomes in surgical patients, especially those who developed sepsis after sustaining massive trauma or burns, a surgical team

---

[1104] Kronke, et al, (1984), "Cyclosporin A inhibits T-cell growth factor gene expression at the level of mRNA transcription," *Proc Natl Acad Sci U.S. A.*; 81:5214-5218

[1105] Granelli-Piperno, A., (1988), "In situ hybridization for interleukin 2 and interleukin 2 receptor mRNA in T cells activated in the presence or absence of cyclosporin A," *J Exp Med*; 168:1649-1658

[1106] Singh, N, (2004), "Mechanisms of glucocorticoid mediated anti-inflammatory and immunosuppressive action" *Ped and Perinatal Drug Therapy*; 6(2): 107

[1107] Maltzman, J.S., Koretzky, G.A.,(2003) "Azathioprine: old drug, new actions," *J Clin Invest*; 111(8): 1122-1124

[1108] Black, CA., (1999), "Delayed type hypersensitivity: current theories with an historic perspective," *Dermatol Online J*; 4(1):7

in Montreal began to record the DTH reaction before and after surgery of all patients for the decade between 1975 and 1985. Despite better surgical techniques and increased life support systems, sepsis continued to be a major cause of morbidity and mortality in this population of surgical patients.[1109]

Two hundred and two patients were tested before surgery. Three to five percent of all patients tested developed sepsis; for patients who needed intensive care postop, the number skyrocketed to more than 30 percent. Of note, 50 percent of the patients were anergic on the third-day postop but regained their reactivity by the seventh postop day. Patients who remained anergic had a higher rate of sepsis. If the skin test failed to normalize, a subsequent sepsis was associated with a higher rate of mortality. The patients were categorized as (1) DTH positive, (2) DTH negative (relatively anergic), and (3) DTH negative (anergic). Of the patients in category 1, 8 percent developed sepsis and 4 percent died; in category 2, 21 percent developed sepsis and 15 percent died; in category 3, 33 percent developed sepsis and 31 percent died. Clearly, a decrease in the functioning of CMI as an expression of a decreased DTH response is an ominous finding, but it is in no way a universal death sentence as AIDSworld has come to believe. It is mediated by the history and antioxidant status of the intra- and extracellular compartments, specifically the availability of both cysteine and glutathione and other reducing equivalents.

It was established that the immunological variables of the surgical sepsis patients had changed in comparison to the nonsepsis patients. As in the above malnourished patients and in the transplant patients, the type 1 cytokine IL-2 was severely inhibited in the sepsis patients. Some antibody classes (IgG and IgA) increased, but other antibody classes decreased. They also found many inhibitors in the serum of sepsis patients and commented, "That inhibitors have a profound effect on T helper lymph cells and polymorphonuclear leukocytes. Teleologically, there is a suggestion that this inhibition post injury may be a normal response related to the 'healing processes' and prevention of autoimmune reactions to self-denatured proteins. The host is, therefore, caught in a dichotomy between healing and sepsis, in the midst of breached defenses."[1110]

Living organisms are autopoetic bioenergetic networks that have the capability of instituting complex regulatory and counterregulatory measures in the face of attacks or damage. Because there are networked cycles that feed into countless other networked cycles, these integrated systems can be up- or downregulated as needed in direct response to environmental signals. New

---

[1109] Christou, NV., (1986), Delayed hypersensitivity in the surgical patient, In: Gallin N, Fauci AS (ed.), Advances in host defence mechanisms, Vol. 6, Raven Press, NY
[1110] Christou, Ibid

homeostatic levels can be attained—to a point. How the cell/organ responds depends on multiple factors.[1111,1112,1113] What is important from the study of surgical patients is that an anergic DTH reaction as an expression of the inhibited cell-mediated immune competence before admission to the hospital was significantly linked to the sepsis results, which, despite massive use of antibiotics, led to a high mortality rate. A decade later, a repeat study confirmed that there is a strongly positive correlation between a reduced DTH response and the risk of dying if sepsis sets in after a surgical event in patients who require observation in an intensive care unit.[1114]

What these surgical (and organ transplant) studies demonstrated is the evolutionary, biologically programmed dual strategy of the immune response: 50 percent of the surgical patients responded to the profound stress to the system with a T helper cell disbalance up to the seventh-day post p after which the system was able to stabilize. Not all the patients who had shown signs of immune disbalance before surgery died. Some continue to live with a longstanding T helper cell disbalance but were still able to overcome the sequelae of the operation, but a small percentage died.[1115]

From the above examples, whether suffering from malnutrition, opiate addiction, or organ failure or simply general surgery patients, a long-lasting T helper cell disbalance (as found in AIDS patients) as a result of external stressors is not uncommon in the population. Data from the surgical studies indicated that not every patient with a T helper cell disbalance developed a lethal infection. Sixty-seven percent of the pre-op anergic patients and 79 percent of the relatively anergic patients did not develop sepsis,[1116] which suggests a high variability of the regulation of the immune response between cell-mediated and humoral immunity, which can change in a way that sepsis is allowed to develop or is halted. A long-lasting cell disbalance under profound stress loads (acquired immunodeficiency = AID) with or without infectious syndrome is by no means a rare or "puzzling" occurrence.[1117]

[1111] Tsong, TY, (1989), "Deciphering the language of cells," *Trends Biochem Sci;* 14(3): 89-92

[1112] Cerami, A., 1992), "Inflammatory cytokines," *Clin Immunol Immunopathol;* 62(1 Pt 2):S3-10

[1113] Martindale, JL, Holbrook, NJ, (2002), "Cellular response to oxidative stress: signaling for suicide and survival," *J Cell Phys;* 192:1-15

[1114] Christou, NY, et al., (1995), "The Delayed hypersensitivity response and host resistance in surgical patients. 20 years later," *Ann Surg;* 222(4):534-546

[1115] Kremer, H.,(2008) *The Silent Revolution in Cancer and AIDS Medicine*, Xlibris, USA p 106

[1116] Christou, (1986) Op cit

[1117] Kremer (2009) Op cit p 106

The Slow Death of the AIDS/Cancer Paradigm and the Apocrypha of the Eukaryotic Cell

In essence, HIV is neither necessary nor required for the development of acquired immunodeficiency, AID, as it is clear that these same immune disbalances are not a rare finding on either surgical or medical in-patient floors. That these disbalances are not automatic death sentences has been proven by years of clinical observation and research, even without knowing the fundamental workings of the immune and energy systems. It is now understood that the redox status of the cell and not the presence of "HIV" that determines the propensity for the system to express either type 1 or type 2 cytokines, and this is controlled by the balance and counterregulation of the glutathione-NO systems. Importantly, what are being called "HIV" characteristics are not found in the cells that are diminishing but in the cells that are proliferating. The HIV/AIDS theory is a total failure and needs to be relegated to trash bin of medical history along with leeching, bleeding, the use of mercury and arsenic, phrenology, and sundry other medical follies.

What in Reality Are the So-Called HIV Characteristics

In Djamel Tahi's 1997 interview with Luc Montagnier, Montagnier claimed isolation of HIV because he was able to "pass on the virus," because he conflated "virus" with the finding of reverse transcriptase in the spun sediment at 1.16 gm/ml along with a lot of cellular material and because he was able to produce EM pictures of particles "budding," etc. However, what Montagnier, Gallo, and other researchers have failed to disclose is that in the HIV experiments, all the so-called HIV characteristics were only able to be demonstrated in cells that were stimulated[1118] by the addition of strong oxidizing agents (PHA, con A., etc.) with the addition of the type 1 cytokine IL-2. This sets in place a chain reaction. IL-2 activates type 1 cytokine IFN-γ, and IFN-γ stimulates cytotoxic NO production. As these cells were taken from homosexual patients who had either AID or AIDS, such patients already demonstrated a Th-2 dominance.[1119] From the above discussion, this indicates that these cells from AIDS patients that were already counterregulated (type 2 dis-symbiosis) were added to a cancer cell line—even more counterregulated. On activation of NO synthesis by interferon-γ, these cells die by either apoptosis or necrosis as IL-2 also stimulates tumor necrosis factor and consequently an increase in the production of ROS. On the other hand, some of the cells had the option

---

[1118] Klatsmann, D., Montagnier, L, (1986), "Approaches to AIDS-therapy," *Nature;* 319: 10-11

[1119] Lucey, DR., et al, (1996), "Type 1 and type 2 cytokine dysregulation in human infectious, neoplastic, and inflammatory diseases," *Clin Microbiol Rev;* 9(4): 532-562

of becoming more counterregulated (hyperpolarization of the mitochondrial membrane, decreased calcium cycling, reversal of the "hybrid impulse," decreased production of ATP by the OXPHOS electron transport chain, and surplus hydrogen diffusion to the cytoplasm) to protect against cell death. In this case, there would be activation of type 2 cytokine profile (IL-4, IL-5, IL-10, etc.). In this scenario, there also could be an upregulation of the cyclooxygenase enzyme (COX-2) with the consequent production of prostaglandin (PGE) and transforming growth factor (TGF). PGE and TGF act as negative feedback on type 1 cytokines, therefore limiting the production of NO synthesis and activation of arginine from the production of NO and redirecting to the path for the synthesis of ornithine decarboxylase and polyamines that stimulate the proliferation of repair mechanisms. The synthesis of reverse transcriptase belongs to this sequence. The counterregulated cancer and lymph cells that have switched to the use of aerobic glycolysis now will extrude highly oxidized packaged cell contents that have been called virus-like particles seen budding from cell surface membranes in the EMs produced by Gallo and Montagnier.[1120] It was the trickery of Gallo's laboratory processes—first the forcing of RT by the addition of hydrocortisone and, subsequently, overcoming the hydrocortisone-induced blockade of cytokine synthesis with the addition of interleukin 2, which activates interferon-γ[1121], which then stimulates cytotoxic NO—that then produced two "HIV characteristics": RT and the apparent destruction of T4 cells by the retrovirus "HIV."

Essentially, what in AIDSworld became a virus was, in fact, the artificial provocation of already-stressed immune cells that were clearly dis-symbiotic with the end result of cells dying by necrosis or apoptosis and/or surviving by increased counterregulation in a lower-energy state. The cell productions, including RT and "HIV proteins," RNA and DNA, as well as the export particles, are all cellular products of highly stressed cells. This is why the HIV antibody tests, HIV cultures, PCR, and cloning are useless money-wasting laboratory prognosticators for use in the prediction of any fatal disease.

[1120] Kremer, Op cit p 200
[1121] Luedke, CE, Cerami, A., (1990), "Interferon-gamma overcomes glucocorticoid suppression of cachectin/tumor necrosis factor biosynthesis by murine macrophages," *J Clin Invest;* 86(4): 1234-1240

CHAPTER 10

Cell Dis-Symbiosis: Reversal of the Trend of the Chimeric Genome, Reassessment of the Appropriate Clinical Marker for an Acquired Energy Deficiency Syndrome

After a few years of the routine of medical practice, the insightful allopath often undergoes a slow transformative process and an awakening, recovering from the onslaught of the minutia that is called medical school and residency, to an astounding realization. Currently, as structured and imagined, the foundational theories, hypotheses, and constructs of the profession allow for the iatrogenic slaughter of two and a quarter million people every decade.[1122] Clearly, in the allopathic catalogue, there is a dearth of understanding about the nature of the living state that allows and accepts this level of carnage. The theories of molecular biology and genetic determinism that inform the basis of the profession are technologically sophisticated yet epistemologically primitive and have long passed being models for successful clinical application. Many of the ideas that are generated from these foundational beliefs are speculative and dangerous both in conceptualization and application. It is the twenty-first century, there is this infantile need to hold tight to nineteenth-century hypotheses as desperately as a three-year-old to his ragged security blanket. There is an urgent need to rework our notion of life processes in a way that

---

[1122] Starfield, B., (2000), "Is US health really the best in the world?," *JAMA;* 284(4): 483-5

makes logical sense in the clinical setting while moving on from the confines of genetic determinism. This can be accomplished by utilizing the principles of evolutionary and quantum biology. These disciplines provide the contextual underpinning of the complex organism operating far from thermodynamic equilibrium.

Life did not arise from the genetic code or a forest of proteins but spontaneously[1123] from the harmonic riffs, the energy, and the vibrations of coherency that gave birth to those proteins. Life has a natural rhythm, and many biomolecules are electric transducers in which acoustic and electromagnetic stimuli are equivalent in their effect.[1124] Mae Wan Ho calls it "quantum jazz"—a fitting metaphor. She states that, "Quantum jazz is the music of the organism dancing life into being, with every single cell, every molecule and atom taking part, emitting light and sound with wavelengths of nanometres to metres and kilometres; spanning a musical range of 70 octaves, each improvising spontaneously and freely, yet keeping in tune and in step with the whole."[1125]

The chimeric nucleus and its music partner, the mitochondria, have been composing ever more complex compositions for two billion years. The music has a predictable rhythm, but when the rhythm is disrupted by a dissonant harmonic in the form of a biological stressor, including specific nutrient deficiencies, the partners no longer constructively interact; and the music gets stuck on the downbeat, the note that begins the unraveling of the evolutionary biological cooperative trend. The chords begin to lose both their harmony and their complexity.

The mitochondrial "music" is in the form of cellwide synchronized oscillations in the $\Delta\psi_m$, NADH, and ROS production with a key role in the oscillating mechanism being played by the balance between superoxide anion efflux through inner membrane anion channels and the intracellular ROS scavenging capacity,[1126] as well as the competition between O_2 and NO at the

---

[1123] http://cenblog.org/the-safety-zone/2011/09/chemical-oscillations-the-belousov-zhabotinsky-reaction/ downloaded 23 March 2015

[1124] Smith, C., (1989), "Coherent electromagnetic fields and bio-communication" in *Electromagnetic Bio-Information* (Ed. Popp, Warnke, Konig, Peschka) 2nd ed. Urban & Schwarzenberg, Baltimore, Md

[1125] Ho, MW., (2007), "Quantum Jazz, The Tao of Biology," http://www.i-sis.org.uk/QuantumJazzTaoofBiology.php downloaded March, 10, 2015

[1126] Cortassa, S., et al., (2004), "A mitochondrial oscillator dependent on reactive oxygen species," *Biophysic J;* 87: 2060-2073

cytochrome c oxidase in complex 4 of the ETC.[1127,1128] Potentially, as much as half of all O_2 inhaled by an adult animal may go to ROS generation.[1129] In one and the same subcellular system, ROS may induce cell division or block it, stimulate or prevent apoptosis, cause either differentiation or dedifferentiation, or enhance or attenuate performance by differentiated cells of their specific functions. ROS are highly unstable, and thus, their action cannot be considered in terms of "dose response"[1130] but must be considered contextually. This is part of the explanation of why the mitochondrial subcellular response to changes in substrate supply is nonlinear and leads to subcellular heterogeneity of mitochondrial energization in intact cells.[1131] This heterogeneity helps explain why the same phenotype can be associated with a number of sequences of cellular events including malignant transformation. The primary cause-initiating phenotypic evolution in this process may be statistically favored but may not be identified unequivocally.[1132] This nonlinear dynamic control of metabolic pathways may offer an understanding of why transformed cells often demonstrate both modes (aerobic glycolysis and oxidative phosphorylation) of energy metabolism.

Mitochondrial Retrograde Signaling

During the course of evolution, the mitochondrial symbiont transferred more than 98 percent of the total protein complement of the organelle to what became the central chimeric nucleus.[1133] Therefore, from the beginning of the endosymbiotic trend, for mitochondria to be able to replicate, function, and respond to external factors, there had to be a coordination and expression of two sets of genes. It is only logical, as in any marriage, that methods of

---

[1127] Moncada, S., Erusalimsky, JD., (2002), "Does nitric oxide modulate mitochondrial energy generation and apoptosis?," *Nature;* 3: 214-220

[1128] Sarti, P., et al., (2012), "The chemical interplay between nitric oxide and mitochondrial cytochrome c oxidase: reactions, effectors and pathophysiology," *Int J Cell Bio;* Volume 2012 (2012), Article ID 571067

[1129] Voeikov, VL., (2006), "Reactive oxygen species—pathogens or sources of vital energy?," *J Alt Complem Med;* 12(2): 111-118

[1130] Voeikov, Ibid

[1131] Romashko, DM, et al., (1998), "Subcellular metabolic transients and mitochondrial redox waves in heart cells," *PNAS USA;* 95: 1618-1623

[1132] Waliszewski, P, et al., (1998), "On the holistic approach in cellular and cancer biology: non linearity, complexity, and quasi-determinism of the dynamic cellular network," *J Sur Onc:* 68: 70-78

[1133] Ryan, MT, Hoogenraad, NJ, (2007), "Mitochondrial-nuclear communications," *Annu Rev Biochem;* 76: 701-722

communication among the central genome, the cytosol, and the mitochondria had to be established to facilitate the evolving and ever-more-complex interacting responsibilities.

However, it was not until 2004 that it was experimentally proved by activating mammalian cells with red and near-IR radiation that mitochondria are able to communicate with the rest of the cell and send signals to the nucleus. This signaling is mediated primarily by $\Delta\Psi_m$, generation of ROS, changes in Ca^{2+} flow, and NO binding to cytochrome c oxidase.[1134]

To facilitate this retrograde signaling, there exists a unique mitochondrial oscillator that depends on oxidative phosphorylation, ROS, and permeability of the mitochondrial inner membrane ion channels, with the harmonics being established by the interplay between the efflux of the superoxide anion through the inner membrane anion channels and the capacity for the intracellular scavenging of ROS. Using near-IR radiation, it was discovered that it only required a local ROS release by ~1 percent of mitochondria to trigger oscillations throughout the entire volume of the cell.[1135]

Given the nature of these oscillatory patterns and frequencies of activation of biomolecules and organelles surrounded by EZ water, it becomes understandable why the so-called specificity of pharmaceuticals is a delusion. Pharmaceuticals are dissonant chords against life's music. No one has an acquired reverse transcriptase excess. Yet if that were indeed the case, since ~-43 percent of the human genome is said to contain retro-elements that are reverse transcribed,[1136] then this "specific" reverse transcriptase inhibitor would in fact, be targeting almost half of the genomic elements during normal cellular functions, especially during cell division, as the amount of cellular DNA would dwarf any potential proviral DNA. However, the "reverse-transcriptase inhibitor" AZT turns out not to be able to accomplish this task as advertised. Not only because it is an azide[1137], acting as a strong oxidizing agent to specifically inhibit the ETC function of the mitochondrial OXPHOS system and disrupt mitochondrial DNA synthesis but also because it is triphosphorylated in vivo

---

[1134] Karu, TI, (2008), "Mitochondrial signaling in mammalian cells activated by red and rear-IR radiation," *Photochem Photobiol;* 84: 1091-1099

[1135] Aon, MA, et al., (2003), "Synchronized whole cell oscillations in mitochondria metabolism triggered b a local release of reactive oxygen species in cardiac myocytes," *J Biol Chem;* 278: 44735-44744

[1136] International Human Genome Sequencing Consortium, (2001), "Human Genome," *Nature;* 409: 860-921

[1137] Umber, J., "Why did HAART improve the prognosis of AIDS?" http://aras.ab.ca/articles/HAART-Nukes-AIDS-Umber/ downloaded 11 April 2015

with less than 1 percent efficiency,[1138] making its touted ability to be a "DNA chain inhibitor" virtually impossible. As a result of the toxicity of this drug, patients develop multiple serious consequences: lipoatrophy, lactic acidosis, cardiomyopathy, myopathy, polyneuropathy, as well as neurotoxicity, cachexia, and death.[1139]

The specificity of "protease inhibitors" is another delusion. The concept claims that these inhibitors will be able to disrupt the viruses' ability to replicate and infect additional cells. Even by the standards set by AIDSworld, this has a low probability of happening considering the low number of what have been called "HIV" found in infected cells[1140] and especially since "HIV" is not, as the theory predicts, found in the cells that are, in fact, decreasing ("infected"), Th 1 CD4+T cells, but in the cells that are increasing (not infected), Th0 and Th2 cells.[1141] Do these protease inhibitors have some special homing device to target (have the right frequency) only the "correct" protease in the right cell? This is hardly the case. What protease inhibitors do, however, is aggravate an already-serious glutathione deficiency[1142] in many of these patients and push cells further into a type 2 counterregulation/type 2 cytokine profile expressed by the decrease in the ability of T helper cells to kill intercellular parasites or to undergo spontaneous apoptosis[1143,1144]—similar to the metabolic pattern found in many cancer cells with hyperpolarized mitochondrial membranes.[1145] At the foundation of this counterregulation is the depletion of GSH, the increase in a type 2 cytokine pattern, and a further feedback inhibition of the type 1 cells and their ability to upregulate iNOS to produce NO, not only as a source for RONS needed to combat the type of infections, which have come to define the AID syndrome, but as an energy activator for multiple biochemical reactions

---

[1138] Hazuda, D., Kuo, L., (1997), "Failure of AZT: a molecular perspective," *Nat Med;* 3(8): 836-837

[1139] Zhang, Y., et al., (2014), "Long-term exposure of mice to nucleoside analogues disrupts mitochondrial DNA maintenance in cortical neurons," *PLOSone;* 9(1): 1-7

[1140] Duesberg, P., (1987), "A Challenge to the AIDS establishment," *Bio Technol;* http://www.virusmyth.com/aids/hiv/pdbiotech87.htm downloaded 11 April 2015

[1141] Romagnani, S., et al., (1994), "Role of Th1/Th2 cytokines in HIV infection," *Immunol Rev;* 140: 73-92

[1142] Arend, C., et al., (2013) "The antiretroviral protease inhibitor ritonavir accelerates glutathione export from cultured primary astrocytes," *Neurochem Res;* 38(4): 732-741

[1143] Phenix, BN, et al., (2001), "Antiapoptotic mechanism of HIV protease inhibitors: preventing mitochondrial transmembrane potential loss," *Blood;* 98(4): 1078-1085

[1144] Peterson, JD, et al., (1998), "Glutathione levels in antigen presenting cells modulate Th1 versus Th2 response patterns," *PNAS USA;* 95: 3071-3076

[1145] Michelakis, ED., (2008), "A new era in medicine opens new windows and brings new challenges," *Circulation;* 117: 2431-2434

and as a specific signaling factor.[1146] Since mitochondria in most cells lack catalase,[1147,1148] they are therefore almost entirely dependent on GSH and its recycling enzymes.

Because type 2 cell dis-symbiosis is characterized by a feedback inhibition of iNOS, there is a significant decrease in the ability of NO and its congeners to participate in the constructive harmony of the cell—in its signaling capacity, in the part it plays in the maintenance of normal cellular structural patterns (amplitude-frequency patterns of electron excited states generation and their relaxation), and in its role vis-à-vis oxygen in determining respiratory rates and ATP production by glucose utilization via the OXPHOS system or enzymatically in the cytosol. However, mitochondria also produce nitric oxide by the activation of a Ca^{2+} sensitive mtNOS. This is particularly important as the NO produced by mtNOS regulates oxygen consumption and thus has the ability to create a localized intramitochondrial "pseudo-hypoxic" state by the displacement of O_2 at the level of cytochrome c. This is especially so if hypoxia is considered, at the level of the ETC, as an O_2 limited energy flux rather than low partial pressure.[1149]

Although the patients who receive these "protease inhibitors" have less risk of developing cachexia than those taking AZT, they have a greater risk of developing other life-altering conditions: insulin resistance and a lipodystrophy syndrome, both as the result of the processing of dysfunctional mitochondrial proteins.[1150] In any case, both NRTI (nucleoside reverse transcriptase inhibitors) and protease inhibitors attack the mitochondrial endosymbiont in such a way to further compromise, in AIDS and pre-AIDS patients, the already-stressed energetic functions of the OXPHOS system and to further unravel the evolutionary biological trend (disrupt the retrograde communication) of the hybrid nucleus and to push immune and nonimmune cells further into a state of disregulation by either type 1 or type 2 cell dis-symbiosis.

[1146] Voekov, V., (2001), "Reactive oxygen species, water, photons, and life," *Rivista Biolo/Bio Forum;* 94: 193-214

[1147] Martin, M, et al., (2000), "Melatonin but not vitamins C and E maintains glutathione homeostasis in t-butyl hydroperoxide induced mitochondrial oxidative stress," *FASEB J;* 12: 1677-1670

[1148] Bal, J., Cedebaum, AI., (2001), "Mitochondrial catalase and oxidative injury," *Biol signals Recept;* 10(3-4): 189-199

[1149] Connett, RJ., et al., (1985), Defining hypoxia: a system view of VO_2, glycolysis, energetic, and intracellular PO_2," *J Appl Physiol;* 1990 68(3): 833-842

[1150] Mukhopadhyay, A., et al., (2002), "In vitro evidence of inhibition of mitochondrial protease processing by HIV-1 protease inhibitors in yeast: a possible contribution to lipodystrophy syndrome," *Mitochondrion;* 1(6): 511-518

A Review: The Hydrogen Hypotheses in the Reversal of the Endosymbiotic Trend

In chapter 7, the hydrogen hypotheses was reviewed in which it was considered that the transformation of eubacterial hydrogen and gene-donating proteobacteria into the mitochondria led to an improved energy yield as a result of the host's energy-rich pyruvate being transferred into the bacterial symbionts for further oxidation. In essence, endosymbiosis was a syntrophic event in which the hydrogen product of the symbiont served as an essential nutrient for its Archaea partner. The flow of hydrogen, which originally was directed out of the symbiont to the Archaea, was now reversed to remain, during most of the cell cycle, with the symbiont, which allowed for an improved energy yield by using the electron transport chain and the hydrogen ion gradient across the inner mitochondrial membrane as an energetic differential to drive the production of ATP, with oxygen as the final electron receiver. It is still not well defined how close to instability this network normally operates, but it can thus be understood that disruptions to the mitochondrial membrane potential and the impaired import/export functions of the mitochondria in pathophysiological conditions reverses not only the flow of hydrogen ions but the oscillatory (electromagnetic frequencies) range that permits the cooperative trend of the endosymbiont.[1151] Mitochondrial membrane disruptions also alter the complex, nonbijective, nonlinear, and quasi-deterministic relationships of the gene(s)-to-protein(s) pathways. Molecular elements of cells do not obey the laws of deterministic physics and chemistry. Because biologists mistakenly considered the effect as the cause, genetic determinists have interpreted genetic disruptions to be a primary cause in initiating cancer changes.[1152] This failure of theory has caused, and continues to cause, substantial harm.

The concept of nonlinearity in cell systems is not a trivial matter. In clinical practice, this approach has to be considered in the initiation of any supportive replacement therapy. Because of the complexity of the cellular network, the same phenotype can be associated with a number of alternative sequences of cellular events.[1153] It is well established that AIDS and pre-AIDS patients have

---

[1151] Kremer, H., (2008), The silent revolution in cancer and AIDS medicine, pp 148-149
[1152] Baker, SG., (2014), "Recognizing paradigm instability in theories of carcinogenesis," *BJ Med Med Res; 4(5):* 1149-1163
[1153] Waliszewski, P., et al., (1998), "On the holistic approach in cellular and cancer biology: nonlinearity, complexity and quasi-determinism of the dynamic cellular network," *J Surg Oncol;* 68: 70-78

severe glutathione and sulfur deficits,[1154] but it also must be considered that selenium is a necessary cofactor in GSH metabolic enzymes (e.g., glutathione peroxidase). T cell proliferation, in response to antigenic stimulation in seleno-protein deficient T cells, is suppressed.[1155] Thus, the nonproliferative T cell response characteristic of AIDS patients may also have its origins in a pronounced selenium deficiency. To highlight this possibility, it has been noted that on the African continent, the highest levels of selenium-enriched soil are found in Senegal. This country was also found to have the lowest numbers of AIDS patients: prevalence at 1.77 percent in the general population and 0.5 percent in antenatal clinic attendees.[1156] Similar consideration must be given to folate and niacin deficiencies. It has also been demonstrated that it is melatonin rather than vitamins C and E that maintain glutathione homeostasis in induced mitochondrial stress.[1157] Melatonin acts as a more efficient scavenger of free radicals than GSH and vitamin E and maintains GSH balance in different models of excitotoxicity.[1158,1159] Melatonin also avoids the damage caused by bacterial LPS on liver and lung.[1160]

Whether analyzing the underlying issues in AIDS or other chronic diseases, these complex relationships of nested and networked metabolic cycles and cycle-limiting nutrients become clinically relevant and essential to understand in order to be able to replace deficits, which can reverse the disregulation of the cell symbiont. It is highly unlikely that this disregulation, which has been explained as a series of nutrient deficits, will be resolved solely by the intervention of pharmaceutical products. Much of what is called chronic disease is the physical manifestation of one or more deficiency states often aggravated by the intervention of inappropriate pharmaceuticals. Using a

---

[1154] Breitkreutz, R., et al., (2000), "Massive loss of sulfur in HIV infection," *AIDS Res Human Retrovir;* 16(3): 203-209

[1155] Shrimali, RK., et al., (2008), "Selenoproteins mediate T cell immunity through an antioxidant mechanism," *J Biol Chem;* 283: 20181-20185

[1156] Burcher, S., (2004), "Selenium conquers AIDS?" http://www.i-sis.org.uk/AidsandSelenium.php downloaded 16 March 2015

[1157] Martin, M, et al., (2000), "Melatonin but not vitamins C and E maintains glutathione homeostasis in t-butyl hydroperoxide-induced mitochondrial oxidative stress," *FASEB J.;* 12: 1677-1679

[1158] Reiter, RJ., (1995), "Oxidative processes and antioxidative defense mechanisms in the aging brain," *FASEB J.;* 9, 526-533

[1159] Melchiorri, D., et al., (1995), "Potent protective effect of melatonin on in vivo paraquat-induced oxidative damage in rats," *Life Sci;* 56 83-89

[1160] Crespo, E., et al., (1999), "Melatonin inhibits expression of the inducible NO synthase II in liver and lung and prevents endotoxemia in lipopolysaccharide-induced multiple organ dysfunction syndrome in rats," *FASEB J;* 13: 1537-1546

systems biochemistry approach, it is necessary to (a) determine the controls (the material aspects of the system) and (b) the regulation (the energetic aspects) that are able to integrate the system over a wide range of frequencies. The idea that there is always a single (generally pharmaceutical) solution to these complex bioenergetic, bioinformation problems is both immature and dangerous.

Genetic Defects Neither Necessary Nor Required for Cancer Transformation Aerobic Glycolysis Necessary for Metastasis

The medical orthodoxy is wedded to the notion that the transformation to cancer occurs as a result of structural defects of DNA sequences in the nucleus caused by any number of initiating agents: viral infections, DNA toxins, chance mutations, radiation, etc. However, there is considerable research that confirms that human cancer may develop without structural defects of mtDNA[1161,1162] or without structural defects in nuclear DNA.[1163,1164] Metabolic studies in a number of cancers have demonstrated that the loss of mitochondrial function preceded the appearance of malignancy and aerobic glycolysis.[1165] Furthermore, while numerous genetic abnormalities have been described in many human cancers, no specific mutation can reliably be used to diagnose any specific type of tumor.[1166,1167,1168] Further, no one has yet identified any consistent genetic changes that can reliably distinguish cancers that metastasize from cancers

---

[1161] Pedersen, PL., (1978), Tumor mitochondria and the bioenergetics of cancer cells," *Prog Exp Tumor Res;* 22: 190-274

[1162] Torroni, A., et al., (1990), "Neoplastic transformation is associated with coordinate induction of nuclear and cytoplasmic oxidative phosphorylation genes," *J Bio Chem;* 265: 20589-20593

[1163] Lijinsky, W., (1973), "Malignant tumours of liver and lung in rats fed aminopyrine or heptamethyleneimine together with nitrite," *Nature;* 244(5412): 176-178

[1164] Lijinsky, W., (2006), "A view of the relation between carcinogenesis and mutagenesis," *Supp: Env Mutagen Soc, 20th Anniversary Issue: Perspectives on Genetic Toxicology;* 14(S16) 78-84

[1165] Roskelley, RC. et al., (1943), "*Studies in cancer.vii. Enzyme deficiency in human and experimental cancer,*" J Clin Invest; 22(5):743-751

[1166] Loeb, LA., (2001), "A mutator phenotype in cancer," *Cancer Res;* 61: 3230-3239

[1167] Nowell, PC., (2002), "Tumor progression: a brief historical perspective," *Semin Cancer Biol;* 12: 261-266

[1168] Dang, L, et al., (2000), "Cancer associated IDH1 mutations produce 2-hydroxyglutarate," *Nature;* 462: 739-744

that have not metastasized, leading one group of researchers to hypothesize that there are no metastasis genes.[1169]

The work of several researchers[1170,1171] has shown that in the transplantation of a nucleus from one cell type to another cell type, the phenotype of a cell is determined by the cytoplasm so that the mutation is not necessary for abnormal cellular behavior, merely a cytoplasm with the wrong signals. Therefore, as has been stressed throughout this text, acquired disease states have their origin in energetic and metabolic aberrations that alter redox signals that inform DNA transcription and translation and change the expressed protein phenotype as each additional fluctuation of energy in this complex cellular system keeps the system further away from the original conformations of macromolecules. A critical number of such fluctuations can result in the rise of persistent structural defects.[1172] Ultimately, at a later phase, unbalanced biological stressors may not only be responsible for sending different activating signals but also damaging the genetic machinery.[1173,1174]

In multicellular organisms, homeostasis is maintained through the balance between cell proliferation and cell death. Cell death can occur by necrosis, which is a passive process characterized by the leaking of intercellular contents followed by inflammation and damage to the surrounding tissue. Apoptosis is an energy-supported, -regulated, and -controlled process that has characteristic alterations in Ca^{2+} metabolism and $\Delta\psi_m$. Apoptosis is also necessary for normal embryo development and regular exchange of worn cells for new ones[1175] and is considered a vital component of various processes including normal cell turnover, immune system development and function, hormone-dependent atrophy, and chemically induced cell death.[1176] Furthermore, apoptosis may play a bioenergetic role as noted in Ervin Bauer's basic process postulated

---

[1169] Vogelstein, B. et al., (2013), "Cancer genome landscapes," *Science;* 339(6127): 1546-1558

[1170] Gurdon, JB., (1968), "Transplanted nuclei and cell differentiation," *Sci Am;* 219: 24-35

[1171] De Robertis, EM, Gurdon, JB., (1977), "Quantitative studies on in vitro transformation by chemical carcinogens"; *PNAS, USA;* 74: 2470-2474

[1172] Waliszewski, P., Op. cit.

[1173] Barzilai, A., Yamamoto, KI., (2004), "DNA damage responses to oxidative stress," *DNA Repair (Amst);* (8-9): 1109-1115

[1174] Cooke, MS, et al., (2003), "Oxidative DNA damage: mechanism, mutation, and disease," *FASEB J;* 17(10): 1195-1214

[1175] HaanenC., Vermes, I., (1996), "Apoptosis: programmed cell death in fetal development," *Eur J Obstet Gynecol Reprod Bio;* 64: 129-133

[1176] Elmore, S., (2007), "Apoptosis: a review of programmed cell death," *Toxicol Pathol;* 35(4): 495-516

more than seventy years ago in which he theorized that the process of transfer of residual energy of a dying part of a living system to the viable one allows the living part to raise its bioenergetic potential, to rejuvenate itself, and to prolong the life cycle of the whole system.[1177,1178] Disregulation of the cell-death pathway (either over- or understimulation of the redox signaling pathways) is involved in the pathogenesis of an increasing number of diseases such as cancer, AIDS, autoimmune diseases, ischemic damage, and neurodegenerative disorders.[1179]

Cancer cells are heterogeneous in phenotypic features including glucose metabolism. In general, transformed cells use aerobic glycolysis as an energy source, but cells with reduced metabolic function may also use the amino acid glutamine or the monosaccharide galactose.[1180,1181]

Varying rates of OXPHOS have been demonstrated to contribute to energy production in cancers and may continue to play a major role in energy production in some.[1182,1183] However, it has been demonstrated that the migration of metastatic cells requires aerobic glycolysis as the energy source for biosynthesis.[1184] This particular metabolic characteristic—the use of aerobic glycolysis to produce up to 90 percent of the cell's ATP—is not unique to cancer cells but is a shared metabolic process with nonmalignant proliferating cells.[1185] What distinguishes cancer cells from normal proliferating cells is that they have lost the ability to respond to the signals that could exit them from the repetitive proliferative cycle. To balance out the low energy yield (~5 percent of the available energy in glucose)[1186] from the enzymatic oxidation of glucose, there is a massive nineteen- to thirty-eight-fold increase in glucose degradation up to

---

[1177] Bauer, E., (1935), "Theoretical biology" Moscow-Leningrad: VIEM Publishers, pp 140-144

[1178] Voeikov, VL, (1999), "The Scientific basis of the new biological paradigm" *21st Century Science & Technology;* 12: 18-33

[1179] Thompson, CB., (1995), "Apoptosis in the pathogenesis and treatment of diseases," *Science;* 267: 1456-1462

[1180] McKeehan, WL., (1982), "Gycolysis, glutaminolysis and cell proliferation," *Cell Bio International Rep;* 6(7): 635-650

[1181] Mazurek, S., et al., (1997), "The role of phosphometabolites in cell proliferation, energy metabolism, and tumor therapy," *J Bioenerg Biomembr;* 29(4): 315-330

[1182] Zu, XL, Guppy, M., (2004), "Cancer metabolism: facts, fantasy, and fiction," *Biochem Biophys Res Commun;* 313: 459-465

[1183] Dewhirst, MW., (2009), "Relationships between cycling hypoxia, HIF-1, angiogenesis and oxidative stress," *Radiat Res;* 172: 653-665

[1184] Mazurek, S., Ibid

[1185] Brand, K., (1997), "Aerobic glycolysis by proliferating cells: protection against oxidative stress at the expense of energy yield," *J Bioenerg Biomembr;* 29(4): 355-364

[1186] Mazurek, S. Op cit.

the pyruvate and lactate stage of the citric acid cycle.[1187,1188] It is of significant interest that there is also evidence that mitochondria, even in solid tumors, continue to retain full oxidative capacities and that aerobic glycolysis can often be reversed, sending pyruvate into the mitochondrial symbiont for further oxidation[1189,1190] (see section on dichloroacetic acid).

Mitochondrial biogenesis in the liver during development furthers the understanding of the dedifferentiation[1191] of cancer cells as the reversal of the chimeric cooperative trend of the eukaryotic nucleus and the endosymbiont mitochondrial biogenesis in the developing rat liver has strong correlations with mitochondrial behavior in liver hepatomas and provides evidence of the reversal of the chimeric cooperative trend of the eukaryotic nucleus and the mitochondrial symbiont under the decreasing availability of hydrogen ions. Indeed, the metabolic and enzymatic analogies that exist between the phenotype of cancer cells and embryonic tissues extend beyond the expression of protein isoforms of glycolytic enzymes. They share a similar trend in the expression of markers of both forms of energy production as well as the same mechanisms that control the biogenesis of mitochondria.[1192] Both are examples in which the upregulation of glycolytic genes and the downregulation of mitochondrial biogenesis coincide with cellular proliferation.

In liver cancer cells (and other cancer cells), there is both a cell proliferation and a reversal of the differentiation that also occurs in the fetal liver during development. In these transformed cells, the number and activity of the mitochondria declines significantly. Yet with this decline, there continues to be, just as in fetal liver cells, a simultaneous and paradoxical increase in the transcripts of RNA messages for the synthesis of the protein complexes of the respiratory chain without being converted to protein synthesis.[1193] It is as if there is a preparatory period and wait for the appropriate performance signals for the normal bioenergetic phenotype to be expressed. It could be called mitochondria in waiting.

[1187] Brand, K., (1997), Op cit.
[1188] Golshani-Hebroni, SG. Bessman SP, (1997), "Hexokinase binding to mitochondria: a basis for proliferative energy metabolism," *J Bioenerg Biomembr;* 29(4): 331-338
[1189] Vaupel, P., Mayer, A., (2012), "Availability, not respiratory capacity governs oxygen consumption of solid tumors," *Int J Biochem Cell Biol;* 44: 1477-1481
[1190] Faubert B., et al., (2013), "AMPK is a negative regulator of the Warburg effect and suppresses tumor growth in vivo," *Cell Metab;* 17: 113-124
[1191] Monk, M., Holding, C., (2001), "Human embryonic genes re-expressed in cancer cells," *Oncogene;* 20(56): 8085-8091
[1192] Cuezva, JM., et al., (1997), "Mitochondrial biogenesis in the liver during development and oncogenesis," *J Bioenerg Biomembr;* 29(4): 365-377
[1193] Cuezva, JM., et al., (1997), Op cit.

In the developing rat liver, corresponding to the evolutionary biological behavior of the mitochondrial symbiont and its relationship to the chimeric nucleus, the existence of two biological programs has been demonstrated. The development of this organ results in an increase in the number of mitochondria per cell (i.e., proliferation, increase in mass),[1194,1195] which is a long-term program controlled both at the transcriptional and posttranscriptional levels of gene expression.[1196] There is also an increase in the functional capability of the preexisting mitochondria (i.e., differentiation). However, this is a short-term program of biogenesis that is controlled at the posttranscriptional levels of gene expression and is responsible for the rapid changes in the bioenergetic phenotype (OXPHOS system) shortly after birth when the mitochondria are no longer "in waiting" and are rapidly conscripted into action.[1197] This process requires the coordination of both the nuclear and mitochondrial genomes, with each coding for different components of the organelle.[1198] The development of a well-defined communication network to coordinate information (energy) flows between the mitochondrial symbiont, and the chimeric nucleus has been evolutionarily conserved over billions of years.

During embryonic development, the liver meets most of its energetic needs by glycolysis as both the number of mitochondria per cell and their bioenergetic activity are low compared to the adult liver cell.[1199] The enzymes in the fetal liver are identical to the isoforms found in cancer cells (e.g., hexokinase II). While there is this increase in glycolytic isoforms in both the fetal liver and liver cancer cell, there is a concomitant decrease in the enzymes that allow for the oxidation of pyruvate and fatty acids, the substrates that are mainly used by the oxidative phosphorylation system in the neonatal and adult liver. Interestingly, as in the case of fetal cells, in cancer cells, there is also an increase in the synthesis of those enzymes and coenzymes associated with the ancestral informational portion of chimeric genomic elements that support cell division. These molecules are synthesized from components of glucose degradation via

---

[1194] Rohr, HP., et al. (1971), "Morphometric analysis of the rat liver cell in the perinatal period," *Lab Invest;* 24(2): 128-139

[1195] Hommes, FA, (1975), in "Normal and Pathological Development of Energy Metabolism," Hommes, FA., Van der Berg, CJ, eds., pp 1-7, Academic Press, London, UK

[1196] Cuezva, JM., et al., (1997), "Mitochondrial biogenesis in the liver during development and oncogenesis," *J Bioenerg Biomembr;* 29(4): 365-377

[1197] Cuezva, Ibid

[1198] Attardi, Giuseppe, (1988), "Biogenesis of mitochondria," *Ann Rev Cell Biol;* 4: 289-331

[1199] Cuezva, Op cit.

the pentose phosphate pathway.[1200] There is also evidence that in adult cells, NO acting, as a cellular mediator, promotes the formation of nitrosylated proteins and the depletion of glutathione followed by the formation of intracellular S-nitrosoglutathione as well as nitrosylation of the cytochrome c oxidase enzyme.[1201] Depletion of intracellular glutathione is then followed by a rapid and concomitant activation of the pentose phosphate pathway.[1202] This "hypoxia" is triggered at concentrations of O_2 that are well above those that are limiting for mitochondrial electron transport.[1203] This can be explained, in some measure, by the action of endogenous NO, which, by increasing the K_m[1204] of cytochrome oxidase for O_2, causes the cell to register hypoxia at higher concentrations of O_2 or, alternatively, as previously suggested, if hypoxia is defined as oxygen-limited energy flux rather than partial pressure, by the change in energy flux at the level of cytochrome c. In effect, the message, "hypoxia," creates a metabolic reaction dependent on both the initial metabolic state of the cell and the severity and duration of the hypoxic event.

Similar to fetal cells, in cancer cells, the transport of hydrogen ions for the mitochondrial OXPHOS system via the glycerol-3 phosphate and malate aspartate shuttles is decreased. In fetal cells, it is the enrichment in adenine nucleotides after birth that contributes to the maturation of the mitochondrial membrane potential. This allows the H+ leaks of the inner membrane of fetal mitochondria to experience a rapid reduction immediately after birth.[1205] In both fetal and cancer cells, there is a redox-dependent alteration in stimulated transcription factors. Promoters are switched on, which initiate the transcription of a particular gene and gene sequences that are sensitive in the adult cell to glucose, hypoxia, pseudohypoxia, insulin, and glucagon.

To underscore the significance of mitochondria/chimeric genome cross-talk, it is useful to compare metabolic patterns that repeat in different processes. The metabolic similarities in the use of the glycolytic pathway for

---

[1200] Petra, KC, Hay, N., (2014), "The Pentose phosphate pathway and cancer," *Trends Biochem Sci;* 39(8): 347-354

[1201] Sarti, P, Op cit.

[1202] Clancy, RM, et al., (1994), "Nitric oxide reacts with intracellular glutathione and activates the hexose monophosphate shunt in human neutrophils: evidence for S-nitrosoglutthione as a bioactive intermediary," *PNAS USA;* 91: 3680-3684

[1203] Jang, BH., et al., (1996), "Hypoxia inducible factor 1 levels vary exponentially over a physiologically relevant range of O_2 tension," *Am J Physiol;* 271: C1172-C1180

[1204] The Michaelis constant K_m is the substrate concentration at which the reaction rate is half of V_{max}, the max. rate at max concentration.

[1205] Valcarce, C., (1990), "Rapid postnatal developmental changes in the passive proton permeability of the inner membrane in rat liver mitochondria," *J Biochem;* 108: 642-645

The Slow Death of the AIDS/Cancer Paradigm and the Apocrypha of the Eukaryotic Cell

ATP production among several types of dividing cells have been noted by a significant number of research teams:[1206,1207,1208,1209,1210] (1) replicating cells in the late S phase of cell division,[1211] (2) regenerating cells during the wound healing process,[1212] (3) liver cells during fetal development,[1213] (4) and tumor cells with varying rates of reproduction.[1214] The differences in the activity states of these various cell types arise from certain metabolic changes particular to the cell: (1) the fetal cells and the cell symbionts before birth have not been regulated by the OXPHOS system, (2) the replicating cells in the late S-phase of cell division and cells in the early regeneration stage of wound healing have not been transiently regulated, and (3) the tumor cells are no longer regulated.[1215] However, the energetic switch from the OXPHOS (proteobacteria) system to the glycolytic (Archaea) system of ATP production is the global constant and common underlying metabolic process. It has been working for ~two billion years.

Thus, under metabolic stress conditions, when the balance between ROS generation and ROS scavenging is disturbed, the mitochondrial network can reach a threshold. On the one hand, the network can be overdriven by an increasing load of ROS leading to the $\Delta\psi_m$ depolarization and apoptosis. Conversely, it can be underdriven as the result of the inability to produce sufficient ROS to maintain the physiological state of required oscillatory frequencies, network interactions, and organizational tensegrity.[1216] This can lead to $\Delta\psi_m$ hyperpolarization (more negative) and the inability to undergo cell death. The former is type 1 overregulation of cell dis-symbiosis, which is

---

[1206] Brand, K., (1997), "Aerobic glycolysis by proliferating cells: protection against oxidative stress at the expense of energy yield," *J Bioenerg Biomembr;* 29(4): 355-364

[1207] Cuezva, Op cit.

[1208] Ostronoff, LK., et al., (1996), "Transient activation of mitochondrial translation regulates the expression of the mitochondrial genome during mammalian mitochondrial differentiation," *Biochem J;* 316: 183-191

[1209] Mazurek, S., et al., (1997), "The role of phosphometabolites in cell proliferation, energy metabolism and tumor therapy," *J Bioenerget Biomembr;* 29(4): 315-30

[1210] Capuano, F., et al., (1997), "Oxidative phosphorylation enzymes in normal and neoplastic cell growth," *J Bioenerg Biomembr;* 29(4):379-384

[1211] Brand, Op cit.

[1212] Capuano, Op cit.

[1213] Cuezva, 1997 Op cit

[1214] Cuezva, Ibid.

[1215] Kremer, H., 2008, "The Silent Revolution in Cancer and AIDS Medicine," Xlibris pp 224-225

[1216] Ingber, DE., (2003), "Tensegrity I. Cell structure and hierarchical systems biology," *J Cell Sci;* 116: 1157-1173

characterized by a cytokine shift to a type 1 profile.[1217,1218] The latter, a type 2 counterregulation of cell dis-symbiosis as seen in cancer, AIDS, and some chronic diseases[1219,1220] is generally characterized by an immune shift to a type 2 cytokine pattern. Both mechanisms are evolutionarily conserved. There is a balancing type 1 regulation (mitochondrial retrograde signaling under homeostatic cellular regulation), which is important for tissue development and homeostasis; however, type 1 overregulation involves an overwhelming increase in oxides leading to an accelerated cell-death pathway. Type 2 counterregulation functions as a cell survival arrangement under decreasing amounts of available energy supplies from the mitochondrial symbiont. This process involves an upregulation of the signals that promote the glycolytic oscillator[1221] as well as antiapoptotic proteins.

Before reviewing the characteristic patterns of type 1 overregulation and type 2 underregulation leading to cell dis-symbiosis, it is import to consider not only the biochemical nature of living tissue but its quantum aspects as well. A discussion of the quantum dynamics of living organisms is beyond the scope of this treatise but can be found elsewhere.[1222,1223,1224,1225,1226] However, it is the opinion of this author that the following list of characteristics play a crucial role in cell communication and homeostasis and cannot be discounted in any hypothesis of disease origin. They provide a context for events that are unexplainable by the scientific materialism of the molecular biology paradigm:

* One of the characteristics of biological tissues is the production of ultraweak photon emissions without any external excitations.

[1217] Santamaria, P.,(2000) "Cytokines and chemokines in autoimmune disease: an overview," *Landes Bioscience;* 1-18 downloaded 3.30.2015 http://www.ncbi.nlm.nih.gov/books/NBK6453/?report=reader

[1218] Lucey, DR., et al., (1996), "Type 1 and type 2 cytokine dysregulation in human infectious, neoplastic, and inflammatory diseases," *Clin Micro Rev;* 9(4): 532-562

[1219] Lucey, Ibid

[1220] Peterson, JD, et al., (1998), "Glutathione levels in antigen presenting cells modulate Th1 versus Th2 response patterns," *PNAS USA;* 95: 3071-3076

[1221] Hess, B., (1979), "The glycolytic oscillator," *J Exp Biol;* 81: 7-14

[1222] Ho, MW, (2008), The Rainbow and the Worm, The physics of organisms, World Scientific New Jersey

[1223] Integrative Biophysics-biophotonics, (2003) Ed. Popp, FA and Beloussov, L., Academic Publishers Boston

[1224] Electromagnetic Bio-Information, (1989) Ed. Popp, Warnke, Konig, Peschka, Urban & Schwarzenberg Baltimore

[1225] Pollack, GH, (2001), Cells, Gels and the Engines of Life, Ebner & Sons, Seattle, Wash.

[1226] Pollack, GH, (2013), The Fourth Phase of Water, Ebner & Sons, Seattle, Wash.

- These photon emissions are weak electromagnetic waves in the optical range (the UV-IR range) and are dependent on reactive oxygen and nitrogen species.
- This light emission is an expression of the functional state of the living organism and may be stored and used (as energy).
- Living systems may be able to amplify these weak signals in such a way that they trigger macroscopic events by coherent excitations in which atoms oscillate in phase.
- Biophoton emissions are able to penetrate the thickness of thousands of cells.
- Mitochondria are the primary source of RONS and thus biophoton emissions.
- Cytochrome c oxidase is considered a photoreceptor and photobiomodulator (other chromophores are porphyrin rings, flavinic, pyridinic rings, lipid chromophores, and aromatic amino acids and several others in the ETC).
- Photons of different wavelengths trigger certain biological functions.
- It follows that there is a correlation of photon intensity and conformational states of DNA.
- Photon emissions provide for a much higher chemical reaction rate than is possible in thermal equilibrium systems.
- Since most photon emissions arise from mitochondria, this then is a method for the retrograde communication network between the mitochondria and the chimeric nucleus and the chimeric nucleus and the mitochondria.
- In normal cells, biophotons are not dissipated in a random manner but are absorbed close to the place where they originated.
- Malignant cells show an exponential increase in light emissions with increasing cell density.
- The difference between normal cells and cancer cells may lie in their capacity for intercommunication, which in turn is dependent on their degree of coherence.
- The inability of the cancer system to reabsorb emitted energy coherently is consistent with the suggestion that tumor cells have a diminished capacity for intercommunication (the dis-symbiosis of the chimeric trend).

Type I Overregulation

In the introduction to this treatise, the observation was made that the eukaryotic cell, while having a dizzying array of interconnected cycles and pathways, has a limited number of global actions. Eukaryotic cells can do what they are programmed to do (i.e., perform the functions of the liver, kidney, heart, blood, etc.): (2) change their specialized function to a different but physiologically normal function (e.g., B cells to plasma cells) or (b) dedifferentiate. Dedifferentiation is generally not a "normal" function and has been described here as type 2 counterregulation. It is characterized by a reversal of the bioenergetic hybrid trend characterized by an alteration of the flow of hydrogen ions from the glycerol-3-phosphate and malate aspartate shuttles to the symbiont, thereby decreasing the availability of hydrogen ions required for the ETC while simultaneously increasing the reducing environment needed for the upregulation of various glycolytic enzymes. This leads to a decrease in the production of ATP by the OXPHOS system and a systemwide redirection of redox signals, which bind to specific DNA cognates in order to upregulate in the transcription and translation of glycolytic enzymes.

Cells can also enter into the mitotic cycle and proliferate. Although the mitotic cycle and proliferation are normal cell responses, without the compensation of the thiol pool and an ability to create an adequate supply of ROS, there is a deranged signaling of biochemical and physiological processes leading to a drop in the mitochondrial membrane potential. The type 2 counterregulated cells enter into a repetitive mitotic cycle. Those cells that do not easily divide may degenerate.[1227] Type 2 counterregulation with a type 2 cytokine profile is characteristic of the diseases, both infectious and neoplastic (KS and lymphomas) that defined the AID syndrome.[1228] These were also the diseases commonly seen in immunosuppressed transplant patients, some surgical patients, drug addicts and patients who suffer from food insufficiency and chronic infections. Finally, cells can also die by the process of either necrosis or apoptosis. Although cell death by apoptosis is a part of the normal process of regeneration and growth in the organism, abnormal rates of cell death by either necrosis or apoptosis have characteristic energetic patterns, which here have been defined as type 1 overregulation.[1229]

[1227] Ward, MW., et al., (2007), "Mitochondrial and Plasma Membrane Potential of Cultured Cerebellar Neurons during Glutamate-Induced Necrosis, Apoptosis, and Tolerance," *J Neuro Sci;* 27(31): 8238-8249

[1228] Lucey, Op cit.

[1229] Igney FH, Krammer PH., (2002), "Death and anti-death: tumour resistance to apoptosis," *Nat Rev;*2:277–88.

Multiple stimuli utilize Ca^{2+} as a second messenger to transmit signals. Mitochondria contribute to the tight spatiotemporal control of this process by accumulating Ca^{2+} and shaping the return of cytosolic calcium to resting levels.[1230] There appears to be a multifactor cross-communication among Ca^{2+}, $\Delta\Psi_m$ and ROS. Biological stressors that uncouple respiration and oxidative phosphorylation can cause an increase in concentrations of cytosolic-free Ca^{2+}. A sustained three- to eightfold increase in steady-state $[Ca^{2+}]_m$ as part of retrograde signaling leads to activation of calcineurin, which then activates NF-κβ (proinflammatory) and other signaling pathways.[1231] In type 1 overregulation, under an acute load of oxidative stressors and the breakdown of the thiol pool and other antioxidant systems, Ca^{2+} is released from mitochondria followed by Ca^{2+} re-uptake (Ca^{2+} cycling).

If the Ca^{2+} release pathway is excessive, it may lead to a loss of $\Delta\psi_m$, opening of the permeability transition pore (PTP)[1232], leakiness of the inner mitochondrial membrane, matrix swelling, and unfolding of the inner membrane followed by release of apoptogenic proteins, inhibition of mitochondrial ATP synthesis, and cell death.[1233] During apoptosis, the $\Delta\psi_m$, which sustains mitochondrial ATP production, decreases. The maintenance of the $\Delta\psi_m$ is one of the mechanisms that prevents apoptosis.[1234]

As the result of an acute overload of biological stressors, both necrosis and apoptosis are triggered by decompensated disregulation of cell symbiosis. Apoptosis is a controlled event involving the action of hydrolytic enzymes, chromatin condensation, and vesicle formation (often mistaken for viral-like particles[1235]) and continues to have a high energy demand and may require active mitochondria.[1236] Under the stimulation of increased calcium cycling, cytochrome c is released into the cytoplasm and acts with cytosolic factors to induce nuclear apoptosis.[1237] NO and its derivatives are key elements

---

[1230] Rasola, A., Bernardi, P, "Mitochondrial permeability transition in Ca2+-dependent apoptosis and necrosis," *Cell Calcium;* 50(3): 222-233
[1231] Karu, TI., (2008), Op cit
[1232] Rasola, A., Bernardi, P, Ibid
[1233] Richter, C., Kass, GEN., (1991), "Oxidative stress in mitochondria: its relationship to cellular Ca^{2+} homeostasis, cell death, proliferation, and differentiation," *Chem-Biol Interact;* 77-1-23
[1234] Richter, C., (1998), "Nitric Oxide and its congeners in mitochondria: implications for apoptosis," *Environ Health Perspec;* 106(5): 1125- 1130
[1235] http://rethinkingaids.com/quotes/test-em.html downloaded 3.29.2015
[1236] Ankarcrona, M., et al., (1995), "Glutamate-induced neuronal death: a succession of necrosis or apoptosis depending on mitochondrial function," *Neuron;* 15: 961-973
[1237] Liu, X., et al., (1996), "Induction of apoptotic program in cell free extracts: requirement for dATP and cytochrome c," Cell; 86: 145-157

in this process. NO binds to cytochrome oxidase and reversibly inhibits respiration[1238,1239] in competition with oxygen. Higher concentrations of NO and its derivatives (peroxynitrite, nitrogen dioxide, or nitrosothiols) can cause irreversible inhibition of the respiratory chain, uncoupling permeability transition, and/or cell death.[1240] The extent and duration of the deenergization of the mitochondrial membrane are determined by the concentration of NO and its congeners as well as the availability of glutathione, protein thiols, and intracellular oxygen tensions or available oxygen energy flux.[1241,1242]

Of note, cytochrome c oxidase is considered as the photoacceptor in photobiomodulation.[1243,1244] It shares control over ATP synthesis with several other components of the OXPHOS system. Even under increasing metabolic demand, cytochrome c rarely has more than 20 percent of the total control over ATP synthesis.[1245] This means that NO mediated changes in oxygen consumption can occur without significant effects on ATP synthesis rate. This property of oxidative phosphorylation has important implications for mitochondrial ROS production and redox signaling because the inhibitor of cytochrome c oxidase, NO, not only affects O_2 consumption but also affects the redox status of the respiratory chain and thus superoxide generation. Therefore, it is possible that a low level of NO can regulate mitochondrial ROS generation without affecting ATP synthesis.[1246]

[1238] Brown, GC, et al., (1995), "Nitric oxide produced y activated astrocytes rapidly and reversibly inhibits cellular respiration," *Neurosci Lett;* 193: 102-204

[1239] Brown, GC., (2001), "Regulation of mitochondrial respiration by nitric oxide inhibition of cytochrome c oxidase," *Biochimica Biophysica Acta(BBA) Bioenerg;* 1504(1): 46-57

[1240] Brown, Ibid

[1241] Richter, C., Op cit.

[1242] Connett, Op cit.

[1243] Karu, T., (1999), "Primary and secondary mechanisms of action of visible-to-near IR radiation on cells," *J Photochem Photobiol;* 49: 1-17

[1244] Wong-Riley, MT., et al., (2005), "Photomodulation directly benefits primary neutrons funcionally inactivated by toxins: Role of cytochrome *c* oxidase," *J Biol Chem;* 280, 4761-4771

[1245] Brookes, PS., et al., (2002), "Mitochondria: regulators of signal transduction by reactive oxygen and nitrogen species," *Free Radic Biol Med;* 33: 755-764

[1246] Brookes, Ibid

Type II Counterregulation: Dedifferentiation and the Warburg Phenomenon

The hypothesis being set forward here is that cellular processes under long-term stress conditions that have been confounded by the century-old focus on the mechanics of genes and proteins are, in fact, operating not only as the result of the evolutionary heritage of the eukaryotic cell but also as the inherent self-ordering aspects of biological systems in a manner that is characteristic of the history of that metabolic evolution. All eukaryotic cells, including those in humans, are the result of the ancient marriage of two ancestral bacteria: the Archaea and the proteobacteria. In the central nucleus, the informational genes are mainly of archaeal origin and the operational genes are primarily of proteobacterial origin.[1247,1248,1249,1250] Initially, the hydrogen transfer from the proteobacteria (hydrogenosomes before the development of the ETC) to the Archaea was used by the Archaea as an improved energy gain for the glycolytic enzymatic production of ATP of which the reduction product was lactate. The genes for the production of glycolytic enzymes are evolutionarily conserved[1251] and, as they were established under strictly anaerobic conditions, perhaps as a consequence, continue to have a requirement for a reducing environment.[1252,1253,1254] In addition to the glycolytic pathway, the glutaminolysis pathway is evolutionarily[1255] conserved but transferred to the TCA cycle to feed into the ETC of the mitochondrial endosymbiont. The oxidation product is glutamate. Thus, a characteristic of type 2 counterregulated cells is the presence of elevated serum levels of lactate and glutamate as the result of

---

[1247] Rivera, MC., et al., "Genomic evidence for two functionally distinct gene classes," *PNAS USA;* 95: 6239-6244

[1248] Cotton, JA., McInerney, JO., (2010), "Eukaryotic genes of archaebacterial origin are more important than the more numerous eubacterial genes, irrespective of function," *PNAS;* 107(4): 17252-17255

[1249] Lopez-Garcia, P., Moreira, D., (1999), "On hydrogen transfer and a chimeric origin of eukaryotes," *Trends Biochem Sci;* 24(11): 424

[1250] Alverez Ponce, D., McInerney, JO., (2011), "The human genome retains relics of its prokaryotic ancestry: human genes of archaebacterial and eubacterial origin exhibit remarkable differences," *Genome Bio Evol; doi:* 10.1093/gbe/evr073: 1-24

[1251] Webster, KA, (2003), "Evolution of the coordinate regulation of glycolytic enzymes genes by hypoxia," *J Experimen Bio;* 206: 2911-2922

[1252] Segerer, A., et al., (1985), "Two contrary modes of chemolithotrophy in the same archaebacterium," *Nature;* 313: 787-789

[1253] Webster, Op cit.

[1254] Brand, Op cit.,

[1255] Lockless, SW., Ranganathan, R., (1999), "Evolutionarily conserved pathways of energetic connectivity in protein families," *Science;* 286: 295-299

decreased energy production by the mitochondrial symbiont and increased cytosolic enzymatic energy production. Both conditions are not uncommon in patients diagnosed with AIDS (and cancer) and, because of a fundamental lack of the understanding of evolutionary and quantum biology, are often worsened by antiretroviral therapeutic intervention.[1256,1257,1258,1259]

The switch in energy production from the OXPHOS system to the glycolytic system is also evolutionarily conserved in the chimeric nucleus. Exposure to oxygen tensions outside of a relatively narrow physiological range activates metabolic switches that turn off mitochondrial electron transport and activate anaerobic glycolysis.[1260] The archaebacterial informational genes use the glycolytic enzymatic pathway while the operational processes, dominated by the proteobacterial portions of the chimeric genome, are more likely to use the OXPHOS system of the endosymbiont.[1261,1262] An interesting feature of the switching from OXPHOS to glycolysis is that the same conditions that regulate energy metabolism also regulate bioenergetic genes so that the enzyme activity and transcription are regulated simultaneously but with different time courses and signaling pathways.[1263] The primary stimulation for the upregulation of glycolytic enzymes is the hydrogen ion diffusion through the mitochondrial membrane.[1264,1265] Again, it must be emphasized that because the fundamental features of genetics, including DNA synthesis, transcription, and translation and their regulation were established on Earth under strictly anaerobic conditions, it follows that these genes, even though they are incorporated into the chimeric genome, continue to require a reducing environment in order to function.[1266] This is not a mystery. These ancient genes are simply doing what

---

[1256] Falco, V., et al., (2002), "Severe Nucleoside-Associated Lactic Acidosis in Human Immunodeficiency Virus–Infected Patients: Report of 12 Cases and Review of the Literature," *Clin Inf Dis;* 34(6): 838-846

[1257] Lonergan, JT., (2000), "Hyperlactatemia and hepatic abnormalities in 10 human immunodeficiency virus-infected patients receiving nucleoside analogue combination regimens," *Clin Infect Dis*; 31(1): 152-166

[1258] Gurwitz, D., Kloog, Y., (1997), "Elevated Cerebrospinal Fluid Glutamate in Patients With HIV-related Dementia," *JAMA;* 277(24) 1931

[1259] Droge, W., et al., (1987), "Elevated plasma glutamate levels in colorectal carcinoma patients and in patients with acquired immunodeficiency syndrome (AIDS)," *Immunobio;* 174(4-5): 473-479

[1260] Webster, Op cit.

[1261] Brand, Op cit.,

[1262] Alvarez-Ponce, D. Op cit.

[1263] Webster, Op cit.

[1264] Kremer, Op cit., 224-226

[1265] Brand, Op cit.

[1266] Segerer, Op cit.

they have always done for billions of years--responding to the cues that drove their evolution.

As a result of the decreased production of ROS and the resultant decrease in the energy of electronic excitation (electromagnetic field) as well as a decrease in water (and microtubule) ordering,[1267] the dynamic functionality of the cell is altered. Cytologically, the cells appear "dedifferentiated." Because normal living cells are self-organizing, self-regulating, self-replicating, catalytic, nonlinear, complex, and thermodynamic, operating on the principle of complementarity with a number of the interconnected variables,[1268] the idea that we can continue to use the principles of deterministic physics and chemistry to resolve knowable abnormalities in these complex arrangements is simply a pipe dream. Dedifferentiation has been shown to be a reversible characteristic under mitochondrial control mechanisms.[1269,1270,1271]

Unlike type 1 overregulated cells, type 2 counterregulated cells, under the influence of long-term chronic stressors, become resistant to apoptosis as a result of hyperpolarization of the mitochondrial membrane. Because of the decrease in available hydrogen ions from the cytosolic shuttles to the symbiont, the energy deficit is compensated by an increase energy production by means of aerobic glycolysis and shift of the glycolytic degradation products into the pentose phosphate pathway.[1272] The cells appear to become dedifferentiated and are unable, as when retrograde signaling was optimally functioning, to spontaneously switch out of the division cycle. Hallmarks of this process are elevated levels of nitrosylated thiol proteins and nitrosated nonprotein thiols, which lead to a feedback decrease in the production of nitrogen oxides, superoxides, and peroxides.

[1267] Pokorny, J., et al., (2012), "Mitochondrial metabolism—neglected link of cancer transformation and treatment," *Prague Med Report*; 113(2): 81-94

[1268] Waliszewski, P, et al., (1998), "On the holistic approach in cellular and cancer biology: nonlinearity, complexity, and quasi-determinism of the dynamic cellular network," *J Surg Onc;* 68: 70-78

[1269] Sun, RC., et al., "Reversal of the glycolytic phenotype by dichloroacetate inhibits metastatic breast cancer cell growth in vitro and in vivo," *Breast Cancer Res Treat;* 120(1): 253-260

[1270] Zhu, YG., et al., (2004), "Curcumin protects mitochondria from oxidative damage and attenuates apoptosis in cortical neurons," *Acta Pharmacol Sin;* 25(12): 1606-1612

[1271] Bonnet, S., et al., (2007), "A mitochondria-K+ channel axis is suppressed in cancer and its normalization promotes apoptosis and inhibits cancer growth," *Cancer Cell;* 11(1): 37-51

[1272] Seyfried, TN, Shelton, LM., (2010), "Cancer as a metabolic disease," *Nutrition Metabol;* 7(7): 1-22

Bcl-2 belongs to a family of proteins that have key regulatory roles in the mitochondrial death pathway involved in the opening and closing of the PTP.[1273] By this method, it regulates cell death by either inducing or inhibiting apoptosis. It is mainly localized to the endoplasmic reticulum, nucleus, and outer membrane of the mitochondria.[1274] Bcl-2 has the unique ability to block apoptosis, which is triggered by multiple cytotoxic agents,[1275] by the sequestration of proapoptotic proteins such as Bax and Bak, thereby blocking PT. The latter two are responsible for the formation of oligomers on the mitochondrial outer membrane, altering the integrity of this membrane and the release of cytochrome c to the cytosol.[1276] Bcl-2 is overexpressed in various cancers and has antiapoptotic functions under the regulation of RONS. Nitric oxide–mediated S-nitrosylation of Bcl-2 prevents its ubiquitination[1277] and subsequent proteasomal degradation, leading to an inhibition of apoptosis.[1278]

Another contributor to this cell-death pathway is the p53 protein, which acts as a sensor for oxidative stress and rapidly translocates from the cytoplasm to the mitochondrial surface where it can directly interact with both the anti- and proapoptotic Bcl-2 family members to inhibit or activate their respective functions. In this way, p53 promotes or inhibits mitochondrial outer membrane permeability.[1279] Nitrosative modification of p53 is a major determinant of p53 subcellular location.[1280]

[1273] Richter, Op cit.
[1274] Chen, ZX, Pervaiz, S., (2008), "BCL-2: pro-or anti oxidant?," *Fron Biosci (Elite Ed.)*; 1: 263-286
[1275] Korsmeyer SJ., (1992), "Bcl-2 initiates a new category of oncogenes: regulators of cell death," *Blood*; 80: 879-886
[1276] Zong, WX., et al., (2001), "BH3 only proteins that bind pro-survival Bcl-2 family members fail to induce apoptosis in the absence of Bax and Bak," *Genes Dev*; 15: 1481-1486
[1277] Ubiquitination (also known as ubiquitylation) is an enzymatic, post-translational modification (PTM) process in which a ubiquitin protein is attached to a substrate protein. http://en.wikipedia.org/wiki/Ubiquitin#Ubiquitination downloaded 6 April 2015
[1278] Azad, N., et al., (2010), "Role of oxidative/nitroative stress mediated Bcl-2 regulation in apoptosis and malignant transformation," *Ann NY Acad Sci*; 1203(1-6): doi: 10.1111/j.1749-6632.2010.05608.x
[1279] Vaseva, AV., et al., (2012), "p53 opens the mitochondrial permeability transition pore to trigger necrosis"; *Cell*; 149: 1536-1548
[1280] Hernlund, E., et al., (2009), "Cisplatin-induced nitrosylation of p53 prevents its mitochondrial translocation," *Free Radic Biol Med*; 46(12): 1607-1613

The Slow Death of the AIDS/Cancer Paradigm and the Apocrypha of the Eukaryotic Cell

Although it has been observed in multiple studies[1281,1282,1283,1284,1285] that low-level induction of intracellular ROS inhibits apoptosis in tumor cells in different systems, none of these studies have considered either (1) the energetic role played by the sustained levels of ROS cycling of electron flows or (2) that in cells that are actively dividing, the loss of a certain required energetic level supplied by ROS will lead to the regression in these cells to a state of proto-cell symbiosis that exhibits characteristics that occurred before the development of the respiratory chain. The evolutionary biological solution after the symbiotic event was the uncoupling of the genomic sections of the nucleus and mitochondria during cell division with lowered levels of ROS and the consequent energy of electronic excitation, which becomes permanently fixed, at the expense of mitochondrial activity, during cell transformation to cancer.[1286] The factor that must be considered in this evolutionary biologically programmed switch in the bioenergetic and metabolic network is the role played by the thiol pool deficit and thus its inability to fulfill its function in counteracting levels of NO that can cause the nitrosylation of vital enzymes and signal proteins at the post-translational stage.[1287]

The biphasic characteristics of the chimeric nucleus have functioned for two billion years. During the cell division phase, the cooperative trend of the chimeric nucleus operates near the margins of instability. This is why multiple medications, whether "antiviral" or "anticancer," which in effect inhibit the ability of the mitochondria to function optimally by creating a "pseudohypoxic" environment, reactivate these evolutionarily conserved biological programs. The survival of metastatic cells is not random. Metastatic cells are produced by specialized subpopulations that preexist in the heterogeneous primary tumor, but they differ energetically. Nonmetastatic cells, in response to type I cytokine or LPS stimulation, are still able to produce high levels of iNOS activity and NO

[1281] Clement, MV., et al, (2003), "Decrease in intracellular superoxide sensitizes Bcl-2 overexpressing tumor cells to receptor and drug induced apoptosis independent of the mitochondria," *Cell Death Differ;* 10:1273-1285

[1282] Suh, YA., et al., (1999), "Cell transformation by the superoxide generating oxidase Mox 1," *Nature;* 401: 79-82

[1283] Clement, MV., Pervaiz, S., (1999) "Reactive oxygen intermediates regulate cellular response to apoptotic stimuli: an hypothesis," *Free Radic Res;* 30: 247-252

[1284] Mannick, JB., et al., (1997), "Nitric oxide inhibits Fas induced apoptosis," *J Biol Chem;* 272: 24125-24128

[1285] Hockenbery, DM, et al., (1993), "Bcl-2 functions in an antioxidant pathway to prevent apoptosis," *Cell;* 75: 245-251

[1286] Kremer, op cit.

[1287] Stamler, JS., (1995), "S-nitrosothiols and the bioregulatory actions of nitrogen oxides through reactions with thiol groups," *Curr Top Microbiol Immunol;* 196" 19-36

production whereas metastatic cells do not. This is consistent with the finding of increased nitrosylation of thiol proteins in tumor cells and the consequent feedback inhibition for inducible NO production in these cells. It has been demonstrated that one of the congeners of NO, peroxynitrite, contributes to apoptosis by the deenergization of the mitochondria and inducing Ca^{2+} cycling.[1288] However, in cancer cells, the decreased production of oxides leads to a hyperpolarization of the mitochondrial membrane potential, a closing of the PT channels, as well as a decrease in Ca^{2+} cycling. This leads to an inhibition of apoptosis as well as a decrease in the biogenesis and proliferation of the mitochondrial symbiont. The hybrid cooperative trend of the nucleus begins to reverse with a decrease in the flow of hydrogen ions from the glycerol-3-phosphate and malate aspartate shuttles to the mitochondria. As a result of the decrease in hydrogen ions available to the ETC process, there is a concomitant decrease in mitochondrial ATP production and a surplus of hydrogen ions diffusing into the cytoplasm, increasing the possibility of the anaerobic conditions and a reducing environment that drives the archaeal portion of the chimeric genome.

Given these conditions, it may be expected that certain biological activities, pathways, and regulatory processes such as glycolysis, which functions preferentially under hypoxia and was established as the first energy generator before being integrated into the oxidative pathway, will be expressed. The suppression of oxidative metabolism under conditions of severe hypoxia reduces oxidative stress, decreases antioxidant levels, and stimulates the primordial reducing environment, even without molecular antioxidants.[1289] According to several studies,[1290,1291,1292] at least eight out of twelve functionally distinct glycolytic enzyme genes are coordinately induced by hypoxia in mammalian cells, the regulation of which involves contributions from at least four separate pathways, some of which have been conserved through four billion years of evolution, dating back to the origin of life. It is thus not unexpected that in many highly malignant rapidly growing tumor cells, type 2 hexokinase is highly

---

[1288] Richter, Op cit.
[1289] Webster, KA., et al., (2001), "Oxidation of zinc finger transcription factors: physiological consequences," *Antiox Redox Signal;* 3: 535-548
[1290] Webster, KA., (1987), "Regulation of glycolytic enzyme RNA transcriptional rates by oxygen availability in skeletal muscle cells," *Mol Cell Biochem;* 77: 19-28
[1291] Webster, KA., et al., (1988), "Regulation of tissue specific glycolytic isozyme genes: coordinate regulation by oxygen availability in skeletal muscle cells," *Can J Zool;* 66: 1046-1058
[1292] Webster, KA., et al., (1990), "Coordinate reciprocal trends in glycolytic and mitochondrial transcript accumulations during the in vitro differentiation of human myoblasts," *J Cell Physiol;* 142: 566-576

expressed.[1293,1294] In liver cancer cells, this isoenzyme has an approximately one-hundred-fold higher affinity for glucose than the glucokinase found in normal liver cells; and when it binds to the outer mitochondrial membrane, there is a reduced sensitivity of this enzyme to feedback inhibition by the product glucose-6-phosphate,[1295] which is an important regulatory property in normal cells.

The role of oxidative and nitrosative stressors in both the maintenance and dissolution of the cooperation of the chimeric nucleus and the mitochondria offers a way out of the retroviral trap and provides for the explanation of the cancers and infectious diseases found in AIDS patients. The outbreak of KS, lymphomas, and opportunistic diseases in noncontiguous clusters of a subset of promiscuous homosexual men who at a particular time in history engaged in a particular set of sexual activities combined with the use of inhaled nitrite gas as well as a plethora of legal and illegal drugs was a metabolic time bomb waiting to explode. By 1985, animal experiments had already demonstrated the tumor-producing effects of the interactions of antibiotics and nitrites.[1296]

It was also discovered early in the AIDS crisis that both HIV positive and AIDS patients presented with alarmingly low levels of cysteine and glutathione.[1297,1298,1299] These patients were found to have an immune shift from the cell-mediated system (Th1) to the humoral system (Th2) as demonstrated by the decrease in circulating CD4+T cells with a simultaneous increase in antibody production, an anergic DTH skin response, and an in vitro failure of response of immune cells to cytokine stimulation. When it was demonstrated

---

[1293] Kikuchi, Y., et al., (1972), "Hexokinase isozyme patterns of human uterine tumors," *Cancer;* 30(2): 444-447

[1294] Thelen, AP., Wilson, JE., (1991), "Complete amino acid sequence of the type II isozyme of rat hexokinase, deduced from the cloned cDNA: comparison with a hexokinase from novikoff ascites tumor," *Arch Biochem Biophys;* 286(2): 645-651

[1295] Bustamante, E., Pedersen, PL., (1977), "High aerobic glycolysis of rat hepatoma cells in culture: role of mitochondrial hexxokinase," *PNAS USA;* 74(9): 3735-3739

[1296] Brambilla, G., (1985). "Genotoxic effects of drug/nitrite interaction products: evidence for the need of risk assessment," *Pharmacol Res Commun;* 17(4): 307321

[1297] Herzenberg, LA., et al., (1997), "Glutathione deficiency is associated with impaired survival in HIV disease," *PNAS USA;* 94: 1967-1972

[1298] Droge, W. et al., (1997), "Role of cysteine and glutathione in HIV infection and cancer cachexia. Therapeutic intervention with N-acety-cysteine (NAC)," *Adv Pharmacol;* 38: 581-600

[1299] Kalebic, T., et al., (1991), "Suppression of human immunodeficiency virus expression in chronically infected monocytic cells by glutathione, glutathione ester, and N-acetylcysteine," *PNAS USA;* 88: 986-990

that it was glutathione levels in antigen-presenting cells and not "HIV" that modulated Th1 versus the Th2 response patterns,[1300] it was noted by AIDSworld but nevertheless did not alter their continuing psychopathic push for more cysteine/glutathione-depleting and mitochondrial toxic pharmaceuticals. The reason it was psychopathic was evident by the production and distribution of second- and third-generation drugs that came to market after the AZT[1301,1302,1303] fiasco was underscored by the Concorde studies.[1304] The Concorde studies demonstrated that the drug AZT neither prolonged life nor staved off the symptoms of AIDS in people who are HIV positive but without symptoms of the syndrome. After the AZT fiasco, the drug companies knowingly[1305] began to add acetal, thioacetal, and aldehyde moieties to their chemical compounds.[1306,1307] This had the benefit of reducing the oxidative stress load of these "antiretrovirals" without acknowledging the real underlying cause of AID: the cysteine/glutathione deficits. The addition of reducing elements to these toxic drugs improved the scorched-body policy of AZT but did not replace sufficiently the antioxidant levels needed to alter the prognosis in many of these patients. Some patients appear to improve, but it is not from killing any "HIV" but from a partial supply of reducing equivalents malevolently added to these poisons. The continued use of these drugs and the genuine lack of adequate replacement therapy have led to numerous "AIDS" deaths that have nothing to do the list of AIDS-defining diseases as a result of the complications of the drugs themselves.

[1300] Peterson, JD., et al. (1998), "Glutathione levels in antigen-presenting cells modulate Th1 versus Th2 response patterns," *PNAS USA;* 95: 3071-3076

[1301] Cretton, E.M., et al., (1991), "Catabolism of 3'-azido-3'-deoxythymidine in hepatocytes and liver microsomes, with evidence of formation of 3'-amino-3'-deoxythymidine, a highly toxic catabolite for human bone marrow cells," *Mol Pharmacol;* 39(2): 258-266

[1302] Eagling, VA., et al., (1994), "The metabolism of zidovudine by human liver microsomes in vitro: formation of 3'-amino-3'-deoxythymidine," *Biochem Pharmacol;* 48(2): 267-276

[1303] Reardon, JE., et al., (1994), "Reduction of 3'-Azido-3'-deoxythymidine (AZT) and AZT nucleotides by thiols," *J Biolol Chem;* 269(23): 15999-16008

[1304] http://www.nytimes.com/1993/04/02/world/new-study-questions-use-of-azt-in-early-treatment-of-aids-virus.html

[1305] Tocher, JH, Edwards, DL., "The interaction of nitroaromatic drugs with aminothiols," *Biochem Pharmacol;* 50(9): 1367-1371

[1306] de Muys, JM, et al., (1999), "Anti human immunodeficiency virus type 1 A activity, intracellular metabolism and pharmacokinetic evaluation of 2'deoxy 3'Oxa 4" Thiocytidine," *Antimicrobi Agents Chemother;* pp. 1835-1844

[1307] Why did HAART improve the prognosis of AIDS? http://aras.ab.ca/articles/HAART-Nukes-AIDS-Umber/ downloaded 6 April 2015

The Slow Death of the AIDS/Cancer Paradigm and the Apocrypha of the Eukaryotic Cell

What the Concorde studies underscored was that many patients who presented with stage 3 thiol deficiency and were already type 2 counterregulated were metabolically devastated by exposure to AZT and had no hope of recovery from this medieval torture. The type 2 cytokine profile can also increase the expression of the cyclooxigenase 2 enzyme (COX 2) and transforming growth factor (TGF-β). COX-2 can induce an increase in the production of prostaglandin E2 (PGE-2) from arachidonic acid.[1308] TGF-β and PEG-2 further suppress the synthesis of iNOS and activate the arginase pathway. Arginase transforms L-arginine into ornithine and polyamines.[1309] The decreasing availability of L-arginine contributes to the diminished production of NO (via iNOS) and peroxynitrite. This aggravates an already type 2 counterregulation by contributing to the closing of the mitochondrial PT and a consequent increased expression of heat shock proteins, Bcl-2 proteins, transformed p53 proteins, ferritin protein, and the enzyme heme oxygenase.[1310,1311] Heme oxygenase can increase the formation of carbon monoxide, which, like NO, can block the enzyme cytochrome c oxidase.[1312] Under the influence of CO, increased polyamines are formed, which activate the repair process and increase the cell division cycle.[1313,1314,1315] The ornithine decarboxylase reaction and polyamine synthesis are important for ATP synthesis via the induction of glycolytic enzymes.[1316] Fundamentally, hundreds if not thousands of patients were killed by the drug AZT.

[1308] Minghetti, L, Levi, G., (1997), "Microglia as effector cells in brain damage and repair: focus on prostanoids and nitric oxide," *Prog Neurobiol;* 54: 99-125

[1309] Kropf, P., et al., (2005), "Arginase and polyamine systhesis are key factors in the regulation of experimental leishmaniasis in vivo," *FASEB J;* 10.1096/fj.04-3416fje

[1310] Lincoln, Op cit.

[1311] Kremer, Op cit.

[1312] Alonso, JR., et al., (2003), "Carbon monoxide specifically inhibits cytochrome c oxidase of human mitochondrial respiratory chain," *Pharmacol Toxicol;* 93(3): 142-146

[1313] Tabor, W, Tabor H., (1984), "Polyamines," *Annu Rev Biochem;* 53: 749-790

[1314] Theiss, C., et al., (2002), "Regulation by polyamines of ornithine decarbosylase activity and cell division in the unicellular green alga chlamydomonas reinhardtii," *Plant Physiol;* 128(4): 1470-1479

[1315] Marton, LJ, Pegg, AE., (1995), "Polyamines as targets for therapeutic intervention," *Annu Rev Pharmacol Toxicol;* 35: 55-91

[1316] Brand, K., (1987), "Role of ornithine decarboxylase on glycolytic enzyme induction during thymocyte proliferation," *J Bio Chem;* 31(5): 15232-15235

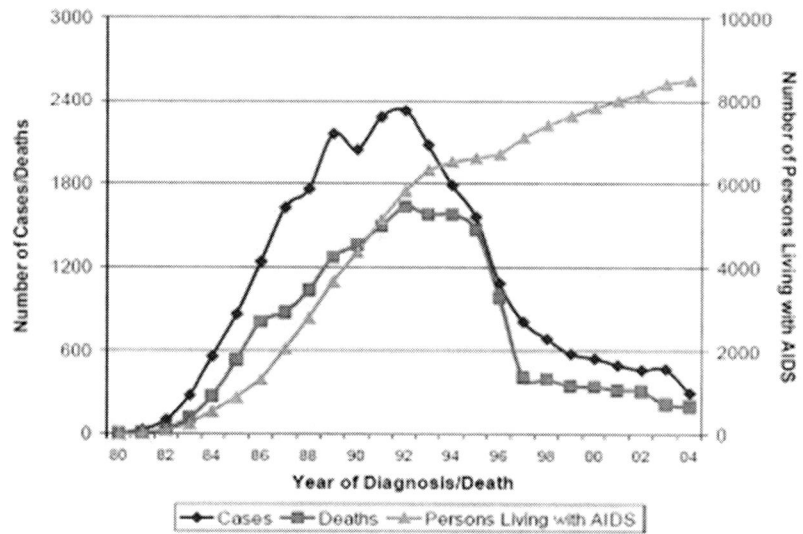

Figure 1.1 AIDS cases, deaths, and prevalence, San Francisco, 1980-2004

The definition of AIDS was modified in 1993 to include people who were HIV positive, had a low CD4+T cell count below two hundred cells/microliter, but were otherwise asymptomatic. Prior to 1993, one of the "AIDS-defining diseases" was required to make the diagnosis. However, the above graph clearly demonstrates that deaths from AEDS began to decline rapidly in 1992-3, and there was an even steeper decline in 1995-6. It should be noted that the incline of the curves coincided with AIDSworld therapeutic intervention: AZT, trimethoprim/sulfamethoxazole, and various antifungals. The decline in deaths occurred with (1) the decline of the use of poppers, (2) the introduction of the second- and third-generation "antiretrovirals" with the noted altered chemical structures, and (3) the widespread use of "HIV antibody" testing, which acted as an AIDSworld dragnet in which frightened people who were never at risk for developing a thiol deficiency syndrome were told they had "HIV disease" and were begun on medicine they never needed.

AIDSworld has been constructed on a tissue of fabrications and fantasies, and like any war, it has been profitable for the few and destructive for the many. The central chimeric nucleus and the mitochondrial symbiont have been functioning in ever more complex and sophisticated ways for two billion years. The cooperation is not fundamentally based on genes or proteins but the bioenergetic/quantum cooperation of these ancient bacteria. What has been called AIDS is actually an acquired energy deficiency disease and can only be understood in that context. In the last century, with the rise of the industrial/war economy, the products and waste products of the society have been unhinging the cooperative trend of this bioenergetic union and pushing cells further into a type 2 counterregulation survival mode. By understanding the metabolic/energetic patterns that drove the symbiotic event, the patterns that unhinge the cooperation are knowable, understandable, and clinically treatable not with more drugs that may push the cell further away from the possibility of a homeostatic balance but by replacement of the deficits and allowing of the "quantum jazz" of the cell to find its own rhythm.

CHAPTER 11

Therapeutic Considerations

Life on Earth emerged from a sea of natural rhythms and an atmosphere of vibratory frequencies that have throughout the evolutionary process been integrated into basic biological responses,[1317] such that living systems are capable of amplifying weak signals including single photons that have the ability to trigger macroscopic events.[1318,1319] Although science has long recognized the physiological correlates of the rhythms of the heartbeat, breath, and brain waves, as well as various diurnal cycles, seasonal and lunar patterns, study of the rhythmic patterns at the subcellular level have only recently gained widespread attention. One of the hypotheses of this text is that there are characteristic nonrandom thermodynamic patterns of subcellular oscillations that are not the consequence but are, in fact, the cause of the underlying basis for intracellular, extracellular, and tissuewide communication networks that establish the innate homeostatic patterns characteristic of the cell or tissue type.[1320] Importantly, all these vital processes occur in an aqueous environment interlaced with numerous polarized filaments that are an intrinsic component of the cells

---

[1317] Persinger, M.A., (2014), "Schumann Resonance frequencies found within quantitative electroencephalographic activity: implications for earth-brain interactions," *Int Letters Chem, Physics, Astorn;* 11(1): 24-32

[1318] Kashimori, Y, et al., (1998), "Effect of syncytium structure of receptor systems on stochastic resonance induced by chaotic potential fluctuation," *Biophys J;* 75: 1700-1711

[1319] Zhang, Dongmei; Györgyi, László; Peltier, William R. (1993). "Deterministic chaos in the Belousov–Zhabotinsky reaction: Experiments and simulations"; 3 (4): 723–745

[1320] Muehsam D. Ventura, C., (2014), "Life rhythm as a symphony of oscillatory patterns: electromagnetic energy and sound vibration modulates gene expression for biological signaling and healing," *Glob Adv Health Med;* 3(2): 40-55

structural reservoir of conserved energy.[1321] The thermodynamic patterns that arise from the fundamental characteristics of oxygen, light, and water are self-organizing, nonlinear, complex, and periodic.

The failure to critically analyze the entirety of the components that contribute to cellular energy processes out of the narrow range of ATP synthesis and function and the morass of genetic sequences and proteins has been a serious oversight. Disease conditions arise as a result of the disruptions in these nonequilibrium frequency/amplitude states. While current biology has chosen to all but ignore water and electromagnetic fields, this has led to the current crisis in modern medicine and the disaster in current AIDS therapy[1322,1323] from AZT to 3TC.

Ca^{2+} waves generating oscillatory Ca^{2+} signals are another type of important wave patterns that can occur repetitively from pacemaker sites from which they may entrain the entire cell.[1324] Other subtle energies that emerge from the cell are the electromagnetic frequencies that result from reactive oxygen species that arise both in the cell and the extracellular matrix.[1325] These processes also spontaneously acquire oscillatory characteristics and act as pacemakers for dependent biochemical reactions.[1326] The oscillatory energies are stored in the space-time structure of the cell to be used for the performance of work.[1327] Because every cell is embedded in a network of interconnected oscillatory

---

[1321] Cifra, M, (2009), "Study of electromagnetic oscillations of yeast cells in kHz and GHz region" *Doctoral Thesis,* Czech Technical Univ., Prague

[1322] mitochondrial DNA toxicity, proximal renal tubular dysfunction, hypersensitivity reactions, multiple metabolic disorders, anemia, leukopenia, skin hyperpigmentation, gastro-intestinal intolerance, mouth ulcers, CNS toxicity (drowsiness, dizziness, confusion, altered dream states, peri-orbital parathesiae, taste perversion, renal calculi and crystaluria, hyperbilirubinemia, alopecia, diarrhea, rash, osteoporosis, progressive weight loss, fatigue, elevated serum lactate, elevated anion gap, myopathy myalgia, muscle wasting, weakness, fatigue, elevated CPK, cardiomyopathy, pain, parasthesias, sensory loss, areflexia, hepatomegaly, elevated liver enzymes, lactic acidosis, pancreatitis, elevated serum amylase, lipoatorphy

[1323]

[1324] Nivala, M, et al., (2013), "The emergence of subcellular pacemaker sites for calcium waves and oscillations," *J Physiol;* 591(Pt 21): 5305-5320

[1325] Covarrubias, L., et al., (2008), "Function of reactive oxygen species during animal development: passive or active?," *Developmental Bio;* 320(1): 1-11

[1326] Voeikov, V., (2001), "Reactive Oxygen Species, Water, Photons and Life," *Rivista de Biologia/ Bio Forum;* 94: 193-214

[1327] Van Wijk, R., (2003," "Cellular and molecular aspects of integrative biophysics" in *Integrative Biophysics Biophotonics* eds. Fritz-Albert Popp and Lev Beloussov, Kluwer Academic Publishers, Boston

patterns that have widespread synchronization with resonating rhythms that allow long-range communication and a high degree of organization into functional groupings that become tissues and organs, and that aberrant cellular oscillatory patterning is associated with severe disease, the goal of any therapeutic intervention is to provide the cell with those things that may be deficient, allowing it to reestablish its own innate biorhythms. While allopathic remedies can be useful under a limited range of conditions, there is generally little need for the extreme force and cell terrorism of many allopathic nostrums. This is especially true of the antiretroviral drugs developed as a thriving industry. There is a considerable body of scientific literature that has addressed the numerous vitamin and nutrient deficiencies commonly found in immunodeficiency states that are consistently overlooked by the emphasis on the promotion of ARTs.[1328,1329,1330,1331]

In our attempts to understand the nature of many disease states, a fit beginning is an examination of the syntrophic nature of the endosymbiotic event that led to the evolution and complexity of the eukaryotic cell. Because the eukaryotic cell is a combination of two organisms that evolved primarily in an anaerobic/reducing environment, many of the basic metabolic processes were developed under these conditions including DNA synthesis, transcription, translation, and their regulation, as well as the glycolytic pathway for energy production.[1332] Once the oxygen crisis occurred and the consequence was a steep thermodynamic gradient of an oxygen environment, there was a need to develop a new set of survival skills. This change in atmospheric conditions allowed for the syntrophic endosymbiotic event, stimulated by the oxygen catastrophe that drove the evolution of the eukaryotic cell and the development of greater and greater multicellular complexity. As such, aerobic metabolism must underlie complex functions at all levels of biological organization. The price for this high-energy nonequilibrium state has to be paid for with an excess of reducing equivalents. With the decreasing availability of reducing equivalents, the ancient part of the genome becomes the guiding force for cell survival.

[1328] Beach, RS, Laura, PF., (1983), "Nutrition and the acquired immunodeficiency syndrome" *Ann Int Med;* 99(4): 565-6

[1329] Gray, RH, (1983), "Similarities between AIDS and PCM," *Am J Pub Health;* 73(11): 1332

[1330] Coodley, GO., (1990), "Nutritional deficiency and AIDS," *Ann In Med;* 113: 809

[1331] Chandra, R.K., (2008), "Interactions of nutrition, infection and immune response," *ACTA Ped;* 68(2): 137-144

[1332] Webster, KA., (2003), "Evolution of the coordinate regulation of glycolytic enzyme genes by hypoxia," *J Exp Bio;* 206: 2911-2922

The Slow Death of the AIDS/Cancer Paradigm
and the Apocrypha of the Eukaryotic Cell

This work has proposed that the etiology of the complex disease patterns that are called AIDS and cancer (as well as others) are characterized by a depressed aerobic capacity punctuated by a reversal of the chimeric trend of the hybrid nucleus and its energetic relationship to the mitochondrial endosymbiont—an evolutionary predictable reversal of the endosymbiotic trend because of an acquired proton deficit. Indeed, large-scale clinical investigations have shown that dysfunctional oxygen and energy metabolism have been found in essentially all complex diseases.[1333] Thus, this pattern is not unique for AIDS and cancer, and these observations can be applied more generally.

Therefore, any evaluation of the patients who have been told that they are "HIV positive" or have AIDS is to assess the level of ROS damage, the thiol status, and any immune imbalance. The therapeutic goal will be to support the ability of the cellular/tissue networks to restore and optimize intrinsic energy functions and to be able to restore intra- and extracellular communication, first at the biomolecular level. This will allow a reordering of the intrinsic oscillatory patterns. An important molecule in the renewal of these rhythms will be nitric oxide release from its state of suppression. The restoration of the flow of this gas plays a key role in the rapid regulation of the microenvironment, inflammatory processes, cell growth, and repair.[1334] The modulation of NO signaling is one manner in which cells and tissues are able to mount a rapid response to changes in environment conditions. Of course, this can only be accomplished in the context of providing sufficient glutathione and relevant antioxidant defenses to maintain sufficient energy production to sustain the necessary redox balance required for complex homeostatic adjustments—the keyword being balance as it is the intracellular redox balance that links various interacting and interlocking cycles of metabolic networks of enzymes, coenzymes, and genetic expression of protein control elements.

These concepts, while not totally eliminating the potential usefulness of allopathic nostrums, call into question the absolute reliance on this mode of therapy for homeostatic restoration. This is not what these drugs are designed to do, and so it is simply an impossibility.

Aside from treating any issue that may be immediately life threatening, the strategy for therapeutic intervention is to evaluate the level of ROS damage,

---

[1333] Myers, J, et al., (2002), "Exercise capacity and mortality among men referred for exercise testing," *NEJM;* 346(11): 793-801
[1334] Seegers, JC., et al., (2001), "Activation of signal transduction mechanisms may underlie the therapeutic effects of an applied electric field," *Med Hypothesis;* 2: 224-230

glutathione/cysteine levels, and degree of immune cell disbalance. The goals of therapeutic intervention are:

1. Restoration of the psycho/spiritual balance toward self-empowerment.
2. Systemic detoxification and hydration.
3. Restoration of cellular homeostatic balance in multiple organ systems. (lung, liver, kidney, immune, hormonal, nervous, muscular and gastrointestinal with special emphasis on the liver and GI systems from mouth to anus).
4. While addressing any acute or life-threatening situations.

The approach has to be systemic and holistic. Thus, a single point of entry by an antibiotic such as Bactrim or Septra into the integrated metabolic cell cycles will generally not be sufficient and may aggravate the overall deficiency state if, as has often been the case in the administration of these double folate inhibitors (in addition to any ART), the patient may already have an underlying folate, niacin, melatonin, and/or selenium deficiency in addition to the glutathione/cysteine problem. In Western countries, physicians often assume that patients have sufficient dietary intake such that these nutrient deficiencies can be discounted. This is a grave error, especially in this era of multiple environmental toxins including EM radiation and GMO foods coupled with nutritionally questionably food choices. Following FDA guidelines would be pure folly. The objective is to provide the cells/tissues with those nutrients that will allow for the reenergization and reintegration of the cooperative trend of the chimeric nucleus and the mitochondrial symbiont. The diagnostic difficulty will be to overcome the internal bias of the patient away from the belief that he/she has a terminal illness that can be sexually transmitted.

Every patient who has been deemed HIV positive will have a different constellation of presenting symptoms depending on ethnicity, pregnancy status, country of origin, drug intake, other infectious diseases (e.g., tuberculosis), nutritional status, and/or anal sexual habits. These are the risk factors not for contracting a virus but for testing HIV positive. I want to emphasize ethnicity especially as it relates to people of African descent. People of African origin have been targeted from the slave era to this current time by the medical complex and most recently by AIDSworld for particular economic and political reasons. The HIV test, which is an antibody test, is a dragnet for African people as genetically they exhibit a heightened antibody response to any given stimulus. Because the HIV test is simply a snapshot of antibody levels at any given time and because all positives are false positives, the likelihood of a black person testing positive is significantly increased. Also, pregnancy and other infectious diseases raise the risk of a heightened antibody response. Recommending that these tests be run on pregnant women is simply criminal negligence and should be regarded and treated as such. Because of the numerous issues of fraudulent science that have been documented in this text, all the recommended AIDS industry tests must be considered as false positives. This means that it is clearly incumbent on the treating physician to establish by way of history (and those lab tests to be considered below) whether or not the patient is indeed currently expressing or is at risk of developing a thiol deficiency and a concomitant problem with cell-mediated immunity. Under the theory of cellular dis-symbiosis, the thiol deficiency state has the following three identifiable stages:[1335]

1. The clinically mute phase: reserve capacity of cell respiration at a critical threshold
2. The clinically compensated phase: type 1 and type 2 cytokine disregulation, Th1 to Th2 cytokine switch, type 1 overregulation of cell dis-symbiosis, and or type 2 counterregulation of cell dis-symbiosis, which is the point of a possible HIV test reaction
3. The clinically manifest phase: Opportunistic diseases, Kaposi's sarcoma, lymphoma, myopathies, encephalopathies, wasting syndrome, etc.

From early in the AIDS crisis, in the context of the immune system, the problem defined itself not as an immune deficiency but a heightened antibody response with a concomitant diminishment in the functioning of cellular immunity. Thus, it is important to establish the level of functioning of the cell-mediated immune (CMI) system, which is not done with an HIV antibody test or viral Load but with:

1. DTH skin testing, which can generally be successfully evaluated with three antigens;[1336]

[1335] Kremer, H., (2008) The Silent Revolution in Cancer and AIS Medicine, Xlibris Corp
[1336] Siripassorn, K., et al., (2006), "Three suitable antigens for delayed-type hypersensitivity skin testing in a tropical country like Thailand," *Asian Pac J Allergy Immunol;* 24(2-3): 143-152

2. Evaluation of the lymphocyte response to mitogenic stimulation (PHA, pokeweed, etc.);[1337,1338]
3. Evaluation of any lymphopenia not in isolation but in the context of immune imbalance expressed as an increase in antibody levels
4. An evaluation of any cytokine switch to a predominant type 2 profile (IL-4, IL-5, IL-6, IL-10)[1339] by use of multiplex cytokine assay[1340] or others.[1341]

Because AEDS is a systemic problem, it is also essential to evaluate the antioxidant system as well as the GSH/GSSH ratio for assessing the level of oxidative stress. The overall antioxidant status can be tested with a serum ORAC (oxygen radical absorbance capacity) assay.[1342] Glutathione levels can be measured in RBCs. The GSH/GSSH ratio can used as another measure of overall oxidative stress and can be used to assess therapeutic effectiveness in maintaining cellular redox potential.[1343]

Since what is being evaluated is neither an infectious nor a contagious disease but a complex metabolic disorder, which may have a number of underlying deficiency issues, this must be communicated to the patient in a concise way to overcome the thirty years of biased propaganda stating otherwise. Clearly, the eradication of any organisms that may be of immediate concern, such as pulmonary infections, intestinal parasites, or candida, while simultaneously intervening to establish a rebalancing of those systems known to be disrupted—lung, liver, kidney, immune cells, nervous system, musculature,

---

[1337] Dupont B, Good RA: Lymphocyte transformation in vitro in patients with immunodeficiency diseases: use in diagnosis, histocompatibility testing and monitoring treatment. Birth Defects Orig Artic Ser 1975;11:477-485

[1338] Stone KD, Feldman HA, Huisman C, et al (2009) "Analysis of in vitro lymphocyte proliferation as a screening tool for cellular immunodeficiency," Clin Immunol;131:41-49

[1339] Committee on Military Nutrition Research, IOM, Methodological Issues in Assessment of Human Immune Function from "Military strategies for sustainment of nutrition and immune function in the field," ISBN: 0-309-55696-1, 722 pages

[1340] Bozza, FA., et al., (2007), "Cytokine profiles as markers of disease severity in sepsis: a multiplex analysis," Crit Care; 11(2): R49

[1341] Olsen, I., Ludvig, M.S., (2013), "Pitffalls in determining the cytokine profile of human T cells," J Immuno Methods; 30: 106-112

[1342] Cao, G. Prior, RL., (1998), "Comparison of different analytical methods for assessing total antioxidant capacity of human serum," *Clinical Chem;* 44(6): 1309-1315

[1343] Serru, V., et al., (2001), "Quantification of reduced and oxidized glutathione in whole blood samples by capillary electrophoresis," *Clinical Chem;* 47(7): 1321-1324

and hormonal system, with special emphasis on the liver and gastrointestinal system from mouth to anus—is the overall strategy to employ.

In the context of evaluating the evolutionary biology of eukaryotic complexity, what has classically been called AIDS here has been redefined as AEDS, an acquired energy deficiency syndrome. This syndrome is the result of a concentrated exposure to alarmingly high levels of certain abiotic and biotic oxidative/nitrosative stressors (as well as dietary deficiencies) and is characterized by a breakdown in the processes involved in cellular energy maximization and thus altered mitochondrial metabolism. The hallmark of the syndrome is a sulfur-deficiency state, specifically the tripeptide glutathione (γ-L-Glutamyl-L-cysteinyl-glycine), which has proven essential for the reduction of the elevated oxidative stressloads and the restoration of homeostatic balance.

While in this particular group of patients it has manifested both as a disbalance in the immune system and by malignant transformation of vascular epithelium and lymphocytes, other consequences that involve the gastrointestinal tract, central nervous system, skeletal muscles, and liver clearly indicate that it has to be considered as a systemic problem that involves rebalancing the glutathione/nitric oxide relationship in multiple cell systems, the cortisol/DHEA-S ratio,[1344,1345] the arginase/nitric oxide synthase ratios in the liver, as well as the cytokine profiles that have balance shifted to a predominant type 2 pattern.[1346,1347]

The health of gut metabolism should not be undervalued in these patients because (1) a large portion of the immune systems resides in this organ system and (2) because the intestinal barrier may have been breached, allowing for the sustaining of a systemic inflammatory response. These problems could arise from multiple factors including poor nutrition, antibiotic use, toxins, poorly digested food particles, local trauma, overgrowth of candida and/or parasites, or alteration of gut flora.[1348,1349] A healthy and functioning intestinal mucosa is

---

[1344] Grillon, C., et al., (2006), "Cortisol and DHEA-S are associated with startle potentiation during aversive conditioning in humans," *Psychopharm;* 186(3): 434-441

[1345] Christeff, N., et al., (1999), "Correlation between increased cortisol:DHEA ratio in malnutrition in HIV positive men," *Nutrition;* 15(7-8): 534-539

[1346] Lucey, DR., et al., (1996), "Type 1 and Type 2 cytokine dysregulation in human infectious, neoplastic, and inflammatory diseases," *Clin Microbiol Rev;* 9(4): 532-562

[1347] Volker, H., et al., (1996), "Abnormal glutathione and sulfate levels after interleukin 6 treatment and in tumor-induced cachexia," *FASB J;* 10: 1219-1226

[1348] Farhadi, A., et al., (2003), "Intestinal barrier: an interface between health and disease," *J Gastroenter Hepatol;* 18: 479-497

[1349] Brenchley JM, Douek DC. (2008) The mucosal barrier and immune activation in HIV pathogenesis. Curr Opin HIV AIDS.;3(3):356-361.

the body's first line of defense against bacteria, inflammatory mediators, and endotoxins. Failure of the gut mucosa can allow both foreign substances and gut bacteria to pass through the system where they can produce both local and remote ongoing inflammation, including organ failure and even death.[1350,1351] Evaluation of leaky gut is done with a zonulin or lactose test or alternatively an IgG food intolerance test.[1352,1353]

In evaluating these patients, it is crucial to keep in mind that what is being dealt with are three specific problems: (1) thiol deficiency, (2) balance shift in the immune system, and (3) fear. Because the organized bureaucracies who are exceedingly well funded and have been able to mount a thirty-year propaganda war against the science of health and healing, this last issue is not minor and can contribute to the long-term stress (and sustained cortisol output) that may be an impediment to health restoration.

Most of the patients that will be encountered will have been told at some point that they have a positive HIV antibody test or elevated viral load. From the previous chapters, the evidence has been substantiated that the tests being currently profitably marketed by AIDSworld give the clinician little practical information with which to assess the present and future metabolic resistance of any patient, especially neither the present nor future status of cell-mediated immunity. After all, it must be stressed that completely submerged in the hyperbole of AIDSpeak is the crux of the pathology of these condition: the status of the CMI. This is the fundamental problem and will continue to be so until physicians can tear themselves away from the pacifiers of meaningless numerical trivia: antibody tests, total CD4+T cell counts, and viral loads. Surely, after thirty years, someone must have spotted the absurdity of using a "diagnostic antibody test," which even the manufacturers assert in the package inserts that these tests cannot be used to diagnose and which are in essence no more than an indirect measure of the humoral immune response. So the question is, how stupid do you have to be to continue for thirty years to use a test that is an indirect measure of the humoral function of the immune system

---

[1350] Swank GM, Deitch EA.(1996) "Role of the gut in multiple organ failure: bacterial translocation and permeability changes" *World J Surg.*;20:411-417.

[1351] Doig CJ, Sutherland LR, Sandham JD, et al. (1998) Increased intestinal permeability is associated with the development of multiple organ dysfunction syndrome in critically ill ICU patients. Am J Respir Crit Care Med.;158(2):444-451.

[1352] Intestinal Permeability Assessment: https://www.gdx.net/core/one-page-test-descriptions/Intestinal-Permeability-Test-Description.pdf downloaded 21 Dec. 2015

[1353] IgG Food Allergy Test: http://www.greatplainslaboratory.com/home/eng/food_allergy_igg.asp downloaded 21 Dec. 2015

The Slow Death of the AIDS/Cancer Paradigm
and the Apocrypha of the Eukaryotic Cell

in patients who by definition of the syndrome have an underlying problem of cell-mediated immunity?

The fundamental question that must be asked and answered is, does this patient have or is this patient at risk of developing a thiol deficiency (or other nutrient deficiencies) and an oxidative stress load that is significant enough to cause long-term disruptions in the metabolic network leading to an energy deficiency?

The most important part of identifying whether or not a particular individual is demonstrating any of the characteristics of thiol deficiency and severe oxidative stress and whether this person is at any stage or no stage at presentation will be to take a thorough health/social/work history that includes drug[1354] intake and sexual habits, including history and frequency anal sex, including such practices as rimming or fisting, as well as levels of exposure to environmental toxins (especially drug intake), antibiotics, psychic stress, vaccines, physical exercise, etc. On the African continent, many patients who have parasitic infections, malaria, vitamin deficiencies and/or tuberculosis, or are simply pregnant have been told that they have AIDS. These problems must be identified and treated appropriately without reference to "AIDS" drugs, especially in pregnant women. In the early years of the crisis, Western patients were known to have had long term exposures to:

1. Nitrate inhalation
2. Uncontrolled antibiotic consumption
3. Analgesics
4. Recreational Drugs
5. Chronic antigen stress as a result of multiple and or recurrent infections (and multiple sexual partners)
6. Allo-antigenic stress via resorption of foreign proteins
7. Gastrointestinal disturbances, including "leaky gut" and
8. Nutritional deficiencies

[1354] I have reviewed charts of numerous HIV+ patients where there was no notation of drug intake including crack cocaine which can mimic many the same symptoms and currently used "diagnostic" lab tests. Physicians also often ignore the side affects and deleterious interactions of multiple drug therapy as well as the role of certain vaccines in contributing to an "HIV+" status

Patients in less developed countries are likely to have a different set of underlying problems

1. Nutritional deficiencies
2. Tuberculosis
3. Parasitic infections
4. Exposure to environmental toxins
5. Poor sanitation
6. Lack of clean water source
7. Pregnancy

After consideration of thiol level and other antioxidant/nutrient levels, it is important to establish a baseline immune status. This is not done by any of the currently marketed HIV antibody or PCR viral load tests or total CD4+T cell count but by assessing whether there has been an immune balance shift from Th1 to Th2. This is done simply by the aforementioned methods to evaluate the status of CMI.

Other tests that may be useful in the evaluation of the activation status of the immune system in this group of patients may include, but not limited to: serology for toxoplasma, herpes I and II, CMV, rubella, mononucleosis, hepatitis A, B, and C as well as rheumatoid factor, antistreptolisins, ESR, C-reactive protein, beta-2-microglobulin, Coombs test, agglutinins, immune complexes, etc.[1355,1356]

Antibiotics use either short or long term in certain individuals can cause a persistent alteration of the normal gut flora,[1357] a condition known as dysbiosis, which alters the defense capabilities of the protective layers of the intestinal lumen and that may result in a consequent leaky gut (see the above discussion). This can be compounded by chronic stress and toxins. The leaky gut then allows foreign proteins and microbes to enter the system, which as foreign antigens can create inflammatory complexes and contribute to ongoing chronic inflammation. The object here is to remove those foods/toxins that may be damaging, repair with specific supplements (glutamine, digestive enzymes,

---

[1355] , (2002), Manual of Clinical Labortory Immunology Ed. Rose, NR, Hamilton, RG, Detrick, B., Washington, D.C., 1322 pp.

[1356] Detrick, B., Hamilton, R.G., Folds, J.D., (2006), "Manual of molecular and clinical laboratory immunology" Am. Soc. for Microbiology, 7th revised edition

[1357] Jernberg, C., et al., (2010), "Long term impacts of antibiotic exposure on the human intestinal microbiota," *Microbiol;* 156: 4216-3223

aloe vera juice, quercetin, ginkgo biloba extract, etc.)[1358] and rebalance with probiotics. This pathology may take months to resolve.

If the patient has been on one of the "antiretroviral" medications, this therapy and its provocation of mitochondrial toxicity must be accounted for. Continuance of these medications (which has been recommended by AIDSworld as a lifetime habit) is counterproductive, but withdrawal of any chronically used drug must be done cautiously while simultaneously balancing the deficits in the antioxidant, immune, nervous, and hormonal systems. Once weaned from ARVs, it is metabolically counterproductive to continue this therapy if there is any hope of obtaining homeostatic balance. Repeated exposure to foreign antigens via intravenous drug use or frequent changes of anal sex partners or other environmental contaminants must be documented (and counseled against) as well as a thorough history of allergies and nutritional intake including gluten intolerance and alcohol consumption. Inhalant drugs, especially both poppers and crack cocaine can mimic, "AIDS" symptoms of pneumonia and low CD4+T cell counts. Alcohol abuse, long-term use of NSAIDs, and exposure to multiple vaccines[1359] can impair glutathione levels and also must be taken into account.

The compendium of AIDS-defining diseases[1360,1361] found on the CDC website include fungal infections, various other viral infections, lymphomas, several types of pneumonia and mycobacterium, as well as Kaposi's sarcoma, are all expressed as a consequence of various inflammatory reactions leading to a switch in the immune profile from a balanced Th1/Th2 to a type 2 predominance.[1362] It has been demonstrated in any number of laboratories that Th-cell function assessed by proliferation or IL-2 production in response to recall antigens was deficient, even in asymptomatic HIV positive

---

[1358] Resnick, C., (2010), "Nutritional protocol for the treatment of intestinal permeability defects and related conditions," *Nat Med J*; 2(3) http://www.naturalmedicinejournal.com/journal/2010-03/nutritional-protocol-treatment-intestinal-permeability-defects-and-related downloaded 14 Dec. 2015

[1359] James, SJ, et al. (2005), "Thimerosal neurotoxicity is associated with glutathione depletion: protection with glutathione precursors," *Neurotoxicology*; 26(1): 1-8

[1360] http://www.cdc.gov/mmwr/preview/mmwrhtml/rr5710a2.htm downloaded 21 April 2015

[1361] http://www.cdc.gov/mmwr/preview/mmwrhtml/00018871.htm downloaded 21 April 2015

[1362] Lucey, D. R., et al., (1996), "Type 1 and Type 2 cytokine dysregulation in human infectious, neoplastic, and inflammatory diseases," *Clin Microbiol Rev*; 532-562

individuals.[1363,1364,1365,1366] Because the DTH test is specifically indicative of a deficiency in cell-mediated immunity,[1367] the DTH skin test[1368] is a low-tech high-value strategy of greater benefit in the assessment of these patients than any "HIV antibody" test or viral load levels.

The optimal intracellular glutathione levels in healthy human subjects who had higher numbers of CD4+T cells than persons with either higher or lower levels was found to be between 20 and 40 nmol/mg protein.[1369] However, the thiol network includes more than cysteine/glutathione and, as indicated in the text, may require the evaluation of selenium, folate, niacin, riboflavin, vitamin C, as well as melatonin[1370] levels.

Defining if a particular patient is at any of the thiol deficiency stages or no stage (as all HIV tests must be regarded as false positive) requires a new set of tests and strategies. The minimal initial testing in all patients under consideration to determine whether the patient is at risk for or already has (1) an acquired mitochondrial dysfunction and/or (2) a disregulation of cell-mediated immunity would be (in addition to the tests for evaluation of CMI):

Measurement of glutathione levels in T helper immune cells, lung mucosal fluid and blood plasma, as well as levels of: cysteine, Vit. B 6, selenium, Vitamin C, niacin, folate and riboflavin. A DTH skin test[1371] and cytokine profile (see below) as well as an in vitro lymphocyte response to mitogen stimulation are

---

[1363] Clerici, M., et al., (1989), "Interleukin 2 production used to detect antigenic peptide recognition by T helper lymphocytes from asymptomatic HIV seropositive individuals," *Nature (London)*; 339: 383-385

[1364] Clerici, M., et al., (1989), "Detection of three distinct patterns of T helper cell dysfunction in asymptomatic, human immunodeficiency virus-seropositive patients: independence of CD4 cell number and clinical staging," *J Clin Invest*; 84: 1892-1899

[1365] Meyaard, LSA., et al., (1994), "Quantitative analysis of CD4+T cell function in the course of human immunodeficiency virus infection," *J Clin Invest*; 94: 1947-1952

[1366] Miedema, F., et al., (1988), "Immunological abnormalities in human immunodeficiency virus (HIV) infected asymptomatic homosexual men. HIV affects the immune system before CD4+T helper cell depletion occurs," *J Clin Invest*; 82: 1908-1914

[1367] Kniker, WT., et al., (1985), "Cell mediated immunity assessed by multitest CMI skin test in infants and preschool children," *Am J Dis Child*; 139(8): 840-845

[1368] Palmer, D., Reed, W., (1974), "Delayed hypersensitivity skin testing. II clinical correlates and anergy," *Clin Inf Dis*; 130(2): 138-143

[1369] Kinschert, R., et al., (1994), "Effect of glutathione depletion and oral N-acetyl-cysteine treatment on CD4+ and CD8+ cells," *FASEB J*; 8(6): 448-451

[1370] Benloucif, S., (2008), "Measuring melatonin in humans," *J Clin Sleep Med*; 4(1): 66-69

[1371] Pallmer, DL., Reed, WP., (1974), Delayed hypersensitivity skin testing. II clinical correlates and anergy," *J Inf Dis*; 130(2): 138-143

recommended. If these levels are normal or near normal, it is unlikely that the patient is at risk for developing the S or syndrome. If the tests (along with the clinical history and presentation) are abnormal, exactly where along the spectrum the patient falls will be determined by another set of variables. If following the above tests, patients are assessed to be at thiol deficiency stage 2 or 3, the following may be included for further evaluation (the arrows indicate expected levels from the norm):

Arginine[1372] ↓ (Because of the feedback inhibition of iNOS and a concomitant increase in arginase activity, L-Arginine may be decreased in these patients.)

Glutamine[1373] ↓ (Along with glucose, it is the primary energy source in lymphocytes and other rapidly dividing cells, including cancer cells.)

Glutamate[1374] ↑ (especially in patients who exhibit neurotoxicity, can be lowered with IV acetylcarnitine, most likely occurs as the result of mitochondrial toxic ARVs)

ferritin[1375] ↑ (another marker for oxidative stress and mitochondrial damage)

niacin and tryptophan[1376,1377] ↓ (as consequence of ROS, helps to reduce ARV-associated dyslipidemia)

polyamines[1378,1379] ↑ (marker for populations of rapidly dividing cells)

urea[1380] ↑ (biomarker for the breakdown of muscle tissue in the low glutathione/cysteine syndrome for use of glutamine as substrate for glycolytic pathway)

[1372] Cloke, TE, et al., (2010), "Increased level of arginase activity correlates with disease severity in HIV-seropositive patients," *J Infect Dis;* 202(3): 374-385

[1373] Newsholme, EA., et al., (1985), "Glutamine metabolism in lymphocytes: its biochemical, physiological and clinical importance," *QJ Exper physiol;* 70: 473-489

[1374] Farmularo, G., et al., (1999), "Reduction of glutamate levels in HIV-infected subjects treated with acetylcarnitine," *J NeuroAIDS;*

[1375] Lopez-Calderon, C., et al., (2015), "Serum ferritin in HIV-positive patients is related to immune deficiency and inflammatory activity," *Int J STD AIDS;* 26(6): 393-397

[1376] Gerber, MT., et al.(2004), "Niacin in HIV-infected individuals with hyperlipidemia receiving potent antiretroviral therapy," *Clin Inf Dis;* 39(3): 419—425

[1377] Taylor, EW., (2010), "The oxidative stress-induced niacin sink (OSINS) model for HIV pathogenesis," *Toxicol;* 278(1): 124-130

[1378] White, EL, et al., (1998), "Polyamine pools in HIV-Infected cells," *J Acquir Immune Defic Syndr Hum Retrovirol";* 17(2): 101-103

[1379] Jänne, J, et al., (1978), "Polyamines in rapid growth and cancer," *Biochim Biophys Acta;* 473(3-4): 241-293

[1380] Dröge, W., Holm, E., (1997), "Role of cysteine and glutathione in HIV infection and other diseases associated with muscle wasting and immunological dysfunction," *FASEB J;* 11(13): 1077-1089

prostaglandin E[1381] ↑ (promotes Th2 and IgE response via the elevation of cAMP in target cells)

transforming growth factor[1382] ↑ (associated with disease progression and Th2 cell dominance)

As early as 1982, a study by Mildvan, et al., first suggested that the immune system of patients with AIDS might involve immune disregulation rather than immune deficiency.[1383] In patients who were symptomatic and had a variety of "opportunistic" infections, the B cell compartment of these patients appeared to be relatively intact compared with T cell function. They suggested (this was before the work of Mosmann and Coffman)[1384,1385] that the immune problem of AIDS patients might be found in a subpopulation of helper cells involved in mainly a cellular response. Thus, the focus should be on T cell function that can be assessed by in vitro cytokine and mitogen stimulation and the DTH skin test. Evaluation of the heterogeneity of the T cell population as well as their functional response patterns is more important than the persistent focus on absolute numbers. While the total CD4+ T cell count may be helpful, it is not useful for assessing if the patient has a predominant cytokine imbalance and thus a problem with CMI. It gives you no information about the functional capabilities of these cells, and further, it is an instantaneous snapshot in time that may be no more than the result of an acute biological stress (recent crack cocaine use) or time of day. T cells may have temporarily left the periphery to return again after the stress event. Also, it must be considered that in those people who may have been on antiretrovirals, there may be bone marrow suppression and a lack of maturation of B cells.[1386] When T cells circulate to the bone marrow and there is a reduced number of cells that can be activated, these Th2 cells then return to the circulation for twenty-four hours but without

---

[1381] Phipps, RP, et al., (1991), "A new view of prostaglandin E regulation of the immune response," *Immunol Today;* 12: 349-352

[1382] Werclinska-Drapalo, A., et al., (2004), "Increased plasma transforming growth factor-beta1 is associated with disease progression in HIV-1-infected patients," *Viral Immunol;* 17(1): 109-113

[1383] Mildvan, D. et al., (1982), "Opportunistic infections and immune deficiency in homosexual men," *Ann Intern Med;* 96(6 Pt 1): 700-704

[1384] Mossman, TR, Coffman, RI, (1989) "TH1 and TH2 cells: different patterns of lymphokine secretion lead to different functional properties," *Annu Rev Immunol;* 7: 145-173

[1385] Mossman, TR., Coffman RI., (1989), "Heterogencity of cytokine secretion patterns and functions of helper T cells," *Adv Immunol;* 46: 111-147

[1386] Max, B., Sherer, R., (2000), "Management of the adverse effects of antiretroviral therapy and medication adherence," *Clin Inf Dis;* 30 (supplement 2): 596-S116

any function. However, this may confuse as the peripheral total T cell count may appear higher, which may be the case in which it has been interpreted that antiretrovirals are killing the virus leading to an increase in circulating T cells. This is an erroneous assumption.

The goal of compensatory therapy is to restore the natural redox homeostasis of cell symbiosis and should be both local and systemic: (1) determination of the underlying causes of thiol deficiency and immune shift, (2) diagnosis using appropriate markers as described, (3) systemic detoxification (may take several months to several years), (4) antioxidation/re-energization and reduction in inflammatory response, (5) acute treatment of relevant clinical manifestations, (6) hydration, and (7) hormonal/nervous system balancing.

This is a not a universal one-size-fits-all protocol but a systematic approach based on the history and clinical presentation of each individual and can be accomplished in a high-tech or a low-tech environment.

Antioxidation and Reenergization

Throughout the text, there has been a focus on the mitochondria and redox balancing and a focus on nutrient deficiencies, the primary being glutathione. An important consideration in using any replacement products is to monitor levels periodically to assess the metabolically normal range. Although there are glutathione products on the market, it is not always well absorbed, and it has been demonstrated that N-acetylcysteine can replenish glutathione in the HIV+.[1387,1388] Recently, a N-acetylcysteine amide[1389] product has become available and, because it is lipotrophic, apparently has a higher absorption and is able to pass the blood-brain barrier and chelate copper,[1390,1391] making it an antioxidant of choice for neurodegenerative

---

[1387] DeRosa, SC, et al., (2000), "N-acetylcysteine replenishes glutathione in HIV infection," *Eur J Clin Invest;* 30(10): 915-929

[1388] Roederer, M., et al., (1992), "N-acetylcysteine: a new approach to anti-HIV therapy," *AIDS Res Hum Retroviruses;* 8(2): 209-217

[1389] Ates, B, et al., (2008), "Antioxidant and free radical scavenging properties of N-acetylcysteine amide (NACA) and comparison with N-acetylcysteine (NAC)," *Free Rad Res;* 42(4): 372-377

[1390] Grinberg, L., et al., (2005), "N-acetylcysteine amide, a novel cell permeating thiol, restores cellular glutathione and protects human red blood cells from oxidative stress," *Free Radic Biol Med;* 38: 136-145

[1391] Offen, D., et al., (2004), "A low molecular weight copper chelator crosses the blood brain barrier and attenuates experimental autoimmune encephalomyelitis," *J neurochem;* 89: 1241-1251

disorders, including "HIV dementia." Other glutathione-supportive products including Immunocal1392 may be useful. Foods that also have been shown to be beneficial include broccoli, cauliflower, brussels sprouts, and cabbage as well as parsley and beets. An excellent source of glutathione is supplied by undenatured whey proteins.1393 Some spices including turmeric, cinnamon, and cardamom may also be helpful.

However, it must be considered that the glutathione/thioredoxin systems require various other nutrient inputs to function optimally: selenium, folate, niacin, riboflavin and vitamin B6, glutamine (40 gm/od), and L-arginine (20–30 gm/od). Alphalipoic acid and methionine have been shown to be beneficial in increasing the plasma ascorbate, total glutathione, and total plasma thiols, as well as circulating CD4+T cells.1394 Melatonin, acting as a powerful antioxidant, has been shown to effectively raise GSH levels in the brain, liver, muscle, and blood serum. The only natural source of melatonin are sour (tart) cherries.

L-carnitine is a nonessential amino acid that regulates cell membrane transport of fatty acids into mitochondria, allowing them to be broken down to acetyl co A via β-oxidation. The production of acetyl CoA is found in high concentrations in leukocytes and PBMs where it acts to support lymphocyte proliferation.[1395] This supplement is especially helpful in patients if they have been treated with AZT as it is a recognized treatment for mitochondrial myopathy and encephalomyopathy.[1396] Supplementation with 800 mg oral L-carnitine, 3,000 mg magnesium chloride, 800 mg L-arginine, and 240 mg glycine daily has shown to increase carnitine levels.[1397]

One of the critical problems that may develop during stage 3 of the thiol deficiency syndrome is cachexia or the wasting syndrome, which is characterized

---

[1392] Baruchel, S., et al., "Anti-HIV and anti-apoptotic activity of the whey protein concentrate: Immunocal," presented at the International Conf. on AIDS, Aug 7-12, 1994 (Abstract no 421A)

[1393] Bounous G., et al., (1989), "The influence of dietary whey protein on tissue glutathione and the diseases of aging," *Clin Invest Med;* 12(6): 343-349

[1394] Fuchs J, et al., (1993), "Studies on lipoate effects on blood redox state in human immunodeficiency virus infected patients," *Arzneimittelforshung;* 43: 1359-1362

[1395] Deufel, T., (1990), "Determination of L-carnitine in biological fluids and tissues," *J Clin Chem Clin Biochem;* 28: 307-311

[1396] De Simone, et al., (1994), "Carnitine depletion in peripheral blood mononuclear cells from patients with AIDS: effect of oral L-carnitine," *AIDS;* 8: 655-660

[1397] Davis, HJ, et al., (1998), "L-Carnitine and magnesium as supportive supplement with anti-retroviral drugs," *Int Conf AIDS;* 12:851 (abstract no. 42384)

by low plasma amino acid levels and notably low cysteine levels.[1398,1399] It can be aggravated by HAART as the drugs used in combination have to be detoxified in the liver, and they notably attack the mitochondrial symbiont as well as worsen any glutathione deficiency. Attention to this problem is particularly crucial as loss of lean body mass is associated with early mortality[1400,1401] as well as increased susceptibility to opportunistic infections.[1402] These patients often have an elevated type 2 cytokine, interleukin 6. This syndrome is characterized by weight loss in the peripheral organs, especially the skeletal muscles, and has often been treated as if it were simply a problem of protein/calorie malnutrition rather than a cellular metabolic imbalance related to low cysteine levels. In the liver, cysteine is required as a control for urea production and protein loss. If cysteine levels are too low, skeletal muscle tissue is broken down to help raise the cysteine or amino acid levels in plasma. In the liver, cysteine is split into sulfate and hydrogen ions, and the hydrogen ions can bond with hydrogen carbonate anions (HCO_3^-), which are required for the formation of carbamoyl phosphate in the first and rate-limiting step of urea synthesis.[1403,1404] If the reducing ions are not available, excess NH_4 from protein skeletal muscle degradation is channeled into liver mitochondria and converted to carbamoyl phosphate and enters the nitrogen into the urea cycle. The urea produced in the liver is released into the bloodstream and filtered out through the kidneys and excreted in the urine. The recruitment of ammonium ions into urea biosynthesis may be increased at the expense of hepatic glutamine synthesis

---

[1398] Droge, W., et al., (1988), "Abnormal amino acid concentrations in the blood of patients with acquired immune deficiency syndrome (AIDS) may contribute to the immunological defect," *Biol Chem Hoppe-Seyler;* 369: 143-148

[1399] Hortin, GL, et al., (1994), "Changes in plasma amino acid concentrations in response to HIV-1 infection," *Clin Chem;* 40: 785-789

[1400] Kotler, DP, et al., (1989), "Magnitud of body cel mass depletion and the timing of death from wasting in AIDS," *Am J Clin Nutr;* 50: 444-447

[1401] Wheeler, DA., et al., (2000), "Weight loss as predictor of survival and disease progression in HIV-infection," *J Acquir Immune Def Synldr Humma Retrovirol;* 18: 80-85

[1402] Kiure, AK, et al., (2002) In: Essex, M et al., *AIDS in Africa,* Kluwer Academic/Plenum Publishers pp 419-435

[1403] Volker, H., et al., (1996), "Abnormal glutathione and sulfate levels after interleukin 6 treatment and in tumor induced cachexia," *FASEB J;* 10(10): 1219-1226

[1404] Andus, T. et al., (1987), "Recombinant human B cell stimulatory factor 2 (BSF-2/IFN-β2) regulates β-fibrinogen and albumin mRNA levels in Fao-9 cells," *FEBS Lett;* 221:18-22

and may account for the elevated glutamate levels commonly found in AIDS patients.[1405]

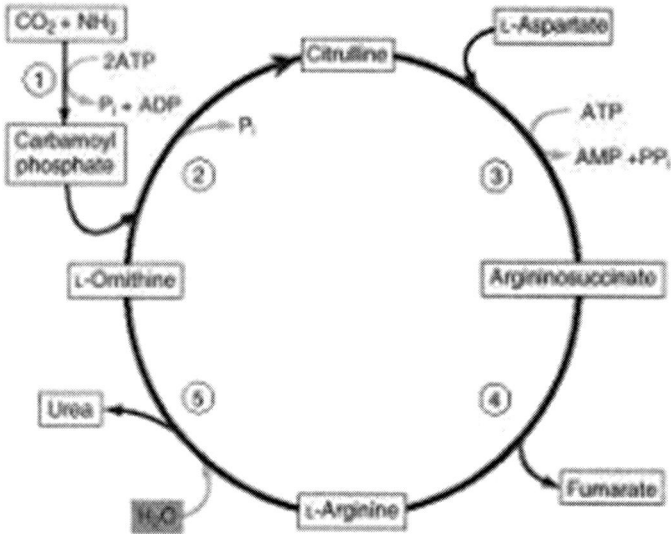

Figure 1

The Urea Cycle

The increased turnover of arginine has further serious consequences as arginine is the substrate for the synthesis of NO and its congeners. If too much arginine is used in the urea cycle, less NO gas can be formed, creating any number of systemic consequences, including the noted type 2 cell dissymbiosis: decrease in production of RONS, closing of mtPT channels, decrease

---

[1405] Famularo, G., et al., (1999), "Reduction of glutamate levels in HIV-infected subjects treated with acetylcarnitine," *J Neuro AIDS;* 2(2): 65-73

in calcium cycling, and switch in energy production from the OXPHOS system to aerobic glycolysis with an increase in demand for skeletal muscle to be converted to glucose and pyruvate to meet the nineteenfold increase in glucose requirement in the glycolytic pathway. If unchecked, this cycle will continue to lead to a negative nitrogen and energy balance.

The electron transport chain in the mitochondria may be supported by CoQ 10 (100–200 mg o.d.), and other mitochondrial activities might be helped with folic acid (5–20 mg o.d.), alpha-lipoic acid (300–600 mg o.d.), L-carnitine, the B vitamins as noted, selenium (200–400 mcg o.d.), zinc (10 mg o.d.), magnesium (threonate seems to have a better absorption), manganese, chromium (100–300 mcg o.d.) and methionine (500-1000 mg o.d.). Other substances for mitochondrial support include trace minerals and unsaturated omega-3 FAs. The evolutionary omega 6/ omega 3 ratio is reported to be 1. In modern Western diets, the ratio is ~17/1 with a clear deficiency in omega 3.[1406]

Before the introduction of antibiotics, vitamin D was (unknowingly) being used as a treatment for tuberculosis as patients were treated in sanatoriums with direct exposure to sunlight. Cod liver oil, which is also high in Vitamin D, was also used to treat tuberculosis as well as a preventative for other infectious agents.[1407] As a result of the continuous hype about the sun and skin cancer and the consequent overuse of sunscreen, as well as a failure of the public health community to address the issue in any meaningful way, there is a global vitamin D deficiency with an estimated one billion people worldwide being affected.[1408] In a recent EUROSIDA study, it was discovered that only 11 percent of HIV positive people had vitamin D levels at more than 30 ng/ml and that levels with 10 ng/ml or less were twice as like to die from an AIDS-related cause and about 40 percent more likely to die of a non-AIDS related cause, particularly cardiovascular disease.[1409] Optimal 25(OH)D levels is 50–70 ng/ml.

Vitamin A is a generic term that includes retinol and retinyl esters. In areas where Vitamin A deficiency is prevalent, especially among children,[1410] supplementation should be considered. A number of clinical trials have

---

[1406] Simopoulos, AP.,(2002) "The importance of the ratio of omega 6/omega 3 essential fatty acids," *Biomed Pharmacother;* 56(8): 365-379

[1407] Williams C. (1849) "On the use and administration of cod-liver oil in pulmonary consumption," *London Journal of Medicine.;*1:1–18.

[1408] Holick, MF., Chen, TC., (2008), "Vitamin D deficiency: a worldwide problem with health consequences," *Am J Clin Nutr;* 87(4): 1080S-1086S

[1409] Viard, JP. eet al., (2011), "Vitamin D and clinical disease progression in HIV infection: results from the EuroSIDA study," *AIDS;* 25(10): 1305-1315

[1410] Caulfield LE, Richard SA, Black RE. Undernutrition as an underlying cause of malaria morbidity and mortality in children less than five years old. Am J Trop Med Hyg. 2004;71:55–63

icated low-serum Vitamin A levels as a risk factor for HIV positive
.ls to progress into the syndrome[1411,1412,1413] and has been found to be a
particular problem in drug addicts.[1414] Vitamin A plays an important role in the
regulation of cell-mediated immunity and humoral antibody response [1415,1416,1417]
and often coexists with an iron-deficiency anemia.[1418] Food sources include beef
liver, cod liver oil, sweet potato, pumpkin, carrots, cantaloupe, spinach, kale,
collards, and butternut squash. It is recommended that supplements for adults
not be greater than 3,000 IU/day.

Ozone, hydrogen peroxide, or UV irradiation of blood

Ozone therapy has been in use in European hospitals and clinics for over fifty years. Ozone, hydrogen peroxide, and UV irradiation of blood have all been found to have positive effects that stimulate the immune system and improve cellular oxygen utilization. This therapy seems counterintuitive as these treatments can increase ROS, which are thought to have harmful effects. As has been discussed in this text, ROS contribute to the cells' energy stores as well as act as signaling molecules as a part of normal cell metabolism. However, aerobic organisms need a regular supply of ROS from the environment in the form of "negative air ions," ROS in drinking water, etc. Intrinsic oscillations resulting from ROS formations and reductions under long-term stress conditions as described in type 2 cell dis-symbiosis tend to decay, which also decreases the

---

[1411] Semba, RD, (1997), "Vitamin A and human immunodeficiency virus infection," *Proc Nutr Soc;* 56: 1-11

[1412] Tang, AM, (1997), "Association between serum vitamin A and E levels and HIV-1 disease progession," *AIDS;* 11: 613-620

[1413] Baum MK, et al., (1995), "Micronutrients and HIV-1 disease progression," *AIDS;* 9: 1051-1056

[1414] Semba, RD., et al., (1994), "Vitamin A deficiency and wasting as predictors of mortality in human immunodeficiency virus-infected injection drug uses," *JIF;* 171: 1196-1202

[1415] Shankar A. Nutritional modulation of immunity and infection. In: Bowman BARR, editor. Present knowledge in nutrition. 8. Washington, DC: International Life Sciences Institute Press; 2001.

[1416] Stephensen CB. Vitamin A, infection, and immune function. Annu Rev Nutr. 2001;21:167–192. doi: 10.1146/annurev.nutr.21.1.16

[1417] Villamor E, Fawzi WW. Effects of vitamin a supplementation on immune responses and correlation with clinical outcomes. Clinical microbiology reviews. 2005;18:446–464.

[1418] Semba RD, Bloem MW. (2002), "The anemia of vitamin A deficiency: epidemiology and pathogenesis," *Eur J Clin Nutr.*;56(4):271-281

availability of stored energy in the space/time cellular structure. With the use of ozone, hydrogen peroxide oxide, or UV irradiation, the increase in ROS may act as a spark to stimulate the required redox reactions to more normal oscillatory patterns;[1419] thus, when even small portions of blood are treated, patients may sense an almost immediate improvement.[1420]

Detoxification

Detoxification is not just a physical process but the process of reintegration of that which the nature of Western culture has sought to divide. The European mythos is based on materialism and disharmony, a disassociation from the spiritual, and a desacralization of the divine. Thus, the logic of this cultural dynamic reduces the nature of "health" to body function. Detoxification is the beginning of the process of making oneself whole, of recreating one's authenticity, and of discharging the inherent alienation that is the logical consequence of this cultural habit. For some, it is easier to linger in the shadow of death than to overcome the fear of evil, which becomes a stronger impetus than the will to live. Overcoming the AIDS paradigm requires moving away from the imposed infantilism of a top-down daddy system that seeks in both overtly harsh and petulantly petty ways to punish those who challenge the inherent absurdities. Emotions are not simply brain chemicals but also electrochemical signals that affect the thermodynamic equilibrium of every cell in the body. There are many ways to calm a raging mental state. An ancient method that has been scientifically (by Western standards) tested is meditation, which has also been found to have a beneficial effect on the immune system after only one month.[1421,1422] Meditation is also a method of self-empowerment to be able to unequivocally walk away from the pseudoscience of the constructed AIDS paradigm. It is a technique of use in calling the spirit back from a world of material distractions.

[1419] Voeikov, VL., (2006), "Reactive oxygen species (ROS): pathogens or source of vital energy? Part 2. bioenergetic and bioinformational functions of ROS," *J Alt Complli Med;* 12(3): 265-270

[1420] Elvis, AM, Ekta, JS., (2011), "Ozone therapy: a clinical review," *J Nat Sci Biol Med;* 2(1): 66-70

[1421] Vera, FM, (2015), "Acute Effects on the Counts of Innate and Adaptive Immune Response Cells After 1 Month of Taoist Qigong Practice," *Int J Behav Med;* (Epub ahead of print) http://www.ncbi.nlm.nih.gov/pubmed/26370102

[1422] Infante, JR., et al., (2014), "Levels of immune cells in transcendental meditation practitioners," *Int J Yoga;* 7(2): 147-151

The presence of heavy metals (including lead, cadmium, mercury, and metalloid arsenic) from environmental sources, dental fillings, and vaccines can have multiple damaging effects on the nervous, immune, cardiovascular systems, gastrointestinal system, lungs, kidneys, liver, endocrine, and bones. Other than acting as oxidizing agents,[1423] they may also cause damage by inhibition of the mitochondrial PT.[1424] They require glutathione for detoxification. This process may take months to years, depending on the level of oxidative stress.

There are several methods to detoxify from heavy metals. Removal of mercury from dental fillings is advisable. The use of reverse-osmosis water filters and water softeners can precipitate much of the lead that may be in drinking water. Chelation therapy may also be utilized. It is the process of removing from the body the undesirable ionic material by the infusion or oral consumption of an organic compound that has suitable chelating properties. The process should only be carried out by qualified practitioners, including dentists who have experience in removing mercury toxins from dental fillings.

The beneficial effect of chelation therapy is the removal of these metal catalysts that can increase the free radical load, thereby reducing the oxidation of lipids, enzyme systems, DNA, and lipoproteins. EDTA (ethylenediaminetetraacetic acid) is typically used and enhanced by several antioxidant nutrients: vitamins A, C, E; alpha lipoic acids; and selenium as well as amino acid complexes such as glutathione peroxidase. There are several other agents available for use including DMPS an oral medication for arsenic, cadmium, and mercury toxicity, and DMSA, an oral medication for mild to moderate lead, arsenic, and mercury toxicity. The combination of cilantro and chlorella are beneficial. Cilantro is a simple kitchen herb that is capable of mobilizing mercury, cadmium, lead, and aluminum in both bones and the central nervous system. Because chlorella has the ability to remove toxins stored in the intracellular space and may mobilize more toxins that can be safely removed from the body, chlorella acts in concert with cilantro to remove the toxins further from storage sites in the extracellular connective tissue.

The liver is the largest gland in the body and should be part of the detox process. It has three main detoxification pathways: (1) filtering the blood to remove large toxins, (2) using enzymes to break down toxic substances, and (3) synthesizing and secreting bile for the excretion of fat-soluble toxins and cholesterol. The longstanding practice of using milk thistle for a variety of

---

[1423] Goyer, RA., et al (1995) Metal Toxicity, Academic Press, New York
[1424] Belyaeva, EA., "Mitochondrial Electron Transport Chain in Heavy Metal-Induced Neurotoxicity: Effects of Cadmium, Mercury, and Copper," *ScientificWorld J;* 2012:136063. doi: 10.1100/2012/136063. Epub 2012 Apr 24.

liver problems has been validated by modern research.[1425] Interestingly, one of the milk thistle extracts, silibinin, was shown in animal studies to increase glutathione levels by up to 35 percent.[1426]

S-adenosyl methionine (SAMe) has also been shown to be effective in the treatment of liver disorders. It occurs naturally in the body where it is concentrated in the brain and liver and acts as a methyl donor in the synthesis of hormones, nucleic acids, proteins and phospholipids, catecholamines, and other neurotransmitters such as dopamine and serotonin. SAMe was found to reduce the markers of oxidative stress in the liver, decrease cytochrome c leakage from mitochondria, and increase the activity of SOD, glutathione peroxidase, and glutathione reductase activity.[1427]

Liver support and detox can also be effected by increasing certain foods. Cilantro, especially if taken as part of a green juice, as well as chlorella is helpful in the excretion of mercury.[1428] Chlorella is also a good source of amino acids and has easily absorbed forms of both B12 and B. It has been shown to be helpful in restoring healthy gut flora. Other foods that support liver health are dandelion, broccoli, collard greens, kale, watercress, pomegranate, and green tea. Onion, broccoli, cabbage, and garlic contain thiocyanates that help activate liver detoxification enzymes.

Colon cleansing and colonics, under guidance, might be considered. Colonics help to break down toxic excrement lodged in the colon that inhibits proper assimilation and elimination. It can also help to eliminate intestinal parasites. Coffee enemas may help with liver detoxification. Probiotics can help restore normal bowel flora. Foods that act as probiotics are plantain, chicory root, jerusalem artichoke, and lacto-fermented food and beverages (unpasteurized sauerkraut, kimchi, etc.) Other substances that may help repair the intestinal lumen after diarrhea, parasites, candida, etc., are N-acetyl-glucosamine, L-glutamine, aloe vera juice, and olive and sesame oils. Two

---

[1425] Dehmlow, C., et al., (1996), "Scavenging of reactive oxygen species and inhibition of arachidonic acid metabolism by silibinin in human cells," *Life Sci;* 58: 1591-1600

[1426] Campos, R., et al., (1989), "Silybin dihemisuccinate protects against glutathione depletion and lipid peroxidation induced by acetaminophen on rat liver," *Planta Med;* 55(5): 417-419

[1427] Brown, MJ, et al., (2012), "Novel protective mechanisms for S-adenosyl-L-methionine against acetaminophen hepatotoxicity: improvement of key antioxidant enzymatic function," *Toxicol Lett;* 212(3): 320-328

[1428] Omura Y, Beckman SL, (1995), "Role of mercury (Hg) in resistant infections & effective treatment of Chlamydia trachomatis and Herpes family viral infections (and potential treatment for cancer) by removing localized Hg deposits with Chinese parsley and delivering effective antibiotics using various drug uptake enhancement methods," *Acupunct Electrother Res;* 20(3-4): 195-229

drops of 100 percent pure gum spirits of turpentine on a sugar cube is an old, cheap, and effective deworming method.[1429]

Both antioxidation and detoxification can be augmented by improved dietary intake, especially of plants and nutrients that containing polyphenols,[1430,1431] which are naturally occurring antioxidants. Curcumin is a polyphenol that has demonstrated anti-inflammatory, antioxidant, immunomodulatory, anticancer potential.[1432] It also has antiangiogenic properties and enhances apoptosis.[1433] Other food sources of polyphenols are cloves, peppermint, star anise, cocoa powder, dried Mexican oregano, and celery seed.[1434]

According to a study reported in 2009, three quarters of U.S. teens and adults are deficient in vitamin D.[1435] This is a major public health problem, and evaluating vitamin D levels should be considered in these patients as vitamin D can modulate both the innate and adaptive immune responses and deficiencies associated with increased autoimmunity as well as susceptibility to infection.[1436] Multiple epidemiological studies have demonstrated an inverse relationship between people who have normal vitamin D levels and cancer.[1437]

Oltipraz—is a dithiothione that has demonstrated abilities to raise blood levels of liver detoxification enzymes as well as possible anticancer effects. It has been shown to induce glutathione S-transferase.[1438] It was originally developed by Johns Hopkins pathobiologist Ernest Buening as an antiparasitic

---

[1429] Mercier, B., et al., (2009), "The essential oil of turpentine and its major volatile fraction (α-and β-pinenes): a review," *Int J Occup Med Environ Health;* 22(4): 331-342

[1430] Perez-Jimenez, J., et al., (2010), "Identification of the 100 richest dietary sources of polyphenols: an application of the Phenol-Explorer database," *Eur J Clin Nutr;* Suppl 3:S112-120

[1431] Manach, C., et al., (2004), "Polyphenols: food sources and bioavailability," *Am J Clin Nutr;* 79(5): 727-747

[1432] Aggarwal, BB., et al., (2003), "Anticancer potential of curcumin: preclinical and clinical studies," *Anticancer Res;* 23(1A): 363-398

[1433] Bar-Sela, G., et al., (2010), "Curcumin as an anti-cancer agent: review of the gap between basic and clinical applications," *Curr Med Chem;* 17(3): 190-197

[1434] Perez-Jimenez, J., et al., (2010), "Identification of the 100 richest dietary sources of polyphenols: an application of the phenol explorer database," *EJCN;* 64: S112-S120

[1435] Ginde, AA., et al., (2009), "Demographic differences and trends of vitamin D insufficiency in the US population, 1988-2004," *JAMA Int Med;* 169(6): 626-632

[1436] Aranow, C., (2011), "Vitamin D and the immune system," *J Investig Med;* 59(6): 881-886

[1437] Garland, CF., (2006), "The role of vitamin D in cancer prevention," *Am J Pub Health;* 96(2): 252-261

[1438] Batist, G., et al., (2003), "Oltipraz Is a Bifunctional Inducer Activating Both Phase I and Phase II Drug-Metabolizing Enzymes via the Xenobiotic Responsive Element," *Mol Pharmacol;* 64(2): 346-44

drug against schistosomiasis. It exerts a protective function in the liver and other cell systems, especially intestinal mucosa. Besides the protective effects against opportunistic germs and endoparasites, it has been shown to have antiviral and anticarcinogenic effects.

Padma 28—is a Tibetan herbal formula containing twenty-two different plants that has been shown to exceed vitamins C and E and beta-carotene in counteracting oxygen and NO radicals and inflammatory mediators from activated macrophages.[1439] It has demonstrated benefits both within the cardiovascular system as well as apoptosis of tumor cells.[1440,1441]

Stabilization of the extracellular matrix—the extracellular matrix is composed of various negatively charged macromolecules possessing polyanionic character, which help to ensure proper protein folding for efficient functioning and as transport chaperones. Some of the polyanions possess antimicrobial activity and are hypothesized to be part of the innate immune system. They appear to be important in supporting the ability of cellular uptake and compartmentalization of proteins.[1442] The extracellular matrix operates in conjunction with the intracellular matrix. The redox potential of the extracellular compartment also functions optimally within a range of potentials and changes in intracellular metabolism alter the status of the extracellular compartment. These changes are correlated with cellular processes: proliferation, differentiation, and cell death. The extracellular matrix is a vehicle for cell-to-cell communication.[1443] For prevention and therapy, this matrix can be reinforced by supplying polyanions in the form of chondroitin sulfates, shark cartilage, macroalgae, and agar-agar. The balance of the redox potential of the matrix synergistically supports the glutathione system and supports cell symbiosis in states of oxidative and systemic stress.[1444]

[1439] Hassig, A., et al., (1997), "Pathogenesis of human suppression in hypercatabolic diseases: AIDS, septicaemia, toxic shock syndrome and protein calorie malnutrition," *Continuum;* 4: June/July

[1440] Navab, R., et al., (2004), "PADMA-28, a traditional Tibetan herbal preparation, blocks cellular responses to bFGF and IGF-I," *Inflammopharmacology;* 12(4): 373-389

[1441] Jenny, M., et al., (2005), "Apoptosis induced by the Tibetan herbal remedy PADMA 28 in the T cell-derived lymphocytic leukaemia cell line CEM-C7H2," *J Carcinog;* doi: 10.1186/1477-3163-4-15

[1442] Jones, LS., et al., (2004), "Polyanions and Proteome," *Mol Cellul Proteomics;* 3(8): 746-769

[1443] Banerjee, R., (2011)," Redox outside the box: linking extracellular redox remodeling with intracellular redox metabolism," *J Bio Chem;* 287(7): 4397-4402

[1444] Banaerjee, R., Ibid

Hydration

Ninety nine percent of the molecules in a cell are water. Yet Western medicine gives scant attention to the water-biomolecule interactions and special properties that allow this relationship to define the "living state." It turns out that electrons in EZ water are much less bound (reside in a higher state of excitation) than electrons in bulk water; therefore, a much lower energy of excitation is needed to free them. Thus, water in what have been called exclusion zones or EZ water becomes a potential electron donor and participates in the energy cycle of the cell. Because it is coherent, the energy stored in these zones cannot be released thermally; and thus, the only possible decay is through chemical channels. When the energy stored in these coherent domains matches the activation energy of the array of guest molecules, the system discharges and completes its oscillation—the interplay between chemistry and electromagnetism.[1445] This energy can be used for growth and development of the organism. MRIs have demonstrated that cancer cells, which operate at lower energy levels, have lost their water ordering. Dehydration has impacts on physical performance, cognitive performance, GI function, kidney function, heart function, and hemodynamic response.[1446] Hydration has been shown to be of relevance for the prevention of certain chronic diseases.[1447] AIDS patients may have symptoms of diarrhea, malabsorption, and oral and esophageal infections that may hinder proper hydration or nutrition; so that while water is not a very flashy therapy, appropriate hydration must be considered as important as any of the other therapeutic modalities. Ionized water, which is very alkaline, has been shown to be beneficial.

Hormonal Balancing

Rebalancing the hypothalamic-pituitary-adrenal (HPA) axis should be considered in these patients. The nervous, hormonal and immune systems are intricately connected through available cell receptors that recognize the products from the others. Stress to the biological system can be toxic, nutritional, electromagnetic, psychological, infectious, etc. The response patterns at the cell level do not say "toxic" or "psychic," but the information

---

[1445] Voeikov, VL, Del Giudice, E., (2008), "Water respiration—the basis of the living state," *Water;* 1:52-75

[1446] Popkin, BM, et al., (2010), "Water, hydration, health," *Nutr Rev;* 68(8): 439-458

[1447] Menz, F., Wenta, A., (2005), "The importance of good hydration for the prevention of chronic diseases," *Nutr Rev;* 63(6 Pt 2): S2-5

is transferred via the redox system. Cortisol has been implicated in the stress response. It counters insulin by stimulating gluconeogenesis, the pathway that synthesized glucose from oxaloacetate. Cortisol blocks T cell proliferation and excessive cortisol can overwhelm the hippocampus, causing atrophy of this area of the brain and memory loss.

The effects of elevated cortisol can be counted with daily exercise, vitamin C (4 gm o.d.), DHEA, gingko biloba, and melatonin. DHEA is especially useful as it helps to improve muscle mass and is involved in the thyroid gland's conversion of T4 to T3.

Melatonin—is a powerful antioxidant. In the animal model of immune dysfunction, melatonin alone or with DHEA was shown to reduce hepatic lipid peroxidation and prevent the reduction of B and T cell proliferation, as well as Th1 cytokine secretion while suppressing elevated production of Th2 cytokines.[1448]

If antibiotics, antifungal, and antiparasitic medications are given, they can be used as temporary measures with the continuance of therapeutic interventions that return the cell to symbiotic balance. Unlike AIDSworld, this is not cookie-cutter therapy and has to be adjusted to the history, disposition, and current state of the individual. Above all, it is important to recall that the problem is systemic, the energy status must be restored, and with that restoration will come a rebalancing of the relationship of the chimeric nucleus and the cell symbiont, followed by a balancing of the immune dysfunction.

The patient should be encouraged to find some daily routine that will help to restore psychic balance. Multiple modes are available: meditation, yoga, tai chi, guided imagery, biofeedback, etc. The object of this time is to learn to be centered and in the present moment. It is also to reduce elevated cortisol production, which may serve to continue to push the balance shift in the immune response.

I have listed numerous ways that the energy and immune systems may be supported. This list is in no way exhaustive; and I have not include other modalities including acupuncture; homeopathic, naturopathic, herbal, and traditional Chinese; and Ayurvedic medicine. It is not because I do not think these modalities to be useful but out of my own ignorance of these old and ancient disciplines and hope that those familiar with these traditions can offer further suggestions to this pressing problem.

[1448] Zhang, Z., et al., (1999), "Prevention of immune dysfunction and vitamin E loss by dehydroepiandrosterone and melatonin supplementation during murine retrovirus infection," *Immunol;* 96(2): 291-297

INDEX

A

actin, 44, 53, 55
AEDS (acquired energy deficiency syndrome), xviii, xxxiv, 242, 250–51
AID (acquired immunodeficiency), 62, 67, 195, 205, 210–11, 230
  cause of, 3, 8, 20, 59, 66, 194–95, 240
AIDS (acquired immune deficiency syndrome), xiii, 2–11, 19–30, 33–39, 47–52, 59–67, 74–79, 96–104, 106–10, 152–55, 188–95, 197–200, 206–8, 216–20, 257–65
  cause of, 22, 24, 34, 194
  definition of, 3–4, 6, 50, 242
  etiology of, 24
  incidence of, 47, 63
AIDS (acquired immune deficiency syndrome) industry, 38, 97, 194
AIDS (acquired immune deficiency syndrome) paradigm, xxv, 66, 81, 116, 199, 265
AIDS (acquired immune deficiency syndrome) patients, xxviii, 4, 22–25, 27, 37–38, 93–94, 98–99, 102–3, 114–16, 132, 153–55, 190–92, 194, 210–11, 220
AIDSpeak, 2, 10–11, 15, 18, 24, 34, 57, 67, 83
AIDSworld, 3–4, 8, 14, 19, 22–23, 25, 36–38, 40, 57, 62, 67, 77, 79, 89, 242
  definition of, x, 2
aldolase, 182–83
amyl nitrite, 86–87, 90, 98, 191
antibiotics, xxviii, 98–99, 107, 156, 210, 239, 248, 253–54, 263, 271
antibodies, xxxiv, 20, 23, 25, 36–37, 39, 43, 46, 49, 57, 62–63, 187, 189–90, 193, 195
antibody tests, 27, 39, 46–47, 67, 76, 106, 115, 193–94, 248, 252
antigens, 6, 26–27, 33, 56, 89, 188, 249
antioxidants, 35, 49, 112, 117, 124, 152, 178, 184, 255, 259–60, 268, 271
antiretrovirals, 129, 133, 234, 240, 242, 258–59
apoptosis, xii, xxxiii, 24, 113–14, 118–20, 141, 153–61, 183–84, 203, 211–12, 215, 222, 230–31, 235–38, 268–69
arginase, 78, 108, 241
arginine, 78, 125, 212, 257, 262
ATP (adenosine triphosphate), xiii–xiv, xxviii, xxx, xxxiii, 54, 92, 109, 122–23, 136, 138–39, 142, 146–48, 168–74, 182, 184
  hydrolysis of, xxvii, xxx, 168–69
  synthesis of, 139, 157, 168, 232, 241, 245
azathioprine, 102, 205–6, 208
azidothymidine, 102, 107, 121

AZT (azidothymidine), 84, 86, 102–3, 105–9, 116, 121, 137, 178, 206, 218, 240–42, 245, 260

B

Bauer, Ervin Simonovich, xxiv–xxv, xxvii, 122
  theory of, xxviii, 122
Béchamp, Antoine, 17–18, 90
biogenesis, 141, 224–25, 238
biology, xv, xix, xxii, xxviii, 17, 83, 118, 181, 245
biomolecules, xxx, 135, 214, 216
Buening, Ernest, 268
Burroughs Wellcome, 86–87, 102–3, 105–6

C

cachexia, 138, 217, 260
cancer, xiii–xiv, xxi, xxxiv, 5, 9, 20, 23, 29, 103–4, 160–63, 176, 205–6, 221, 223, 247
  cause of, 20, 23, 70
  spread of, 9
carcinogens, 22, 35, 62, 86, 96, 194, 222
cardinal adsorbent, 170–71
CD (coherent domains), xxxi–xxxii, 122, 136, 169, 171
CDC (Center for Disease Control), x, 36, 39, 46, 57, 76, 88–89, 93–95, 189–91, 193, 195, 255
cell death, xxxiii, 9, 16, 30, 37, 101, 107, 111, 113, 120, 137–38, 141, 222, 230–32, 236
cells
  APC (antigen presenting), 187, 208
  cancer, xiii, xxi, 20–21, 29–30, 34, 40, 44, 69, 107, 157–58, 160–61, 176, 179–80, 223–26, 238–39
  death of, 9, 37, 101, 107, 111, 113, 138, 141, 145, 156, 212, 222, 227, 230, 232
  definition of, xv
  dis-symbiosis of, xii, xiv, xxxiii, 30, 44, 80, 84, 101, 108, 124, 134, 156–57, 178, 218, 227–28
  endothelial, xxxv, 114, 132
  eukaryotic, xii, 52, 72, 144, 185
  fetal, 225–27
  immune, xviii, xxv, xxix, xxxiv–xxxv, 3, 62, 77, 81–82, 100, 102, 111–12, 115–16, 122, 131–32, 154–55
  infected, 35, 72, 106, 217
  lymph, 82, 209, 212
  mammalian, 97, 113, 122, 238
  metabolism of, 4, 8, 14, 66, 70, 72, 80, 90, 95, 98, 129, 145, 162, 172, 264
  metastatic, 223, 237–38
  mononuclear, 66, 77, 79, 106, 121, 155, 260
  muscle, 54, 109, 180, 238
  proliferating, 102, 134, 151, 182
  stressed, 10, 157, 212
  Th (T helper), 4, 27–29, 56, 60–62, 77, 104, 114–15, 156, 187, 193, 198–99, 201, 203, 217
  Th1 (T helper 1), 61, 63, 115, 127, 187, 196–97, 199–200
  Th2 (T helper 2), 52, 63, 127, 187, 196–97, 258
  tumor, 33, 82, 130–31, 136, 176, 179–80, 227, 229, 237–38, 269
  uninfected, 10, 21–22, 105
  vascular endothelial, xxxiv, 88, 112, 122, 126
cloning, 5, 82–83, 212
CMI (cell-mediated immunity), 43, 57, 61, 65, 97–98, 109, 186–87, 193, 196, 198, 200, 209, 249, 252–54, 256

counterregulation, xxxiii–xxxiv, 35, 101, 112, 124, 155–57, 163, 178, 184–85, 211, 217, 228, 230, 241, 243
Craddock, Mark, 60
cyclosporine, 205–7
cysteine, xvi, xviii, 49, 108, 117–18, 127, 132, 138, 209, 239, 256, 261
cysteine residues, 117–18, 151, 158, 183
cytochrome, 101, 109, 120, 123, 139–40, 146, 157–58, 215–16, 218, 226, 231–32, 236, 267
cytokines, 6, 10, 23, 29, 78, 107, 130, 153, 155, 187, 196–98, 204, 211
   type 1, 11, 30, 44, 78, 112, 114, 197, 208, 212, 237
   type 2, 78, 108, 111, 187, 261
cytoplasm, xii–xiii, 54, 118, 122–24, 142–43, 147, 155, 157, 212, 222, 231, 236, 238
cytoskeleton, xxv–xxvi, xxx, 52–55, 169, 171

D

DCA (dichloroacetate), 161
diseases, 3–5, 16, 18, 34, 37–38, 57, 65, 70, 88–90, 94–95, 97–98, 190–91, 194–95, 203–4, 230
   chronic, 163, 185, 220, 228, 270
DNA (deoxyribonucleic acid), xi, 5, 10, 12–14, 28, 40, 52, 55, 65, 68, 70, 72–74, 77–78, 82–83, 106
DNA (deoxyribonucleic acid) polymerase, 11, 13, 28, 106, 108
DNA (deoxyribonucleic acid) synthesis, 72, 79, 85, 98, 100, 102, 197
drugs
   (ARV) antiretroviral, xxix, 4, 59, 62, 77, 121, 206, 246
   addictive, 192
   antiparasitic, 268

   immune-suppressing, 95, 102–4, 206, 208
   nitrite, 87, 94
   recreational, xxxiv, 192
DTH (delayed-type hypersensitivity), 187, 195, 199, 208–9
Duesberg, Peter, 207

E

EIA (enzyme immunoassay) tests, 43–44
Eichmann, Adolf, x
ELISA (enzyme-linked immunosorbent assay), 43, 45, 47
EM (electron micrographs), 22, 31–33, 212
endosymbiosis, xi, xvi, 143–45, 147, 219
endosymbiotic theory, 143–44, 150
energy
   activation, 130, 137, 164–65, 270
   metabolism of, xi, xviii, 93, 95, 120, 132, 134, 148, 150, 215, 224, 234, 247
   structural, xxii, xxv–xxviii, xxx, xxxii–xxxiii, 80
enzymes
   glycolytic, xiii, 79, 128, 151, 180–81, 183, 224, 230, 233, 241
   reverse transcriptase, 8–11
evolution, xvi–xvii, xxiv, 13–15, 68, 97, 142, 162, 215, 235, 238, 246

F

FADH2 (flavin adenine dinucleotide), 139, 143
FDA (Food and Drug Administration), x, 39, 49, 57, 67, 83, 86, 103–4

G

genes
   eubacterial, 150, 152

mitochondrial, xi, 15, 105
genetic determinism, x, xiv–xv, 72–73, 161, 213–14
genetics, xiii, xix, 66–67, 181, 234
genome, xiii, 9, 12–14, 67, 71–75, 82–83, 141, 149, 162, 180, 246
  central, xi, xv–xvi, 67, 152, 155–56, 161, 184
  chimeric, xvi–xvii, xxvii, xxxiv, 151, 181, 213, 226, 234, 238
  HIV (human immunodeficiency virus), 5, 74–75, 82
  human, xvii, 12–14, 60, 66, 69, 71–73, 76, 149–50, 181, 216, 233
  nuclear, 141, 143
glucocorticoids, 27–29, 155, 208
glucose, 14, 92, 142, 146, 180, 182, 223, 226, 239, 257, 263
glutamine, 254, 257, 260
glycolysis, xii, xxviii, 93, 95, 109, 122, 131, 142, 160–62, 172, 180, 182, 184, 225, 234
  aerobic, xxv, xxix, 142, 147, 150–52, 157, 162, 178–81, 212, 215, 221, 223–24, 227, 235, 239
  anaerobic, 234
GSH (glutathione)
  deficiency of, xxix, xxxiv, 79, 99, 121, 134, 261
  intracellular, 96–97, 132, 226
  levels of, 61, 129, 134, 240, 250, 255, 267
  oxidized, 92
GSH (glutathione) depletion, 34, 63, 226, 255–56, 267
GSH (glutathione) reductase, 92, 98, 116
GSSG (glutathione disulfide), 92, 98, 118–19, 132

H

HAART (highly active anti-retroviral therapy), 77–80, 261
Harman, Denham, 164
hemoglobin (Hgb), 90–91, 123, 125, 171
HIV (human immunodeficiency virus), 2, 6–8, 14–16, 24–25, 30–39, 41–43, 45–49, 51–52, 66–67, 69–70, 74–77, 83, 106, 194–95, 199–200
HIV (human immunodeficiency virus) antibody tests, xiv, 2, 27, 38, 42–43, 49, 51, 57, 59, 212, 249, 256
HIV (human immunodeficiency virus) disease, 4, 121, 134, 195, 239, 242
HIV (human immunodeficiency virus) DNA, 30, 32–33, 69, 106
HIV (human immunodeficiency virus) infection, 6, 31, 47, 81–82
HIV (human immunodeficiency virus) isolation, 24, 26, 37, 42–43, 83
HIV (human immunodeficiency virus) proteins, 15, 30, 38, 44–45, 52, 57, 212
HIV (human immunodeficiency virus) tests, 36, 38–39, 42, 46–49, 76, 248, 256
homosexuals, 9, 20, 84, 88, 96, 189, 191, 194
HTLV (human T-lymphotropic virus), 2, 22–24, 28–30, 33, 50, 74, 194
hybrid impulse, xii, 155, 162–63, 184–85, 212
hydration, 259, 270
hydrogen hypothesis, 146–49, 219
hydrogenosomes, 146–47
hydrolysis, xxvii, xxx, 137, 168–69
hydroxylamine, 85, 100
hypergammaglobulinemia, 190, 204
hyperpolarization, 157–58, 160, 212, 227, 235, 238

hypoxia, 141, 183, 218, 226, 238

I

immune suppression, 87, 102, 129, 190–91, 199
immune system, xiv–xv, xviii, 28, 35, 43, 48, 114–15, 153–54, 190, 199, 201–3, 207–8, 251–52, 264–65, 268–71
immune theory, 190, 193
immunity
 adaptive, 195–96
 cellular, 103–4, 203, 249
infections, xiii, 21–22, 27, 31, 36, 50, 56, 62, 64–65, 67, 72, 200, 204, 207, 264
 opportunistic, xxv, 84, 96, 102, 112, 114, 122, 132, 154, 189, 191–92, 194, 205, 258, 261
 parasitic, 131, 253
infectious agents, 4–5, 14, 49, 95, 114–16, 189, 193, 263
infectious diseases, xiii, 8, 46, 239, 248
iNOS (inductible nitric oxide synthase), 61, 115, 117, 126–28, 130, 132, 159, 197, 241
isolation, xxvi, 2, 16–17, 19–23, 26–27, 31, 42–43, 66–67, 82–83

K

Kay, Lily, xx
kinesin, 54–55
Koch, Robert Heinrich Hermann, 17–18, 21, 23, 90, 208
 postulates of, 17–18, 21, 23
Kremer, Heinrich, xi, xiv, xxvi, xxxiii, 27, 29–30, 63, 100, 154, 173, 179, 210, 212, 219, 227
 theory of, xi, xiv

KS (Kaposi's sarcoma), xxxiv, 33, 84, 88, 94–96, 102–3, 112, 114, 122, 132, 179, 189, 191–92, 194, 205–6

L

Levy, Jay, 10
Ling, Gilber, xxvi, xxx, 170–71, 173
LTR (long terminal repeats), 14, 69
lymphocytes, 40, 48, 52, 61, 127, 186–87, 190, 192, 199–200, 203, 208, 251, 257
lymphomas, xxxiv, 102–3, 179, 205, 230, 239, 249, 255

M

malnutrition, 4, 156, 192, 202–4, 210, 251
McClintock, Barbara, 12, 68–70, 74
melatonin, 100, 218, 220, 248, 256, 260, 271
mercury, 120, 211, 266–67
methemoglobinemia, xxix, 88, 90, 94, 96
mitochondrial biogenesis, 141, 224
mitochondrial endosymbiont, 162, 164, 183, 218, 233, 247
mitochondrial matrix, 139, 158
mitochondrial membrane, xii, xxix, 109, 118–20, 137, 140, 153, 157–58, 160, 184, 212, 219, 226, 230, 234–35
 inner, 119–20, 139, 141, 219, 231
 outer, 120, 141, 158, 160, 239
mitochondrial symbiont, xiii, 143, 153, 215, 224–25, 228, 234, 238, 242, 248, 261
mitogens, 6, 10–11, 20, 23, 28–29, 34–35, 44, 89, 97, 188, 190, 193
mitosis, 53, 150, 176, 184
mitosomes, 146–47
mitotic cycle, xii, xxxiii, 132, 230
mutations, 12, 68, 112, 179, 221–22

gene, xxiii, 71, 179
myosin, 54–55, 169–70

N

necrosis, xii, xxxiii, 63, 80, 109, 114, 118, 120, 132, 153–54, 156, 158, 184, 211–12, 230–31
nervous system, 97, 100, 201, 203, 250
niacin, 79, 248, 256–57, 260
nitric oxide, xiv, xvi, 96–97, 110–11, 113–14, 122, 124, 165, 193, 208, 218
nitric oxide synthase (NOS), xvi, xxix, 61, 63, 100, 108, 115, 125–27, 251
nitrites, 84, 86, 93, 96–97, 128, 156, 189, 192
  volatile, 84, 87, 95, 189
nucleus, chimeric, xi, xiv, 143, 150, 153, 162–63, 214, 225, 229, 234, 237, 239, 248, 271
nutrition, 204, 235, 246, 250–51, 264, 270

O

Oltipraz, 268
oncoviruses, 5, 9, 19, 70
opioids, 202–3
Orwell, George, 1
overregulation, xii, xxxiii, 155, 163, 184–85, 228, 230–31
oxidation, xxv, 85, 92, 124, 126, 139, 147, 151, 166, 181, 183, 219, 224, 266
OXPHOS (oxidative phosphorylation), xiii, xvii, xxv, xxvii–xxix, 85, 109, 123, 139–40, 156, 161, 172–74, 180, 183, 215–16, 231–32
OXPHOS (oxidative phosphorylation) system, 108, 142–43, 147, 152, 218, 227, 230, 232, 234, 263

oxygen, reactive, xiv, xxiii, xxx, 110–11, 117, 120, 122–23, 129, 136–37, 148, 151, 165, 173–75, 214–16, 245
oxygen availability, 95, 180, 238

P

Padma 28, 269
Pasteur, Louis, 17, 21, 90
PCP (pnuemocystis), xxxiv, 85, 88, 98, 122, 189, 204–5
PCR (polymerase chain reaction), xv, 59, 76, 79, 212
peroxynitrite, 113–14, 127, 129–30, 232, 238, 241
PGE (prostaglandin), 212
PGL (persistent generalized lymphadenopathy), 31, 38
phosphorylation, xiii, xvii, xxv, xxvii–xxix, 55, 85, 97, 105, 109, 123, 139–40, 172–74, 182–83, 215–16, 231–32
photon emissions, xxiii, 136, 175–76, 229
pneumonia, 4, 88–89, 96, 99, 108, 114, 187–89, 203–5, 255
  plasma-cell, 204
polyamines, 78, 107, 212, 241, 257
poppers, 86, 88, 90, 93, 95, 103, 110, 112, 129, 131, 242, 255
protease inhibitors, 60, 65, 79, 121, 217–18
proteins
  charged, 170
  cytoskeletal, 31, 54, 57
  degradation of, 138, 140, 172
  mitochondrial, xii, 147, 157
proteobacteria, xi, xvi, 100, 184, 227, 233
PTP (permeability transition pore), 141, 231
pyruvate, 119, 137, 142, 147, 151–52, 160–61, 180, 182, 184, 224, 263

R

RBC (red blood cell), 49, 88, 90–92, 109, 138, 250, 259
redox, 97, 117–18, 129, 139, 150, 259, 269
retrotransposons, 12–13, 15
reverse transcriptase, 5, 9–13, 15, 19–24, 24n207, 27–31, 34, 50, 63, 69–70, 72–74, 81–82, 104–6, 194, 211–12
RNA (ribonucleic acid), 5–6, 9, 13–15, 21, 26, 31, 40, 52, 65–66, 68, 70, 72, 77, 79–80, 82–83
ROS (reactive oxygen species), 110, 119–21, 129–30, 136–37, 147, 152, 157, 164–66, 174–75, 184, 215–16, 227, 230–31, 237, 264–65
   production of, 137, 161, 172, 174, 211, 214

S

sepsis, 4, 137, 182, 209–10
SOD (superoxide dismutase), 91, 129–30, 165, 267
STD (sexually transmitted diseases), 48, 89, 96, 191
stress, 9, 12, 79, 151, 153, 201, 270
   alloantigenic, xxxiv
   chronic, 203, 254
   long-term, 162, 199, 202, 233, 252, 264
   oxidative, 37, 49, 74, 79–80, 92, 100, 114, 122–23, 129–32, 150–52, 181, 222–23, 250, 257, 266–67
   psychological, xxxiv, 4, 153
Szent-Györgyi, Albert, xxii, 176

T

telomeres, 10, 81
tensegrity, 136
TGF (transforming growth factor), 212, 241, 258

therapy
   antibiotic, 97
   antiretroviral, 77, 109, 117, 257–58
   cancer, 108, 157, 184
   chelation, 266
   compensatory, 259
   ozone, 264
   radiation, 16
   replacement, 16, 63, 99, 121, 219, 240
thiol deficiency, 20, 172, 182, 241, 249, 252–53, 259
thiols, 108, 111–12, 126, 128, 132, 183
Thomas, Lewis, 103
tumors, 116, 158, 179, 206, 221

V

vaccines, xviii, 6, 9, 16–17, 43, 156, 193, 197, 253, 255, 266
virology, xxi, 5, 8, 12, 19, 32, 34

W

Warburg, Otto, xiii, 95, 179
water, xix, xxii–xxiii, xxxi–xxxii, 17, 122, 126, 139, 162, 167–69, 174, 182, 235, 245, 270
   bulk, xxxi–xxxii, 270
   EZ (exclusive zone), xxxi–xxxii, 169, 216, 270
   interfacial, 169–70
Weaver, Warren, xix

Voeikov, V p136 fn 764